ENVIRONMENTAL CANCER

Advances in Modern Toxicology

Editor
Myron A. Mehlman

Vol. 1, Part 1—Myron A. Mehlman
    Raymond E. Shapiro, and
    Herbert Blumenthal

New Concepts in Safety
Evaluation

Vol. 2—Robert A. Goyer and
    Myron A. Mehlman

Toxicology of Trace Elements

Vol. 3—H. F. Kraybill and
    Myron A. Mehlman

Environmental Cancer

Vol. 4—Francis N. Marzulli and
    Howard I. Maibach

Dermatotoxicology and
Pharmacology

IN PREPARATION

Vol. 1, Parts 2 and 3—Myron A. Mehlman,
    Raymond E. Shapiro, and
    Herbert Blumenthal

New Concepts in Safety
Evaluation

Gary Flamm and Myron A. Mehlman

Mutagenesis

Advances in Modern Toxicology

VOLUME 3

ENVIRONMENTAL CANCER

EDITED BY

H. F. KRAYBILL
NATIONAL CANCER INSTITUTE

MYRON A. MEHLMAN
NATIONAL INSTITUTES OF HEALTH

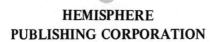

HEMISPHERE
PUBLISHING CORPORATION
Washington   London

A HALSTED PRESS BOOK

JOHN WILEY & SONS

New York   London   Sydney   Toronto

Hemisphere Publishing Corporation
1025 Vermont Ave., N.W., Washington, D.C. 20005

Distributed solely by Halsted Press, a Division of John Wiley & Sons, Inc., New York.

1 2 3 4 5 6 7 8 9 0   D O D O   7 8 3 2 1 0 9 8 7

Library of Congress Cataloging in Publication Data
Environmental cancer.

    (Advances in modern toxicology; v. 3)
    Includes bibliographical references and index.
    1. Carcinogenesis.   2. Environmentally induced
diseases.   I. Kraybill, Herman Fink, 1914–
II. Mehlman, Myron A.   III. Series.
RC268.5.E58   616.9′94′071   77-1776
ISBN 0-470-99117-8

Printed in the United States of America

CONTENTS

PREFACE

Human beings are, as is all life, the manifestation of balancing genetic and environmental influences, where the interfaces of life with the environment are the atmosphere, the hydrosphere, and the geosphere.

In recent decades there has been an increasing awareness of the importance of the interaction of mammalian systems with their environment. Such appreciation has led to cognizance of the myriad of environmentally attributable risks that confront humans. This ever-increasing awareness of environmental hazards is evidenced by the existence of activist groups and by the zeal of environmentalists who campaign for corrective measures. However, it must be recognized that achieving a proper balance between humans and the multiple environmental stressors is a complex matter, having as its goal health protection, with preventive measures, to ensure survival in this advanced technological era.

Legislative authorities and regulatory actions are structured and promulgated to attain these goals in human health protection pursuant to the diminution of chronic disease and/or amelioration of debilitating effects. Clearly, to be effective, actions in antipollution projects concerned with either the atmosphere, the hydrosphere, or geosphere must assume national and international scope. In the conduct of such actions it must be recognized that evaluating the impact of environmental effects on human health is a complex and ever-continuous process; it requires the problem be put in proper perspective, that is, that an equitable assessment be made in terms of probable benefits and possible risks to society.

A widely held view is that modern technology is exclusively responsible for introducing into the environment a host of pyrolytic products and other chemical agents that are directly or indirectly responsible for all adverse effects on humans attributed to environmental insults. However, many of these insults and potential insults are the result of substances that are of natural origin. Examples such as the radionuclides ^{40}K, ^{14}C, ^{3}H, and ^{226}Ra are worth mentioning. Plant materials contain mycotoxins (aflatoxin), safrole and oil of calamus in spices and essential oils (both flavorants now banned as food additives), and thiourea in certain seeds. Metal and metalloid elements from the geologic strata, such as asbestos, selenium, lead, cadmium, mercury, chromium, iodine, and fluorine, also enter the biosphere. Therefore, risk assessment of a particular agent must be considered in terms of the total background with an additional consideration of the added risk from a specific industrial component. Some persons may rely on and take complete solace in regulatory processes leading to the banning of environmental chemicals, while others may show complacency on these issues. Both extremes in many instances constitute gross oversimplification and misunderstanding of the problem.

The concepts set forth in this book are intended to provide an overview of the complex problems faced in environmental carcinogenesis. The relative contribution of endogenous to exogenous factors and the added stress from occupational exposure to chemical carcinogens are factors important to an understanding of environmental carcinogenesis. While the contribution of environmental agents to the induction of human cancer is not known with any precision, it appears likely that a high percentage of cancers may be preventable through application of reasonable environmental controls. The National Cancer Program is dedicated to such a goal.

H. F. Kraybill
Myron A. Mehlman

Chapter 1

HIGH-PRESSURE LIQUID CHROMATOGRAPHY: A NEW TECHNIQUE FOR STUDYING METABOLISM AND ACTIVATION OF CHEMICAL CARCINOGENS

James K. Selkirk

Carcinogenesis Program, Biology Division
Oak Ridge National Laboratory
Oak Ridge, Tennessee

INTRODUCTION

The human population is being exposed to polycyclic aromatic hydrocarbon (PAH) carcinogens at an increasing rate, as a consequence of industrial growth. Pott's observation in 1775 that scrotal cancer found in chimney sweeps was probably caused by some agent in soot was the first suggestion that cancer could be caused by environmental contaminants. However, it was not until more than a century later that skin tumors were produced experimentally in rabbits by painting with coal tar extracts (Yamagiwa and Ichikawa, 1918). This marked the beginning of the search for the active carcinogenic substance in soot, culminating in the isolation and identification of benzo[a]pyrene by British investigators two decades later (Cook and Hewett, 1933; Heiger, 1933). Synthetic dibenz[a,h]anthracene had been shown to be a carcinogen (Kennaway and Heiger, 1930), and the structural similarities between both molecules implicated polycyclic aromatic hydrocarbons as potential carcinogens in man. Many other PAH were synthesized subsequently, most of which proved to be poor carcinogens (Public Health Service, No. 149). Nevertheless, many PAH were discovered that are routinely used as tumorigens in laboratory animals. Elucidation of the metabolic mechanism by which these compounds transform normal cells into malignant cells

The author would like to give very special thanks to Dr. H. V. Gelboin, Chief of the Chemistry Branch, National Cancer Institute, Bethesda, Maryland. Thanks also go to Dr. J. P. Whitlock for editorial comment and to Carole Selkirk for tireless assistance in preparation of the manuscript.

necessarily rests in a complete description of their physicochemical similarities and the molecular conformation formed between the carcinogen and target site inside the cell. Although the ultimate species of these chemical carcinogens and the target site or sites where transformation to malignancy occurs is now unknown, it is hoped that complete assemblance of the metabolic pathway will illuminate the mechanism of the activated carcinogenic species in transformation, thus explaining the reason for the aberrant cell behavior we term malignancy.

Polycyclic hydrocarbons are metabolized by the microsomal mixed-function oxidase aryl hydrocarbon hydroxylase (AHH), which is predominantly found in liver. This enzyme has been studied extensively in rodents and is the subject of several excellent reviews (Conney, 1967; Gelboin, 1967; Gelboin et al., 1972). While it is known that this enzyme complex is involved with detoxification of xenobiotics in conjunction with cytochrome P-450 (Lu et al., 1972), it is not yet apparent whether some part of the complex is also directly involved with the activation process, whereby the molecule forms its active species. A second microsomal enzyme, epoxide hydrase, converts epoxides into vicinal glycols. Since epoxides are more active carcinogens than the parent hydrocarbon, this enzyme may play a critical role in carcinogenesis. While epoxide hydrase has been investigated using noncarcinogens and is the subject of a comprehensive review (Oesch, 1973), its activity has also been demonstrated in the formation of the three known dihydrodiols of the carcinogen benzo[a]pyrene (Selkirk et al., 1974b; Leutz and Gelboin, 1974).

Other intermediates currently under investigation in several laboratories, primarily using benzo[a]pyrene, are transient free radicals. This type of intermediate is known to be easily generated chemically and enzymically (Nagata et al., 1972; Ts'o et al., 1972). Because it is too unstable to isolate and study, it is not yet possible to determine if this labile species is involved in the carcinogenic activity of benzo[a]pyrene.

It seems clear that subtle mechanisms and fast reactions are important steps in carcinogen activation, detoxification, and the physiochemical binding to the transformation receptor(s) in the cell. It is therefore critical to develop equally sensitive methodology to efficiently trap, isolate, and identify these elusive intermediates in order to determine their proper place in tumorigenesis.

METABOLISM OF BENZO[a]PYRENE

Polycyclic aromatic hydrocarbon metabolites are arbitrarily divided into two groups based on solubility. In the first group are those metabolites that can be extracted from an aqueous incubation mixture by an organic solvent, e.g., ethyl acetate. This group consists of ring-hydroxylate products such as phenols and dihydrodiols (Kinoshita et al., 1973; Selkirk et al., 1974a; Sims, 1970) and hydroxymethyl derivatives for those polyaromatics with aliphatic side chains such as dimethylbenz[a]anthracene (Boyland and Sims, 1965) and methylcholanthrene (Sims, 1966). In addition to the hydroxylated metabolites are quinones that are produced enzymically by microsomes and non-enzymically from air oxidation of phenols. Labile metabolic intermediates such as epoxides can also be found in this fraction using special isolation conditions (Selkirk et al., 1975a).

In the second group are the water-soluble products that remain after extraction with an organic solvent. While it is believed that many of these derivatives are formed by conjugation of the hydroxylated products to glutathione (Booth et al., 1961; Nemoto and Gelboin, 1975) or other moieties that would render the compound more hydrophilic and presumably less toxic, this group of derivatives has not been rigorously studied.

The known metabolite profile of benzo[a]pyrene (BP), seen in Fig. 1, consists of three groups of positional isomers. There are three dihydrodiols, three quinones, and two phenols. The major benzo[a]pyrene metabolite found in 3-hydroxybenzo[a]pyrene, with 9-hydroxybenzo[a]pyrene present in lesser amounts. The BP-4,5-epoxide has been isolated and identified as a precurser of the BP-4,5-diol. Other studies suggest that epoxides are the precursors of the 7,8-diol and 9,10-diol as well. There have been no intermediates isolated as phenol precursors; however, evidence exists for epoxide involvement in the formation of 9-hydroxybenzo[a]pyrene (Selkirk et al., 1974a). There is little

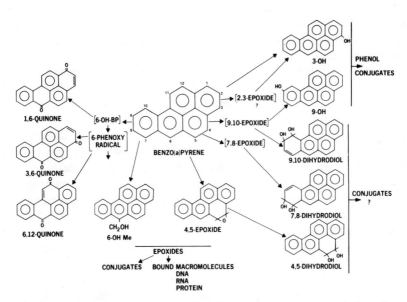

FIGURE 1 Benzo[a]pyrene metabolism. Drawn structures are metabolites that have been isolated and characterized. Bracketed compounds are projected intermediates that have not yet been isolated or need further characterization. Molecular species bound to macromolecules and conjugated derivatives have not been characterized.

further knowledge of the order and kinetics of metabolite formation. The effect of various metabolites on microsomal enzyme activity has not been thoroughly studied. However, it has been demonstrated that there are two different types of hepatic oxygenase induction (Alvares et al., 1967, 1968; Wiebel et al., 1971) that are dependent upon the chemical nature of the inducer. This may have significant influence on an active intermediate species of carcinogen formed and its probability of reaching a target site. In addition, there appear to be a number of sulfur-conjugation enzymes that possess specificities for diols, phenols, and epoxides (Boyland and Chasseaud, 1969). Removal of reactive intermediates and toxic metabolites are certain to affect the probability of cell survival, both normal and transformed.

Considerable progress has been made in the isolation and characterization of the aryl hydrocarbon hydroxylase enzyme complex (Lu and Coon, 1968; Lu et al., 1972), and similar work is in progress for epoxide hydrase (Dansette et al., 1974). We can therefore expect considerable advances in the next several years in assembling the dynamic scheme of metabolite formation for carcinogenic polycyclic hydrocarbons.

METABOLIC ACTIVATION OF POLYCYCLIC HYDROCARBONS

Polycyclic aromatic hydrocarbons are relatively inert chemically and quite hydrophobic, and cell lipids are probably needed for these compounds to be dispersed in the cytoplasm. Autoradiographic studies *in vitro* indicate that PAH possess access to all parts of the cell, although at present there is no evidence for active transport (Allison and Mallucci, 1964; Shires and Richter, 1966). It was apparent in 1950 that due to the stability of the polyaromatic molecule, some form of biochemical action was necessary to raise the molecule to a higher reactive state for metabolism to occur (Boyland, 1950). Since dihydrodiols and phenols were the major polyaromatic metabolic products, it was suggested that reactive epoxides were likely precursors that could then be hydrated to dihydrodiols or opened nonenzymically to form phenols. Twenty-one years later the first demonstration was made that an epoxide was an obligatory intermediate in microsomal metabolism of the carcinogen dibenz[*a,h*]anthracene (Selkirk et al., 1971). This observation has been followed by the discovery of epoxide intermediates for many other polycyclic hydrocarbons (Selkirk et al., 1975a; Sims and Grover, 1974).

Since epoxides are now the most likely candidate for the carcinogenic form of polycyclic aromatic hydrocarbons, there have been several studies to test this hypothesis. Early *in vivo* studies showed polyaromatic epoxides to be less carcinogenic than the parent hydrocarbon in mouse skin (Miller and Miller, 1967). However, the current knowledge of epoxide lability suggests that these intermediates will alkylate most nucleophilic sites with a low probability of the epoxide reaching a critical target site. A recent study, using an inhibitor of epoxide hydrase, which would be expected to impart a greater half-life to intermediate epoxides, has yielded more significant tumor data than the earlier studies (Bürki et al., 1974). It was with tissue culture systems where the possibility of nonspecific alkylation was reduced with the absence of cell debris that epoxides were shown to be more active in malignant transformation than the parent hydrocarbon or any of the hydroxylated metabolites. Utilizing hamster embryo cells (Huberman et al., 1972) and mouse prostate cells (Marquardt et al., 1972), it was demonstrated that epoxides of dibenz[a,h]anthracene, benz[a]anthracene, and methylcholanthrene were better transforming agents than the parent hydrocarbon. Other hydroxylated derivatives were also shown to be even less carcinogenic than the parent hydrocarbon.

Table 1 shows the results of a transformation assay with dibenz[a]-anthracene and several derivatives. The 5,6-epoxide showed considerably greater transforming activity than the K-region phenol or diols. The phenol yielded the most cytotoxicity, and only the epoxide was active in producing transformation with short-term treatment (4 hr).

There is also a good correlation for increased mutagenicity in bacteria (Ames et al., 1972) and mammalian cell systems (Huberman et al., 1971) for polycyclic aromatic epoxides. While this report will not debate the question of transformation as a mutagenic event, a small caveat should be mentioned at this juncture. At some point in the development or discovery of even more reactive epoxides or other intermediates, we may find them to be less carcinogenic or mutagenic than the more stable intermediates. This will most likely be due to the fact that current test systems add the compound exogenously to the tissue or culture media where it is likely to react randomly with available nucleophilic sites. In such cases, structure–activity relationships will not be valid, and the assay will not produce the intended measurement. A recent report measuring mutagenesis in *Salmonella typhuimurium* with several labile BP epoxides appears to indicate this point may already be reached (Wood et al., 1975). This may be in contrast to the *in vivo* situation where the same derivative is biochemically synthesized within the protective confines of the cell or tissue and holds a greater probability of hitting a target site to cause malignant transformation.

While epoxides of polycyclic aromatic hydrocarbons are the major form of reactive intermediates being investigated as the proximate carcinogenic species, there are several other possible mechanisms. The free radical 6-oxo-BP has been proposed as the reactive form of BP (Nagata et al., 1972). Tumor incidence in rat forestomach (Wattenberg, 1966) and mammary gland (Marquardt et al., 1974) has been reduced by treatment with chemicals acting as radical scavengers, suggesting this reactive intermediate is an active form of the carcinogen. Use of radicals as tumor agents will become feasible when more direct analysis of their metabolism can be achieved. Until then, it will not be possible to accurately confirm their role in tumorigenicity.

There has also been a report of a 6-hydroxymethylbenzo[a]pyrene metabolite (Fig. 1) from rat liver microsomes (Flesher and Sydnor, 1973) in which the hydroxymethyl moiety may be substituted at the 6-position of

TABLE 1 Transformation and Cytotoxicity Produced by DBA and Its K-Region Derivatives[a]

Concentration of compounds (μg/ml)	7-Day treatment of cells seeded on a feeder layer				4-Hr treatment of cells seeded in CM			
	Total no. of colonies	Cloning efficiency (%)	No. of transformed colonies	% transformation	Total no. of colonies	Cloning efficiency (%)	No. of transformed colonies	% transformation
Control (0.5% acetone)	922	4.6	2	0.2	952	5.3	2	0.2
DBA								
2.5	760	4.2	4	0.5	NT[b]			
5	690	3.8	4	0.7	911	5.0	5	0.5
10	790	4.4	7	0.9	882	4.9	3	0.4
15	796	4.4	0		952	5.4	2	0.2
DBA-5,6-epoxide								
2.5	598	3.3	3	0.5	722	4.4	8	1.1
5	601	3.3	12	2.0	740	4.1	14	1.9
7.5	395	2.5	31	7.8	637	4.0	15	2.4
10	350	1.9	14	4.0	550	3.4	19	3.5
15	278	1.5	NT					

5-Hydroxy-DBA

				0	796	4.4	4	0.5
1	242	1.3	0		668	4.2	2	0.3
2.5	0				522	2.9	2	0.4
5	0							

DBA-5,6-cis-dihydrodiol

				1.3	892	5	3	0.3
2.5	399	2.0	5		879	4.9	3	0.3
5	104	1.0	NT		727	4.4	3	0.4
10	0							

DBA-5,6-trans-dihydrodiol

				0	1016	5.1	2	0.2
5	646	3.6	0		1041	5.2	5	0.5
10	236	1.3	NT		947	4.7	3	0.3
15	35	0.4	NT					

[a]From Huberman et al. (1972).
[b]NT, not tested.

benzo[a]pyrene as a single unit independent of the tetrahydrofolate one-carbon pool (Sloane and Heinemann, 1970). This compound is also carcinogenic, forming sarcomas when injected subcutaneously in rats (Natarajan and Flesher, 1973). Substitution at the 6-position of benzo[a]pyrene as an activation for the benzo[a]pyrene molecule has been postulated from chemical studies that have shown this site to be the most chemically reactive (Cavalieri and Calvin, 1971). However, 6-hydroxybenzo[a]pyrene has not been found in extracts of microsomal incubations; and it has been postulated that the 1,6-, 3,6-, and BP-6,12-quinones are produced only as oxidation products of the 6-oxo-radical (Nagata et al., 1972).

Another possible mechanism is suggested by a recent report of keto–enol tautomer formed from unstable polycyclic aromatic phenols (Newman and Olsen, 1974). In this scheme, an epoxide intermediate would open non-enzymically to form an unstable phenol that tautomerizes to its ketone form, during which it would be a suitably reactive electrophile for alkylation of target macromolecules.

One of the most intriguing problems confronting the study of chemical carcinogenesis is the target site(s) with which the carcinogen reacts to begin the process that we recognize phenotypically as cancer. The working hypothesis has been centered around the fact that polycyclic aromatic hydrocarbons covalently bind to cellular macromolecules: DNA, RNA, and protein (Brookes and Lawley, 1964; Gelboin, 1969; Heidelberger and Moldenhaur, 1956; Kuroki et al., 1971; Miller and Miller, 1951). The amount of hydrocarbon bound is proportional to the concentration of macromolecule in the tissue, with cellular portein taking up most of the hydrocarbon, followed by RNA and then DNA. Although there is no unequivocal evidence that carcinogenesis is a mutagenic event and epigenetic mechanisms are theoretically feasible (Pitot and Heidelberger, 1963), much of the current search for the critical target site(s) is with DNA (Irving, 1973).

Major emphasis in this area lies in determining which polycyclic derivatives are most efficiently bound to DNA, including what type of chemical bond is formed and which DNA bases are involved. Early studies showed that the hydrocarbon was probably bound covalently since rigorous solvent extraction failed to remove all the hydrocarbon from the macromolecules (Brookes and Lawley, 1964; Goshman and Heidelberger, 1967). Currently, there is much activity in comparative binding of parent hydrocarbons and epoxides to DNA, as an attempt to ascertain which are more relevant to carcinogenesis (Baird and Brooks, 1973; Baird et al., 1973, 1975).

METHOD OF ANALYSIS FOR POLYCYCLIC HYDROCARBONS

Many polycyclic aromatic hydrocarbon metabolites were reported isolated before the advent of finely resolving analytical techniques, resulting in incomplete separation and either partial or tentative structural characterization.

Thin-layer chromatography was the major analytical technique and required no special instrumentation. A glass plate was simply covered uniformly with a layer of slurried silicic acid or alumina (0.25 mm) that, when dry, became fixed to the plate. The compounds were spotted, and the plate placed in a solvent tank. Separation was accomplished when the solvent ascended the plate by capillary action. Although this form of chromatography has a limited number of theoretical plates, indicative of a low-resolving capacity, it has the advantages of the stationary phase (e.g., silicic acid) and the solvent phase, aiding in the separation of the solutes by a combination of absorption and partitioning. This combination has enabled fairly good separation for groups of derivatives containing different functional groups (e.g., dihydrodiols and phenols) but is relatively ineffective for resolving isomers (e.g., 9-OH-BP from 3-OH-BP) (Sims, 1970) and is destructive to labile metabolites (Borgen et al., 1973). In addition, neither the quantitative data nor the migration data possess a high degree of reproducibility. Recent modifications using packed columns and less acidic alumina have reduced the destruction of some labile polycyclic intermediates but have not improved resolution or quantitation (Grover et al., 1972).

The major analytical technique used for drugs, pesticides, and other nonpolar organic molecules during the last decade has been gas chromatography. This method contains a high number of theoretical plates (ca. 2,000), yielding good peak resolution with highly reproducible retention time that qualifies it as both a superior qualitative and quantitative analytical system. However, gas chromatography use in polycyclic hydrocarbon analysis has been confined almost exclusively to the nonpolar parent hydrocarbon and has been the method of choice for the study of benzo[a]pyrene as an environmental pollutant (Committee on Biologic Effects of Atmospheric Pollutants, 1972). Since the major requirements for successful gas chromatographic analysis are a reasonable degree of volatility and thermal stability, most oxygenated polycyclics are eliminated from analysis without prior protection of functional groups. Formation of silyloxy derivatives and subsequent gas chromatography for one polycyclic epoxide have been reported (Stoming et al., 1973). However, this overall technique is time-consuming and results in the thermal destruction of the epoxide.

Since reactive intermediates are usually quite labile and short-lived, a rapid and nondestructive assay is necessary that can yield as good or better resolution for positional isomers as gas chromatography. It is also necessary that such a system be far more sensitive and rapid than conventional forms of chromatography. In addition, it must be a single-step process since it is quite probable that more labile polycyclic metabolites will, for the most part, be lost during separation or subsequent work-up for structural analysis.

High-pressure liquid chromatography (HPLC) has many distinct advantages over other forms of chromatography and is ideally suited for the study of reactive intermediates in metabolism and carcinogenesis. Resolution of isomers is equivalent to gas chromatography with a greater number of theoretical plates (ca. 5,000). Retention times are highly reproducible due to tightly packed small-bore columns with microparticle stationary phases (5–30 μm), which reduce meniscus effects and ensure the best chance of resolving closely eluting compounds. Unlike gas chromatography, there is no requirement for volatility or thermal stability. It is only necessary that the compounds be soluble in some solvent—aqueous or organic. The HPLC system is completely amenable to biologic systems since the column packing can be neutral, anionic, or cationic. In aqueous systems salt concentration, salt anion, and pH can be readily manipulated. Two important features in mechanistic studies are the rapidity of the analysis and the gradient elution. In most cases, HPLC analysis takes less than 1 hr with the sample completely recoverable for further reaction or structural analysis. HPLCs contain gradient devices that allow several gradient modes to facilitate separation of mixtures of very similar compounds.

One HPLC system currently used is schematically represented in Fig. 2. This system is the basis of the Dupont model 830 and can be operated either in an isocratic mode, using a constant mixture of solvents (A) and (B), or with a gradient mode where solvent (B) is added to solvent (A) either linearly, slowly (concave), or rapidly (convex) by means of preset proportioning valves. The design of this system also uses solvent (A) as a pressure head to drive solvent (B) from the holding coil to form the gradient mixture. A mixing chamber placed immediately in front of the column ensures uniform solvent composition; the injection port, which is located immediately after the mixing chamber, allows injection close to the front of the column and directly into the solvent flow. Separation of benzo[a]pyrene metabolites accomplished by HPLC using gradient elution and a solvent mixture of water–methanol is seen in Fig. 3.

A small unidentified peak is eluted first, then three clearly separated vicinal glycols (9,10-diol, 4,5-diol, and 7,8-diol) and three quinones (1,6-quinone, 3,6-quinone, and 6,12-quinone), two of which are not completely separated. These are followed by two phenols, 9-OH-BP and 3-OH-BP. The unused BP elutes considerably behind the metabolites, thus minimizing tailing effects common to thin-layer chromatography. Table 2 shows the retention times and molecular weights of the metabolites, which were determined from the peaks collected after passage through the flow cell.

Comparison of BP metabolite profiles between thin-layer chromatography and HPLC is seen in Fig. 4, in which (A) shows the [^{3}H]BP metabolite pattern with the uv absorbance (254 nm) superimposed. There is no discernible lag between the appearance of a peak and collection of the compound, given the small volume size of the flow cell (8 μl) and the bore size of tubing carrying the eluate (0.019 in.). Individual metabolites in (B) through (G) were from a [^{14}C]BP microsomal incubation that was chromatographed on

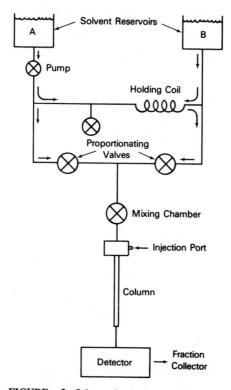

FIGURE 2 Schematic representation of HPLC system. This flow diagram utilizes a single pump to drive both solvents as in the Dupont model 830. Proportionating valves regulate solvent mixtures that are passed through a mixing chamber near the head of the column. Detectors routinely used with HPLC are ultraviolet, fluorescence, and re-fractometry.

silica-gel thin-layer plates. The spots were eluted and further purified by HPLC. The two peaks in (C) show 9-OH-BP and 3-OH-BP, neither of which was resolved by thin-layer chromatography. This was the first unequivocal demonstration that 9-OH-BP was a metabolic product (Selkirk et al., 1974a).

EFFECT OF ENZYME INHIBITORS ON BP METABOLISM

7,8-Benzoflavone (7,8-BF) is a strong inhibitor of aryl hydrocarbon hydroxylase (AHH) (Wiebel et al., 1972), as determined by fluorescence studies measuring formation of phenolic metabolites. However, monitoring the entire metabolic profile with HPLC can accurately measure the specificity of 7,8-BF. Table 3, showing the effect of 7,8-BF on BP metabolite formation,

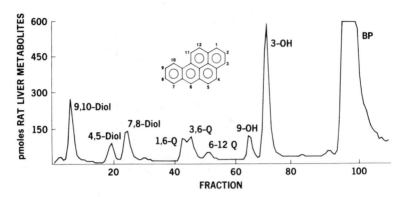

FIGURE 3 Separation of metabolites of benzo[*a*]pyrene. Male Sprague-Dawley rats (160–180 g) were injected intraperitoneally with 5 mg 3-methyl-cholanthrene in 0.5 ml corn oil; 40 hr later the rats were killed. Liver microsomes were prepared as described in Kinoshita et al. (1972). The metabolites were formed by incubating rat liver microsomes with [³H]benzo[*a*]-pyrene (sp. activity, 200 mCi/mmol) or [¹⁴C]benzo[*a*]pyrene (sp. activity, 21 mCi/mmol) (Amersham/Searle, Arlington Heights, Illinois), as follows: each flask contained a total volume of 1.0 ml: 100 µg microsomal protein, 0.36 µmol reduced nicotinamide adenine dinucleotide phosphate, 3 µmol MgCl$_2$, 50 µmol Tris-HCl buffer (pH 7.5), and 100 µmol benzo[*a*]pyrene dissolved in 0.040 ml methanol. The flasks were incubated for 10 min at 37°C under red light illumination, and the reaction was stopped by the addition of 1.0 ml acetone. The mixture was then extracted with 2.0 ml ethyl acetate. Five extracts were pooled and dried over 1.0 g anhydrous magnesium sulfate, the solvent was evaporated under vacuum, and the residue (metabolites) was dissolved in 0.1 ml methanol. The metabolite separation was performed on a high-pressure liquid chromatograph (Dupont model 830) fitted with a Zipax permaphase column (1-m ODS). The metabolites were eluted with a reverse-phase gradient system (methanol–water, 30:70 initially and 70:30 at final composition). The gradient rate of change was 3%/min; the column temperature, 50°C; the pressure, 350 psi; flow rate, 0.6 ml/min. The eluate was monitored by uv absorption at 254 nm. Fractions were collected at 20-sec intervals, and the radioactivity was determined in a Beckman 350 scintillation counter with Aquasol (New England Nuclear) as the counting medium (Selkirk et al., 1974b).

confirms a large inhibitory effect on phenol formation as measured by HPLC. However, the broad analytic range of HPLC shows inhibition of diol and quinone formation. Furthermore, there is a decrease in the amount of BP metabolized (5.9%), as compared with the control (18.3%). It is clear from this type of analysis that 7,8-BF apparently interacts with the enzyme complex to inhibit oxygenation at all sites of the benzo[*a*]pyrene molecule. However, diol formation was inhibited by 7,8-BF to a relatively greater extent than the phenol (76–79%) and quinone formations (55–68%). Since diols represent the products of hydrase action on epoxide intermediates, 7,8-BF would seem to have somewhat greater effect on epoxide formation than on phenol formation.

1,2-Epoxy-3,3,3-trichloropropane (TCPO) is a potent inhibitor of the epoxide hydrase enzyme (Oesch et al., 1971). In contrast to 7,8-BF, TCPO had a more selective effect on the metabolism of BP. As shown in Table 3 and Fig. 5, TCPO completely inhibited the formation of all three diols and reduced total BP metabolism by almost 50%, suggesting that TCPO may interfere with BP oxygenation as well as with epoxide hydration. The formation of 3-OH-BP was not affected by 2 mM TCPO as determined by total radioactivity of each metabolite formed. This result has been confirmed by fluorescence studies (Yang and Strickhart, 1975), suggesting that the enzymic mechanism for phenol formation at position 3 follows a more complicated kinetics or may utilize a different enzymic mechanism.

In the presence of TCPO, the ratio of 9-OH-BP relative to 3-OH-BP was increased to greater than twice the control value. It is probable that the increase of 9-OH-BP resulted from a nonenzymic rearrangement of the BP-9, 10-epoxide. Using selective enzyme inhibition and HPLC analysis, it should be possible to isolate portions of the metabolic scheme and determine the number of steps involved in the activation and detoxification of carcinogenic polyaromatics including precursor metabolites for later enzymic steps or rearrangements.

EFFECT OF 7,8-BF AND TCPO ON BP-DNA FORMATION

Microsomes convert BP to an intermediate that binds covalently to DNA (Gelboin, 1969). Since epoxides are more chemically reactive than the parent

TABLE 2 Retention Time and Molecular Weight of Benzo[a]pyrene Metabolites Separated by High-Pressure Liquid Chromatography[a]

Metabolite	Retention time (min)	m/e[b]
9,10-Dihydrodihydroxy-BP	8.5	286
4,5-Dihydrodihydroxy-BP	15.5	286
7,8-Dihydrodihydroxy-BP	18.0	286
1,6-Quinone-BP	25.5	282
3,6-Quinone-BP	26.0	282
6,12-Quinone-BP (tentative)	28.0	c
9-Hydroxy-BP	35.0	268
3-Hydroxy-BP	37.0	268
BP	48.0	252

[a]From Selkirk et al. (1972a).
[b]Molecular weight determinations performed on a JeoL JMS-01SG-2 at 70 eV with a solid probe. Temperature ranged from 90 to 150°C.
[c]Insufficient material for complete analysis.

TABLE 3 Effect of 7,8-BF and TCPO on BP Metabolite Formation[a],[b]

	9,10-Diol	4,5-Diol	7,8-Diol	Quinones	9-OH-BP	3-OH-BP	Total metabolites	BP	% metabolism[d]
Control	215.0	81.4	146.4	172.2	51.2	248.8	915.0	4035.0	18.3
7,8-BF	48.5	19.6	31.5	77.7	15.7	95.8	288.8	4650.8	5.9
	(22.5)[c]	(24.1)	(21.5)	(45.1)	(30.7)	(38.5)			
TCPO	0.0	0.0	0.0	95.8	123.1	250.8	469.4	4360.4	9.4
	(0.0)	(0.0)	(0.0)	(55.6)	(240.0)	(100.8)			

[a]From Selkirk et al. (1974b).
[b]Data expressed as pmol $\times$ 10^{-2}. Each experiment consisted of five pooled incubations containing a total of 5,000 $\times$ 10^2 pmol BP as substrate.
[c]Numbers in parentheses represent percent of control value.
[d]Ethyl acetate extractable material. The water-soluble radioactivity was 1% in all three incubations.

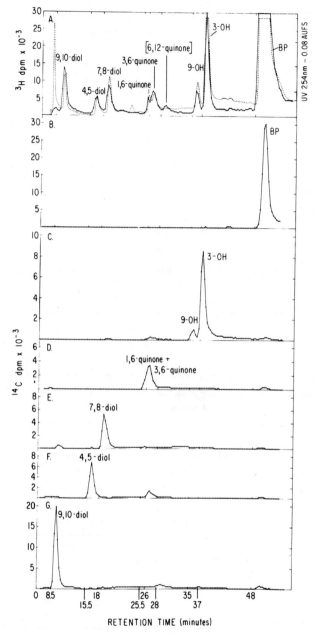

FIGURE 4 HPLC identification of total and individual BP metabolites (Selkirk et al., 1974a). See text for discussion.

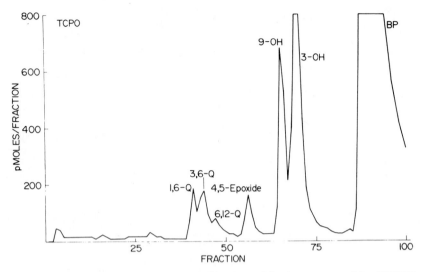

FIGURE 5 HPLC pattern of BP metabolites formed in the presence of 2 m*M* TCPO
(Selkirk et al., 1975).

hydrocarbon, they are better alkylating agents and have been shown to bind
more efficiently to DNA in tissue culture (Kuroki et al., 1971). Thus, epoxide
hydrase inhibition should increase the half-life of intermediate epoxides and
make them more available to nucleophilic sites. At the same time, an inhibitor
of phenol formation and metabolism in general, such as 7,8-BF, would be
expected to form less epoxide and therefore reduce the amount of compound
available for binding. Table 4 shows 7,8-BF inhibited both BP–DNA binding
and diol formation, suggesting that diols were precursors to other reactive
species that are also bound to DNA (Sims et al., 1974).

In contrast to 7,8-BF inhibition, there was a stimulation of BP–DNA
formation in the presence of TCPO. Inhibition of all three diols further
suggested that BP–DNA was largely through an epoxide intermediate and that

TABLE 4 Effect of 7,8-BF and TCPO on Activity and BP–DNA Formation[a]

Additions	AHH units[b]	Percent	BP–DNA (cpm/mg)[c]	Percent
None	11,617		1,724	
7,8-BF	5,643	(49)	938	(54)
TCPO	9,128	(79)	2,478	(143)

[a]From Selkirk et al. (1974b).

[b]Picomoles of hydroxylated BP with the fluorescence equivalent to 3-OH-BP formed
in 30 min.

[c]The pmol equivalents to [³H]BP are 10.7, 4.4, and 12.7 for no addition, 7,8-BF,
and TCPO, respectively.

although TCPO inhibited overall oxygenation of BP as indicated by a reduction in BP utilization, it probably raised the effective level of reactive epoxide by inhibiting epoxide hydrase and increased the amount of epoxide available for binding to DNA.

EPOXIDES AS INTERMEDIATES IN BENZO[*a*]PYRENE METABOLISM

One of the keystones in the reactive intermediate theory of benzo[*a*]-pyrene carcinogenesis is proof that epoxides are, indeed, metabolic intermediates. In the preceding discussion it was quite apparent that epoxides were present in microsomal incubation mixtures. Although epoxides were not isolated from incubations containing an epoxide hydrase inhibitor, the relative increase of 9-OH-BP suggested that the BP-9,10-epoxide was being produced but was unstable and rearranged to 9-OH-BP. Also, a BP metabolite characteristic of an epoxide had been partially characterized (Grover et al., 1972; Wang et al., 1972).

Utilizing the water–methanol solvent gradient with alkaline buffering to pH 9.0 to help stabilize epoxides and inhibit epoxide hydrase, it was possible to trap the BP-4,5-epoxide. Figure 5 shows the BP metabolite spectrum in the presence of 2 mM TCPO. As was previously seen, there was complete inhibition of dihydrodiol formation and an increase in 9-OH-BP. In addition, the adjusted solvent system revealed a new peak (retention time 29.2 min) between the quinone and phenol regions. This peak was isolated and characterized.

Table 5 summarizes the analytical data. The metabolite formed in the presence of TCPO migrated on HPLC with a retention time identical to authentic BP-4,5-epoxide. The uv spectra of the metabolite and standard BP-4,5-epoxide were almost identical (Fig. 6), as was the molecular weight and mass spectral fracture pattern. The epoxide metabolite was then incubated with liver microsomes and the products analyzed on HPLC, together with a mixture of known [^{14}C] BP metabolites.

TABLE 5 Characterization of a Metabolite of BP as BP-4,5-Epoxide[a]

	Metabolite	Synthetic BP-4,5-epoxide
Mass spectrum *m/e*	268	268
Major fragments	252, 239, 134, 119.5	252, 239, 134, 119.5
uv absorbance (max)	328, 315, 303	328, 315, 303
	275, 265 nm	275, 265 nm
HPLC retention time	29.2 min	29.2 min
HPLC retention time of dihydrodiol product	13.2 min	13.2 min

[a]From Selkirk et al. (1975a).

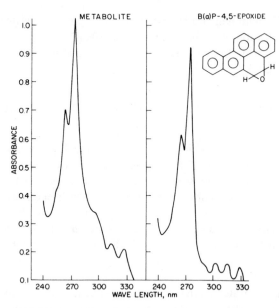

FIGURE 6 Ultraviolet spectra of metabolite and synthetic BP-4,5-epoxide (Selkirk et al., 1975).

Figure 7 shows that the metabolite was converted to a [^{3}H]-diol product that cochromatographed with [^{14}C] BP-4,5-dihydrodiol. No [^{3}H] peak was found that corresponded to the 7,8-dihydrodiol or the 9,10-dihydrodiol.

TCPO inhibition of the three dihydrodiol and the appearance of the 4,5-epoxide suggested that the other two diols passed through epoxide

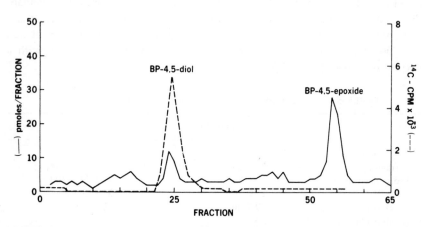

FIGURE 7 Conversion of metabolite to BP-4,5-dihydrodiol by liver microsomes. Dashed line represents [^{14}C] BP-4,5-diol added to the organic extract (Selkirk et al., 1975a).

intermediates but were too unstable to be isolated under the conditions used. This hypothesis was reinforced by the fact that synthetic BP-7,8-epoxide was unstable to those analytical conditions (unpublished results).

The isolation and characterization of an epoxide of BP lends additional support to the role of epoxides as significant intermediates in polyaromatic hydrocarbon metabolism.

The renewed interest in carcinogenic polyaromatic hydrocarbons as a major environmental contaminant (Committee on Biologic Effects of Atmospheric Pollutants, 1972) has produced a host of new polyaromatic derivatives synthesized by new and innovative chemistry (Dansette and Jerina, 1974; Goh and Harvey, 1973), with structural analysis based on more reliable analytical procedures than used even a decade ago. It is therefore probable that in the near future carcinogenesis experiments and tumorigenesis screening will be performed on these new chemical species, resulting in a clearer picture of which components of the metabolite spectrum are the reactive forms critical to malignant transformation.

METABOLISM OF BENZO[*a*]PYRENE IN HUMAN TISSUE

The ultimate goal of mechanistic studies in carcinogenesis is to understand and prevent the malignant process in humans. Armed with the increasing encyclopedia of tumorigenesis information in animal (Public Health Service, No. 149) and cell systems (Heidelberger, 1973), it has become possible to measure some of the chemical and biochemical components known to be associated with either detoxification or activation of chemical carcinogens. Such studies are timely and extremely important since carcinogenic polyaromatic hydrocarbons are known to be ubiquitous pollutants of the atmosphere, waterways, oceans, and soil. Sources of these hydrocarbon emissions include heat and power generation, refuse burning, transportation, industrial processes, and oil spills.

Aryl hydrocarbon hydroxylase has been found in human liver (Kuntzman et al., 1966), skin (Levin et al., 1972), placenta (Nebert et al., 1969; Welch et al., 1969), lymphocytes (Busbee et al., 1972; Whitlock et al., 1972), monocytes (Bast et al., 1974), and lung macrophages (Cantrell et al., 1973). Exposure to cigarette smoke, pesticides, and polycyclic hydrocarbons induces the metabolizing activity of AHH and makes some of these compounds increasingly suspect as human carcinogens. In addition, recent lymphocyte studies in human population samples suggest there may be genetic variation of AHH in humans (Kellerman et al., 1973). Identification of polycyclic hydrocarbon metabolite patterns in high-risk populations, compared with control populations, may assist in identifying the active carcinogenic metabolite(s) and differentiate between activation and detoxification pathways in humans.

A comparison between the metabolism of BP by microsomes from human liver and rat liver is shown in Fig. 8. The human liver profile presented

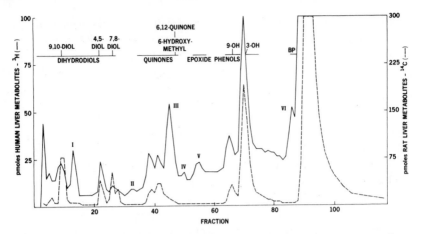

FIGURE 8 Pattern of BP metabolites formed by incubation with human liver microsomes. (———) pmol hydrocarbon formed by human microsomes with [³H]-BP. (- - - -) pmol hydrocarbon formed by rat liver microsomes with [¹⁴C] BP. Roman numerals indicate metabolites produced only by human microsomes.

additional metabolites not observed in the rodent metabolite pattern. In the diol region, a large peak (I) appeared just after 9,10-diol (fractions 13–15), and a small peak (II) appeared after 7,8-diol (fractions 31–34). The quinone region presented a major peak (III) at the region of the 6,12-quinone. We found synthetic 6-hydroxymethyl-BP cochromatographed with 6,12-quinone in the system, and peak (III) may have contained that derivative (Flesher and Sydnor, 1973). A small peak (IV) followed immediately after (fraction 49–51) with a peak (V) in the epoxide region (fractions 53–56) where the BP-4,5-epoxide was isolated. However, peak (V) probably represented another type of derivative since the known epoxides were unstable under such conditions. The increasing background (fractions 31–80) results from a small quantity of BP leaching from the column, which occurred using reversed-phase elution when low metabolism created a large unmetabolized BP residue. The background was removed by elimination of most of the BP before analysis (Fig. 9).

Lymphocyte metabolism over a 30-min period (Fig. 9) also showed some marked differences from both human and rat liver. All three dihydrodiols were absent, and with the exception of small peaks II and IV, which were also absent, the metabolites (I, III, V, VI) were present as with human liver. However, the relative amount of peak III in the quinone region was reduced, the 3-OH-BP to 9-OH-BP ratio was altered, and there was a relative increase in peak VI.

The metabolite profile (Fig. 10) for a 24-hr incubation of [³H] BP and human lymphocytes in culture showed the presence of all three dihydrodiols with the 7,8-dihydrodiol as the major peak. This result agreed with those previously reported (Booth et al., 1974), although the authors neither reported the presence of quinones nor resolved phenol peaks with their mode of separation. Peaks I–III and V represented the new material seen in human liver and were present with peak IV possibly hidden between peaks III and V. Peak VI and most of the BP were removed before HPLC analysis.

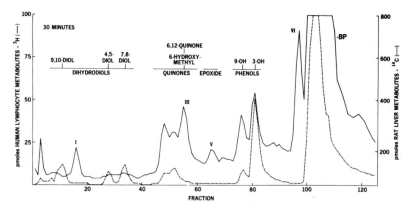

FIGURE 9 Pattern of BP metabolites formed by incubation with human lymphocytes for 30 min. Lymphocytes were isolated by the shock-lysing procedure of Severson et al. (1969). The buffy coat was collected from 500 ml fresh heparinized blood and the red cells lysed with two treatments of a hypotonic salt solution (0.2% EDTA/0.26% NaCl), the lymphocytes centrifuged at 800 rpm, and the supernatant removed. The entire shock-lysing procedure was repeated a second time. The lymphocytes were resuspended in Eagles minimal essential medium (Grand Island Biological Company, New York) supplemented with 10% fetal calf serum, penicillin 100 unit/ml and streptomycin 100 μg/ml. The suspended cells were divided into two equal parts. The first portion was treated with 1% phytohemagglutinin and pokeweed mitogen for 72 hr, followed by benz[a]anthracene (1 μg/ml) for 24 hr; the cells were collected for incubation with [^{3}H]BP.

Metabolites were formed by incubating the lymphocytes with [^{3}H]BP and rat liver microsomes with [^{14}C]BP in the following manner: each flask contained in a total volume of 1.0 ml: 7.0–8.0 × 10^6 lymphocytes or 100 μg liver microsomal protein; 0.36 μmol NADPH for liver; 0.79 μmol NADPH and NADP for lymphocytes; 3 μmol MgCl$_2$; 50 μmol Tris–HCl buffer (pH 7.5); and 100 nmol [^{3}H]BP dissolved in 0.04 ml methanol. The flasks were incubated 30 min for lymphocytes and 10 min for liver at 37°C under red light illumination. The reaction was stopped by adding 1.0 ml acetone; the metabolites were extracted with 2.0 ml ethyl acetate. [^{14}C]BP metabolite standards and [^{3}H] incubation extracts were mixed and injected simultaneously into the column. Ten ethyl acetate extracts were combined and dried over 2.0 g anhydrous MgSO$_4$, evaporated under vacuum to dryness, and the metabolites dissolved in 0.1 ml methanol for analysis by HPLC.

The second portion of lymphocytes was also treated with phytohemagglutin and pokeweed mitogen for 72 hr (Fig. 10), but benz[a]anthracene was omitted and [^{3}H]BP (2 μg/ml) added directly to the medium. After 24 hr in the dark, the medium was extracted with 2 volumes of ethyl acetate, which was evaporated to dryness. The metabolites were dissolved in 0.1 ml methanol for HPLC analysis (Selkirk et al., 1975b).

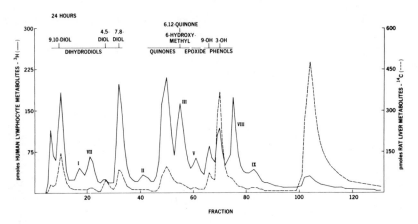

FIGURE 10   Pattern of BP metabolites formed by incubation with human lymphocytes for 24 hr (Selkirk et al., 1975b).

In addition to peaks I–VI, several new peaks were observed during the longer incubation period: one peak in the diol region (VII) and two more peaks in the phenol region (VII, IX). Peak VII was large enough to allow partial analytical characterization and had a molecular weight (m/e 268) corresponding to a phenol, with its spectrum similar to, but distinct from, the other known BP phenols.

Human tissue studies of polycyclic aromatic hydrocarbons have been largely confined to determining amount, specificity, and inducibility of the drug-metabolizing enzymes. The fluorometric analysis, which measures conversion of BP to 3-OH-BP, is sensitive and adequate to discriminate slight variations in enzyme content. However, it cannot determine the flux of the total metabolite profile with time, nor can it differentiate pattern changes of metabolites between various tissues and species. While the human studies reported above did not completely characterize the new metabolites, they nevertheless show salient differences between human and rat tissue metabolism of BP. This finding may be especially important since most carcinogenesis data have been derived from rodent studies.

Lymphocyte metabolism of BP, which produced relatively the same metabolites as human liver, also showed the epoxide hydrase activity in the cells not to be as rapid as the rat epoxide hydrase during short-term incubation; rather, longer exposure to the hydrocarbon was required to reach an active level of hydration activity.

It is anticipated, based on the known lability of reactive epoxides, that reduced epoxide hydrase activity could allow epoxides in lymphocytes to possess a greater potential to alkylate target sites. This has already been shown for binding to DNA and for enhancing tumor formation in mouse skin (Kinoshita et al., 1973).

CONCLUSION

The importance of understanding polycyclic aromatic hydrocarbon carcinogenesis cannot be overstated, since the widespread occurrence of these chemicals as environmental contaminants presents a very real health hazard for humans.

The advent of HPLC should result in a burgeoning of knowledge concerning metabolism of all forms of chemical carcinogens. The efficiency of this new technique, with its superior utility for the study of labile reactive molecules, has made the task of understanding chemical carcinogenesis more approachable than envisioned using previous methods with less analytical capacity.

Note added in proof: Since the writing of this report there has appeared considerable evidence that the diols of benzo[*a*]pyrene are capable of acting as substrates for the monooxygenase system and are remetabolized to form a diol-epoxide. Current evidence shows that the diol-epoxide intermediate is more mutagenic and appears in some systems to be the predominant species of the molecule that binds to macromolecules in the cell. The reader is referred to the following references for a discussion of this subject: Sims et al. (1974), Huberman et al. (1976), and Yang et al. (1976).

REFERENCES

Allison, A. C. and Mallucci, L. 1964. *Nature* 203:1024.

Alvares, A. P., Schilling, G. R., Levin, W. and Kuntzman, R. 1967. *Biochem. Biophys. Res. Commun.* 29:521.

Alvares, A. P., Schilling, G. R. and Kuntzman, R. 1968. *Biochem. Biophys. Res. Commun.* 30:588.

Ames, B. N., Sims, P. and Grover, P. L. 1972. *Science* 176:47.

Baird, W. M. and Brookes, P. 1973. *Cancer Res.* 33:2378.

Baird, W. M., Dipple, A., Grover, P. L., Sims, P. and Brookes, P. 1973. *Cancer Res.* 33:2386.

Baird, W. M., Harvey, R. G. and Brookes, P. 1975. *Cancer Res.* 35:54.

Bast, R. C., Jr., Whitlock, J. P., Jr., Miller, H., Rapp, H. J. and Gelboin, H. V. 1974. *Nature* 250:664.

Booth, J., Boyland, E. and Sims, P. 1961. *Biochem. J.* 79:516.

Booth, J., Keysall, G. R., Kalyani, P. L. and Sims, P. 1974. *FEBS Lett.* 43:341.

Borgen, A., Darvey, H., Castagnoli, N., Crocker, T. T., Rasmussen, R. E. and Wang, I. Y. 1973. *J. Med. Chem.* 16:502.

Boyland, E. 1950. *Symp. Biochem. Soc.* 5:40.

Boyland, E. and Chasseaud, L. F. 1969. *Adv. Enzymol.* 32:173.

Boyland, E. and Sims, P. 1965. *Biochem. J.* 95:780.

Brookes, P. and Lawley, P. D. 1964. *Nature* 202:781.

Bürki, K., Stomung, T. A. and Bresnick, E. 1974. *J. Natl. Cancer Inst.* 52:785.

Busbee, D. L., Shaw, C. R. and Cantrell, E. T. 1972. *Science* 178:315.

Cantrell, E. T., Warr, G. A., Busbee, D. L. and Martin, R. R. 1973. *J. Clin. Invest.* 52:1881.

Cavalieri, E. and Calvin, M. 1971. *Proc. Natl. Acad. Sci. U.S.A.* 68:1251.

Committee on Biologic Effects of Atmospheric Pollutants. 1972. *Particulate polycyclic organic matter*, Washington, D.C.: National Academy of Sciences.

Conney, A. H. 1967. *Pharmacol. Rev.* 19:317.

Cook, J. W. and Hewett, L. 1933. *J. Chem. Soc.* 398.

Dansette, P. and Jerina, D. M. 1974. *J. Am. Chem. Soc.* 96:1224.

Dansette, P., Yagi, H., Jerina, D. M., Daly, J. W., Levin, W., Lu, A. Y. U., Kuntzman, R. and Conney, A. H. 1974. *Arch. Biochem. Biophys.* 164:511.

Flesher, J. W. and Sydnor, K. L. 1973. *Int. J. Cancer.* 11:433.

Gelboin, H. V. 1967. *Adv. Cancer Res.* 10:1.

Gelboin, H. V. 1969. *Cancer Res.* 29:1272.

Gelboin, H. V., Kinoshita, N. and Wiebel, F. J. 1972. *Fed. Proc.* 31:1298.

Goh, S. H. and Harvey, R. G. 1973. *J. Am. Chem. Soc.* 95:242.

Goshman, L. M. and Heidelberger, C. 1967. *Cancer Res.* 27:1678.

Grover, P. L., Hewer, A. and Sims, P. 1972. *Biochem. Pharmacol.* 21:2713.

Heidelberger, C. 1973. *Adv. Cancer Res.* 18:317.

Heidelberger, C. and Moldenhaur, M. G. 1956. *Cancer Res.* 16:442.

Heiger, I. 1933. *J. Chem. Soc.* 395.

Huberman, E., Aspiras, L., Heidelberger, C., Grover, P. L. and Sims, P. 1971. *Proc. Natl. Acad. Sci. U.S.A.* 68:3195.

Huberman, E., Kuroki, T., Marquardt, H., Selkirk, J. K., Heidelberger, C., Grover, P. L. and Sims, P. 1972. *Cancer Res.* 32:1391.

Huberman, E. et al. 1976. *Proc. Natl. Acad. Sci. USA* 73:607.

Irving, C. C. 1973. *Methods Cancer Res.* 7:189.

Kellerman, G., Lyten-Kellerman, M. and Shaw, C. R. 1973. *Am. J. Hum. Genet.* 25:327.

Kennaway, E. L. and Heiger, I. 1930. *Br. Med. J.* 1:1044.

Kinoshita, N., Shears, B. and Gelboin, H. V. 1973. *Cancer Res.* 33:1937.

Kuntzman, R., Mark, L. C., Brand, L., Jacobson, M., Levin, W. and Conney, A. H. 1966. *J. Pharmacol. Exp. Ther.* 152:151.

Kuroki, T., Huberman, E., Marquardt, H., Selkirk, J. K., Heidelberger, C., Grover, P. L. and Sims, P. 1971. *Chem. Biol. Interact.* 4:389.

Levtz, J. C. and Gelboin, H. V. 1974. *Arch. Biochem. Biophys.* 160:722.

Levin, W., Conney. A. H. and Alvares, A. P. 1972. *Science* 167:419.

Lu, A. Y. H. and Coon, M. J. 1968. *J. Biol. Chem.* 243:1331.

Lu, A. Y. H., Kuntzman, R., West, S., Jacobson, M. and Conney, A. H. 1972. *J. Biol. Chem.* 247:1727.

Marquardt, H., Kuroki, T., Huberman, E., Selkirk, J. K., Heidelberger, C., Grover, P. and Sims, P. 1972. *Cancer Res.* 32:716.

Marquardt, H., Sapozink, M. D. and Zedeck, M. S. 1974. *Cancer Res.* 34:3387.

Miller, E. C. and Miller, J. A. 1951. *Cancer Res.* 11:108.

Miller, E. C. and Miller, J. A. 1967. *Proc. Soc. Exp. Biol. Med.* 124:915.

Nagata, C., Tagashira, Y. and Kodama, M. 1972. In *Chemical carcinogenesis*, ed. P. O. P. Ts'o and J. A. DiPaolo, part A., pp. 87–111. New York: Marcel Dekker.

Natarajan, R. K. and Flesher, J. W. 1973. *J. Med. Chem.* 16:714.

Nebert, D. W., Winker, J. and Gelboin, H. V. 1969. *Cancer Res.* 29:1763.

Nemoto, N. and Gelboin, H. V. 1975. *Arch. Biochem. Biophys.* 170:739.

Newman, M. S. and Olsen, D. R. 1974. *J. Am. Chem. Soc.* 96:6207.

Oesch, F. 1973. *Xenobiotica* 3:305.

Oesch, F., Kaubisch, N., Jerina, D. M. and Daly, J. W. 1971. *Biochemistry* 10:4858.

Pitot, H. C. and Heidelberger, C. 1963. *Cancer Res.* 23:1694.

Public Health Service survey of compounds which have been tested for carcinogenic activity. Publ. No. 149.

Selkirk, J. K., Huberman, E. and Heidelberger, C. 1971. *Biochem. Biophys. Res. Commun.* 43:1010.

Selkirk, J. K., Croy, R. G. and Gelboin, H. V. 1974a. *Science* 184:169.

Selkirk, J. K., Croy, R. G. and Gelboin, H. V. 1974b. *Cancer Res.* 34:3474.

Selkirk, J. K., Croy, R. G. and Gelboin, H. V. 1975a. *Arch. Biochem. Biophys.* 168:322.

Selkirk, J. K., Croy, R. G., Whitlock, J. P. and Gelboin, H. V. 1975b. *Cancer Res.* 35:3651.

Severson, C. D., Frank, D. H., Stokes, C., Seepersad, M. F. and Thompson, J. S. 1969. *Transplantation* 8:538.

Shires, T. K. and Richter, K. M. 1966. *Exp. Cell Res.* 44:617.

Sims, P. 1966. *Biochem. J.* 98:215.

Sims, P. 1970. *Biochem. Pharmacol.* 19:795.

Sims, P. and Grover, P. L. 1974. *Adv. Cancer Res.* 20:165.

Sims, P., Grover, P. L., Swaisland, A., Pal, K. and Hewer, A. 1974. *Nature* 252:326.

Sloane, N. H. and Heinemann, M. 1970. *Biochem. Biophys. Acta* 201:384.

Stoming, T., Knapp, D. and Bresnick, E. 1973. *Life Sci.* 12:425.

Ts'o, P. O. P., Caspary, W. J., Cohen, B. I., Leavitt, J. C., Lesko, S. A., Lorentzen, R. J. and Schechtman, L. M. 1972. In *Chemical carcinogenesis*, ed. P. O. P. Ts'o and J. A. DiPaolo, part A, pp. 113–147. New York: Marcel Dekker.

Wang, I. V., Rasmussen, J. F. and Crocker, T. T. 1972. *Biochem. Biophys. Res. Commun.* 49:1142.

Wattenberg, L. W. 1966. *Cancer Res.* 26:1520.

Welch, R. W., Harrison, Y. E., Govaini, B. W., Poppers, P. T., Ernster, M. and Conney, A. H. 1969. *Clin. Pharmacol. Ther.* 10:100.

Whitlock, J. P., Jr., Cooper, H. L. and Gelboin, H. V. 1972. *Science* 177:619.

Weibel, F. J., Leutz, J. C., Diamond, L. and Gelboin, H. V. 1971. *Arch. Biochem.* 144:78.

Wiebel, F. J., Gelboin, H. V., Buu-Hoi, N. P., Stout, M. G. and Burnham, W. S. 1972. In *Chemical carcinogenesis*, ed. P. O. P. Ts'o and J. A. DiPaolo, part A, pp. 249–270. New York: Marcel Dekker.

Wood, A. W., Goode, R. L., Chang, R. L., Levin, W., Conney, A. H., Yagi, H., Dansette, P. and Jerina, D. M. 1975. *Proc. Am. Assoc. Cancer Res.* 14:435.

Yamagiwa, K. and Ichikawa, K. 1918. *J. Cancer Res.* 3:1.

Yang, C. S. and Strickhart, F. S. 1975. *Biochem. Pharmacol.* 24:646.

Yang, S. K. et al. 1976. *Proc. Natl. Acad. Sci. USA* 73:2594.

Chapter 2

CONCEPTUAL APPROACHES TO THE ASSESSMENT OF NONOCCUPATIONAL ENVIRONMENTAL CANCER

H. F. Kraybill
National Cancer Institute
National Institutes of Health
Bethesda, Maryland

INTRODUCTION

Man's interaction with the environment is a complex one, well-recognized but not fully comprehended. Some interactions are beneficial while others impose a risk. Involved in this benefit-risk equation are biological, physical, and chemical agents; the latter may be the chemical itself, a metabolite, or a pyrolytic and/or degradation product. Among a spectrum of biomedical responses to environmental stresses imposing a cytotoxic effect are those with carcinogenic, mutagenic, or teratogenic activities. Many chemicals may originate in the environment and through technological processes be dispersed into and pollute the air, soil, water, and food. Natural sources may contribute toxins that cannot always be avoided unless preventive measures are applied for their control. Both organic and inorganic chemicals are associated with cytotoxic effects and effects on target organs. Variation in biological activity with structure and valence, or physical properties, especially volatility, solubility, and stability, are factors that must be fully recognized in an assessment of relative toxicity within a general class of compounds or a single compound with specific elements.

The kinds of environmental agents to which humans can be exposed are illustrated in Fig. 1.

In the natural environment, cytotoxic agents originate in the atmosphere from plants and bacteria, or they are transmitted by animals or insects. In the atmosphere are gaseous and particulate matter, such as nitrous oxide, sulfur dioxide, chemical effluents, silicates, asbestos, lead, nitroso compounds, radionuclides, and combustion products. In plant and bacterial systems, there are mycotoxins, cycasin (from cycad nuts), bracken fern, tannins, and bacterial-fungal metabolites, such as ethionine and antibiotics. Animals and insects transmit certain parasites and viruses.

27

Through exploitation of natural resources for the purposes of industrialization, humans have created certain unwanted environmental stress agents. The list of these chemicals is quite extensive, including many inorganic and synthetic organic chemicals. It is estimated that there are about 4 million chemicals in the universe. Industrial technology introduces thousands of new ones each year. One can cite food chemicals (additives, preservatives, etc.), pesticides, detergents, dyestuffs, drugs, petroleum products, nuclear products, and a host of other synthetic chemicals manufactured by industry.

No part of the world is free of environmental stress agents, such as pesticide contaminants, fallout radionuclides, mycotoxins, marine toxins, and the large group of industrially produced synthetic chemicals. Monitoring systems have revealed that the distribution of pollutants prevails on a global basis via the sea or via atmospheric and stratospheric transport through distillation from the earth's crust. It is estimated, for example, that by the year 2000,

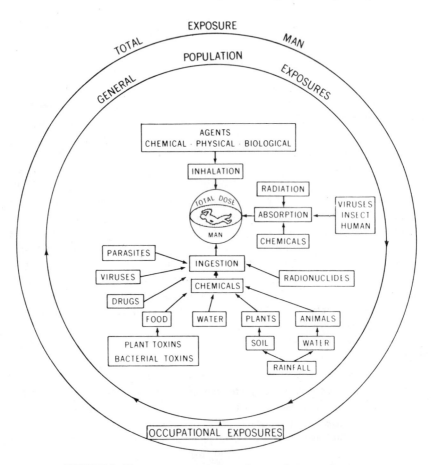

FIGURE 1 Human exposure to hazardous environmental agents.

man-made sources of tritium, if uncontrolled, will equal the natural production rate; thus the steady-state equilibrium of tritium between humans and the biosphere would be doubled (Rose, 1971). In some countries the environmental stress situations are unique. However, as more and more data accrue, one realizes that many of these problems are international in scope.

Carcinogenic insult to humans and animals may come from chemical, physical, or biological agents, all of which increase the probability of tumor formation or induction of neoplasia. The impact of these cytotoxic materials on humans, as shown in epidemiologic studies, may be an increase in the number of tumor-bearing individuals, an increase in number of tumors per individual, or a reduction in the latency period for induction of tumors. Depending on which report one reads, environmental agents are said to be involved in from 75 to 90% of all human cancers (Boyland, 1969; Epstein 1970; Higginson, 1969; World Health Organization, 1964). Boyland (1969) estimates that 90% of human cancers are evoked by chemical agents. Despite such a variation in estimates, it is generally recognized that environmental stresses are involved in cancer induction, and hence, preventive measures could and should be instituted. It is also suspected that oncogenic viruses and/or physical agents (radiation) and bacterial and parasiticological agents may be involved in cancer causation or may interact with chemicals in such causation (Epstein, 1974).

According to the American Cancer Society (1974), more than 25% of the 200 million people living in the United States will develop some form of cancer. In 1969, 323,000 people died of cancer in the United States; in 1972, 610,000 cases of cancer were diagnosed and about 1 million people were under treatment for cancer (Department of Health, Education, and Welfare, 1973). Thus, cancer is the second leading cause of premature deaths, exceeding casualties in war, auto accidents, and other disease states. The economic impact of cancer deaths in terms of hospitalization, medical care, loss of earnings during illness, and reduction of life span has been estimated to be $15 billion for the year 1971 in the United States (Department of Health, Education, and Welfare, 1973). Certainly, aggressive measures are indicated for allocation of resources for the prevention of cancer.

Against this background, it is evident that national legislative measures are required to prohibit the intentional introduction of chemicals, new and old, into the environment without some prior assessment of their probable impact. Environmental impact statements have captured the attention of legislators and public policy analysts. With the introduction of new chemicals into the environment, it becomes prohibitively expensive, if not logistically impracticable, to prove out the safety and risk of each compound (Lewin, 1974). New methods will have to be developed to permit a more rapid evaluation of the carcinogenic potential of whole classes of compounds.

ENVIRONMENTAL INTELLIGENCE NETWORK

Monitoring and Surveillance of Carcinogen Exposure

Monitoring and *surveillance* are terms used almost synonymously. Monitoring environmental contaminants and/or carcinogens is, essentially, gathering data on both the intentional and inadvertent additions of these chemical contiminants to the air, water, and diet. In occupational situations, monitoring assesses the levels of chemicals that are released and are inhaled or absorbed. Surveillance involves an overview of such data by an intelligence network, which follows trends on a geographical basis and documents alterations in environmental levels of contaminants.

Just as it is important to evaluate dose-response relationships in experimental animal studies, so is an estimate of exposure values requisite in making epidemiological assessments.

General Population Monitoring

Federal and state agencies have operated environmental intelligence networks for many years. There is a plethora of published information and data that relate to the toxicity and epidemiological aspects of various environmental contaminants (Berg and Burbank, 1972; Committee on Biologic Effects of Atmospheric Pollutants, 1972a, b).

The U.S. Public Health Service was probably the first federal agency to establish extensive networks for the monitoring of contaminants in water (Water Quality Program) and pollutants in air (Air Pollution Program). In the early 1960s, they set up an extensive network to monitor fallout radionuclides in air, water, foods, and diet. Monitoring of food and milk was done on a regional basis to show trends in the movement of radioactive material through the stratosphere and its ultimate localization in areas where food crops and forage were produced (Kraybill et al., 1962). The regions covered in this collation of data on ^{137}Cs and ^{90}Sr included New York, Chicago, St. Louis, Atlanta, Dallas, Denver, Seattle, and Los Angeles. Similar radiological monitoring was conducted in the United Kingdom and Germany (Agricultural Research Council, 1960; Merten and Knoop, 1960). Almost all of these studies were concerned with food radioactivity measurements in population groups of a certain age, socioeconomic status, geographical location, and religious and ethnic identification. Special attention was given to children as a group, since they could be exposed to radioactive material for a long time and probably would have lengthy disease-induction periods. Dietary patterns were found to influence the intake and exposure to radionuclides on a geographic basis. Ancillary studies were also conducted in the 1960s by the Food and Drug Administration and the Atomic Energy Commission in the United States. The studies by the Atomic Energy Commission and other institutions also concentrated on measurements of radionuclides in people (Sadarangani et al., 1973; Kulp et al., 1960; Comar and Georgi, 1961).

The principal problem with monitoring for contaminants, noncarcinogenic or carcinogenic, and assessing the minimum, maximum, and average intakes by the general population is the lack of precise values for intake of specific foods and food classes. If such a compendium of data were available for all foods consumed by different groups (categorized by age, ethnic origin, and geographical location, revealing variation in diet patterns), then a scale of values could be derived for calculating the exposure range for each environmental contaminant, drug, or food chemical. Instead, tabular values must be taken from food survey reports, which are only estimates on what canvassers believe people eat. These estimates are derived from a recall procedure. Other data come from nutritional surveys, in which the U.S. Army has excelled. In these Army surveys, average values are used based on the consumption patterns of 100–400 men for 7 days to 1 month. The only accurate procedure is to actually quantitate intakes of all foods, as has been done in some surveys on pesticide exposure (Dunham et al., 1965; Walker et al., 1954). An exact procedure would be to accumulate data as is done by dietitians in hospitals; there, food consumed is quantitated from amount given and the unconsumed amount returned. However, this procedure is not feasible for large population surveys. But the point is that a better handbook of data is needed in this area. It may be asked why the emphasis is on accurate data on food and diet. The answer, of course, is that for the general population, food and diet may represent the major component in environmental exposure to a carcinogen. For example, in the case of DDT and DDE, 85% of the total exposure of the general population is via food (Kraybill, 1969; see Fig. 2).

Pesticides, some of which are suspect carcinogens on the basis of studies in mice and rats, have been monitored perhaps more extensively than any other environmental contaminant. Levels of the organochlorine insecticide DDT (recently banned except in malaria control of the vector mosquito) have been monitored worldwide in air, water, food, and humans. Many investigators have published in this field; an excellent treatise on the epidemiology of DDT by Davies and Edmondson (1972) illustrates how extensive monitoring can be with humans including their blood, urine, and body tissues, especially for those occupationally exposed. The environmental sources of DDT exposure and the population groups by occupation involved in DDT exposure are illustrated in Figs. 2 and 3. The same general format could be used to delineate and quantitate the level of exposure of other environmental contaminants.

Both the federal and state governments have devised air pollution health warning systems, which alert the public when certain levels of air pollution are reached. A wide array of pollutants, including gaseous and particulate elements and compounds of carcinogenic potential and activity, are monitored continuously. Other contaminants now being monitored are the polycyclic aromatic hydrocarbons, organic synthetic pesticides, carcinogenic metallic elements and compounds such as arsenic and asbestiform minerals (the amphiboles and chrysotiles), and many industrial plant effluents. In this latter

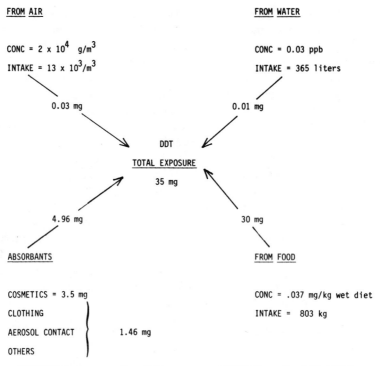

FIGURE 2 Sources of pesticide exposure (DDT) (from Kraybill, 1969).

class are some of the aliphatic and aromatic hydrocarbons and their derivatives, including azo-, nitro-, and amine organic compounds.

Extensive monitoring for inorganic and organic contaminants has been
conducted, and the effort has been expanded recently, since it has been
shown that raw water pollutants migrate through the treatment processes used
in securing potable water for municipalities. The discovery that these biorefractories are increasing in types and amounts, and include either recognized
or suspect carcinogens, has caused much concern. Federal and state water
quality programs have focused on this problem. Symposiums have been held
both nationally and internationally, directing attention not only to aquatic
carcinogens but also to their epizootic effect in finfish and shellfish, in which
neoplasms have been observed. In a recent paper by Kraybill (1974c), the
classes of compounds and specific chemical carcinogens in raw and potable
water and their distribution in geographic regions are described, and the levels
of each chemical are delineated in some cases.

Monitoring Carcinogens in the Work Place

Exposure to carcinogens in the work place represents a stress beyond
that received from general environmental exposure (air, water, diet, drugs,

radiation, tobacco smoke, automobile exhausts, etc.). Thus, persons occupationally exposed to carcinogens represent the population groups at risk. It is from this group that many causal effects have been elicited in epidemiological studies. Percivall Pott, a perceptive Irish physician, noted an association between cancer of the scrotum in his adult male patients and their exposure to soot as chimney sweeps (Pott, 1775). No one will question that this observation by Pott is the first excursion into chemical epidemiology.

No attempt will be made to recount all the observations that Pott sparked as a result of his early studies, but a few may be worth mentioning. Of significance are the observations of bladder cancers from occupational exposure to amines and amides (Goldblatt, 1947, 1958; Walpole and Williams, 1958), based on well-documented cases of β-naphthylamine exposure. There

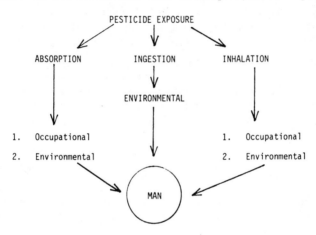

Occupational Exposure

1. Pest Control Operations
2. Agricultural Applications
3. Formulation Operations
4. Mosquito Abatement Operations
5. Pesticide Manufacturing

Environmental Exposure

1. Air
2. Water
3. Food
4. Cosmetics - Drugs
5. Contact Exposure
6. Aerosol Uses
7. Soils
8. Automatic Dispensing Devices
9. Pesticide Strips

FIGURE 3 Types of pesticide exposure of various populations (from Kraybill, 1969).

has been concern for 50 yr about mining and milling workers because ore dust from chromate, talc, and nickel smelting is associated with lung and nasal cancers. Shimkin (1969) speculated that the high death rate from lung disease in Schneeberg miners might be due to their inhaling ore dust and to the radioactivity from uranium in the mines. Between 1876 and 1939, there were 400 cases of lung cancer (Lorenz, 1944). This led to intensive studies in the United States that confirmed that uranium miners were at high risk and at an even greater risk when cigarette smoking was an additive exposure (Lundin, 1969).

Hueper (1969), in his excellent monograph on occupational and environmental cancers of the urinary system, describes the epidemiology of aromatic amine cancers. Also worth mentioning are the skin cancers induced by creosote oil, coal tar pitch, and asphalt (Heller and Henry, 1930). More recently, excellent studies by Egbert and Geiger (1936) and Selikoff et al. (1968) draw attention to the effect of long-term exposures in mines and fabrication plants to asbestos, which induces lung cancer and other respiratory diseases. Many of these causal agents are described by Hueper (1969), but one would be remiss not to mention here the recent observations on the vinyl chloride monomer that induced the rare lesion of angiosarcoma of the liver in experimental animals (Maltoni, 1974), which was simultaneously reported in vinyl chloride workers (Creech and Makk, 1975). This latter episode is significant since it delineates the hazard in the work place and the potential health effect of dispersal of this chemical into the atmosphere and the aquatic environment.

If workers are to be protected from either acute or long-term exposures, the work environment must be monitored continuously. Standards relating to control must be promulgated and enforced. Monitoring must include a spectrum of preventive procedures, such as analysis of aerial effluents in the work place and wipe samples from surfaces where chemical carcinogens may settle out. Since many carcinogenic chemicals may be resorbed through the skin as well as inhaled or ingested, the levels of these carcinogens in or on wearing apparel, wash water from hands, filter presses, wood floors, hand rails, and valve handles must be determined (Vigliani and Barsotti, 1962). A comprehensive medical protection program would also include wipe samples or smears from the skin of workers, urine and blood samples, and expired air samples from workers potentially exposed to chemical carcinogens. Wherever indicated, a battery of biochemical and clinical chemistry analyses should be routinely performed to monitor any physiological, pathological, and morphological changes resulting from carcinogen exposure.

As evidenced by the increase in occupationally induced cancers and deaths therefrom in statistical reporting of these occupational cancers, it is apparent that precautionary measures, including worker protection to exposures and adequate monitoring, is lacking in many industrial operations.

Exposure data from a sophisticated monitoring system is an essential requirement in the conquest of cancer.

Data and observations on exposure-response relationships are derived from two sources: (1) experimental studies on the chemical in laboratory animals, revealing tumor incidence, time-to-tumor formation, and organ site involved; and (2) associated epidemiologic pursuits dealing with human population laboratories. There is a great need for a "crosswalk" between these two areas of exploration since that would provide the basis for making meaningful scientific appraisals as to the relative carcinogenic hazards of chemical, physical, and biological factors with respect to induction of neoplastic disease. Continuous surveillance thus provides some assessment of the extent of exposure with time and place and trends in escalation or diminution.

EXPOSURE-RESPONSE RELATIONSHIPS

The term *exposure* is commonly used to define the quantitative aspects of environmental insults to humans. While the term *dose* is used in the quantification of a stress in animal experimentation, the term *exposure* as an indicator of the degree of toxic challenge has relevance for observations in experimental animals and human population laboratories. While dose- or exposure-response relationships can be readily assessed qualitatively and quantitatively in animal experiments, unfortunately such information awaits completion of extensive epidemiological studies in the human population. Such studies are time-consuming and frequently unrewarding, unless a sufficiently long induction period has elapsed and human cancers are evoked by the particular agent under observation and study.

Relevancy of Experimental Exposures

Many problems have been encountered in extrapolating data on animal exposures to human exposures and in translating carcinogenic response in the animal to the human, where exposure conditions are not comparable. A common practice in experimental studies is to exaggerate the exposure to achieve a so-called MTD (maximum tolerated dose). This exaggerated dose is imposed upon the rodent for 18-24 months to establish a carcinogenic response, if possible. Quite frequently, these endeavors are failures since overdosing produces overt toxicity, which invariably produces organ refractoriness, such as a swamping of the liver microsomal enzymes. In addition, metabolic overloading may either result in a chemical being metabolized by an alternate pathway, not necessarily comparable to metabolic stress in human exposure situations, or the chemical may be unmetabolized, stored in the body or excreted unchanged.

For most every chemical, pollutant, or nutrient, the mammalian system has a finite value for a threshold or tolerance level that the well-defined biochemical and metabolic pathways can accommodate. In essence, *toxicity* is a relevant term, and any useful chemical, if taken in excess, will lead to untoward effects (for example, excessive amounts of vitamins A and D result in hypervitaminosis). The small margin of safety for some common chemicals in our dietary are given in Table 1.

Realizing that there are small margins of safety for allegedly innocuous compounds essential for physiological processes, one must conclude that any acutely toxic chemical is certainly bound by such limitations. This essential pharmacologic threshold principle appears to be forgotten when attempts are made to maximize the response, either carcinogenic or noncarcinogenic, by administering excessive doses of a chemical. Consequently, the end result frequently is that high mortalities occur in animals under study; for those surviving the metabolic overload, the overt toxicity obscures, if not circumvents, the appearance of neoplastic disease that could be induced at the cellular level. The rationale for adopting the practice of a maximum tolerated dose has its basis in statistical approaches. Specifically, one assumes that measurement of an increase in tumor incidence may be achieved by administering a high stress (high dose) to a limited number of experimental animals where the alternative of assessing the incidence and risk to thousands or millions of persons exposed to the chemical in question is not feasible. Therefore, the principle of using high doses is a substitute for the inability to utilize a "mega"-animal experiment. Furthermore, it is maintained that low orders of exposure may yield some false negatives in a tumorigenic evaluation. As convincing as the mathematical explanation may be, there must be some recognition of the fact that false negatives or false positives will result in any event. Furthermore, the ultimate biomedical effect observed may not be at all biochemically or pharmacologically consistent with and relevant to environmental exposures, including occupational exposure, as they occur in human situations.

There are many examples that could be cited on the exposure-response problem and the practice of overdosing. One example is the study of the

TABLE 1 Some Limiting Values for Intake of Nutrients
and Chemicals[a]

Chemical or nutrient	Daily intake (allowance)	Chronic toxic dose (limit value)	Safety factor
Nicotonic acid	20.0 mg	100.0 mg	5
Vitamin A	5000 units	90,000 units	18
Vitamin D	400 units	2,000 units	5
Fluoride	1.0 mg	5.0 mg	5
Sodium chloride	5 g	10.0 g	2
Selenium	0.5–1.0 mg	10 mg	10

[a]Reprinted from Kraybill (1974d), by courtesy of Marcel Dekker, Inc.

fungal metabolite and potent hepatocarcinogen aflatoxin, which failed to induce liver cancer in the monkey at high dose but did do so after a dose was selected that approached comparable environmental levels in man (Kraybill, 1974b).

In some work by Innes et al. (1969), the experimental dose of DDT given to mice, according to calculations made by Kraybill (1969, 1974b), amounted to 853 times the average dietary exposure to DDT for humans and was about three times the occupational exposure for this pesticide (Table 2). Loomis (1969) has claimed that the experimental dose of DDT given to mice in the Innes study was 160,000 times the amount of DDT that humans receive in their daily diet; this calculation has not been confirmed. But this example does show how exaggerated dose schedules have been applied that do not parallel human exposures and so introduce difficulties in the evaluation of findings on a toxicological basis. Some attention is now being given to designing experiments with a dose schedule that has comparative significance to human situations of toxic stress.

Toxicologists have recently examined a group of chemicals shown experimentally to produce a carcinogenic response at exceedingly high doses; the human intake equivalence levels per day would be beyond imagination. Such correlations in experimental exposures versus human exposures through dietary intake are shown in Table 3.

An interesting treatment of the subject of exposure-response relationships has been set forth by Jones (1974). In the discussion of concepts, he stresses the linearity of dose-effect relationships. While it is true in many cases that tumor incidence, at least experimentally, increases with dose and time-to-tumor formation decreases with increase in dose, there are exceptions to this observation. The exposure–response relationship is circumscribed by many factors, such as influence of overloading on metabolism, alternate pathways of metabolism, breakdown of compound in the gut by bacterial systems, and the appearance of noncarcinogenic lesions with increasing dose of the toxic agent that may terminate the response by death of the animal prior to tumor formation. Aflatoxin dosing in monkeys, mentioned above, is an exception to Jones's assumptions on linearity. Jones (1974), in discussing certain environmental agents such as radiation and a group of chemicals including nitrosamines, emphasizes the importance of time-to-tumor formation in terms of exposures. His mathematical data purport to show that exposure to some environmental agents at extremely low doses extends the induction period for cancer far beyond the life span of humans. Thus, it may appear that there is an "apparent threshold" that can be demonstrated under the particular conditions of an experiment (strain of animal, diet, environment, etc.). Alterations of these conditions could elicit, however, a positive response within the life span. Such alteration could come about, for instance, from the influence of other chemicals on a carcinogenic cellular imprint that could prevail from prior challenge, and thus potentiators could alter the milieu, or cellular

TABLE 2 DDT Exposures: Correlation of Experimental Doses in Mouse to Calculated Equivalent Experimental Exposure in Humans and Actual Environmental and Occupational Exposures in Humans

Species	Exposure period	Daily dry diet consumed (g)	Daily average intake DDT (mg)	Total intake DDT per year (mg)	Total intake DDT per lifetime (mg)	Dose rate DDT per annum or lifetime (mg/kg)
Mouse—experimental bioassay[a]	569 days	4	0.527	192.6	316.6	140.0
Human—experimental equivalent to mouse exposure	70 yr	500	70.0	25,500.0	1,788,500.0	140.0
Human—actual environmental exposure (dietary only)[b,c]	70 yr	500	0.0821	30.0	2,100.0	0.164
Human—occupational[d,e]	70 yr	500	25.0	9,125.0	638,750.0	50.0

[a]Data from Innes et al. (1969) (calculations based on 20-g mouse living 18 months and 50-kg man living 70 hr).
[b]Environmental exposure in diet = 30 mg/yr (Kraybill, 1964).
[c]Ratio of experimental to environmental exposure = 853:1.
[d]Estimated occupational exposure by W. J. Hayes = 0.5 mg/kg body weight (unpublished data).
[e]Ratio of experimental to occupational exposure = 2.8:1.

TABLE 3 Some Correlations of Experimental Doses to Probable Equivalent
Human Exposure for Demonstration of Chemical Carcinogenesis

Chemical	Experimental dose	Equivalent human intake levels per day
Cyclamates	5% in diet or 2.188 g/day	138–522 bottles of soft drink (80–240 times human intake)
Oil of calamus	500–5000 ppm in diet	250 quarts of vermouth
Saccharin	0.5% in diet	40 times human intake
	5.0% in diet[a]	400 times human intake
	7.5% in diet[a]	500 times average sugar consumption[b]
Diethylstilbestrol (DES)	One clinical treatment	5×10^6 lb liver for 50 yr
Safrole	5000 ppm	613 bottles of root beer
4,4′-Methylenebis-(2-chloroaniline)	1000–2000 ppm in diet	100,000 times the amount migrating daily in a packaged diet

[a]Only a few bladder tumors were found at high dose, using a contaminated product.
European studies based on the 0.5% intake produced no tumors.
[b]A dose of 3.75 mg/kg body weight is equivalent to the sweetness of 135 kg sucrose
per day.

environment. Despite these possibilities, the extended time-to-tumor formation
would be a factor in risk assessment in societal decisions on carcinogenic
hazards. It is interesting in the calculations made by Jones that he, too,
emphasizes the nonrelevancy of experimental exposure-response relationships
to the human exposure situation.

Another important aspect in exposure-response considerations is the use
of pharmacokinetic data. There have been many reports that clearly show that
the toxicity of a chemical is proportional to the capacity of the body to
handle the chemical or dose applied, the rate of administration and excretion,
and the rate of accumulation in the body. If the dose is excessive, protective
mechanisms (cellular enzymes) are neutralized and a toxic response may be a
noncarcinogenic lethality rather than a neoplastic lesion.

Role of Contaminants and Interactants

Barnes and Denz (1954) pinpointed the weaknesses in studies of chronic
toxicity: "A chronic toxicity test is always a make-shift affair to be replaced
as soon as possible by a more permanent structure of knowledge built on the
foundations of physiology, biochemistry and other fundamental sciences."
However, as Zbinden (1973) has observed, these admonitions have not been
heeded, and in many cases for the demonstration of toxic effects, the proper
methods are not available. The impact of hormonal balance and disturbances
in physiologic behavior caused by inordinate stress on metabolic pathways by
improper dosing certainly confounds the problem of assessment of toxicity.

The requirement for amassing routine toxicity data, including data on carcinogenic activity, obscures the need for acquisition of more meaningful data using test methods based on fundamental sciences (biochemistry, pharmacology, physiology, etc.).

Another parameter often missed in the biological assessment of exposures to chemicals is the role of interactants and contaminants in exposure to the chemical alleged to be a carcinogen. Comprehensive analyses using the most sophisticated methods and instrumentation are necessary prior to a biological assay. In the work place, interactants may be the potentiator or cocarcinogen. For example, the role of cigarette smoking in exposure to asbestiform materials was mentioned above. Diesel fumes, ore dust, cigarette smoke, and inhaled radon daughters all influence the induction of bronchiogenic carcinoma in uranium miners.

Saccharin, a nonnutritive sweetener and food chemical, has been used for over 50 yr without any reports of an adverse toxic effect; but recent studies have indicated it as a potential carcinogen. The fact that about nine out of ten laboratories in the United States and Europe failed to demonstrate any carcinogenic activity for saccharin directed attention to the protocol and conditions in a laboratory where a positive finding, albeit of minor importance, was revealed. An intensive survey for contaminants was made of the test animals' drinking water and their commercial laboratory diet. The most instructive lead was the discovery of three contaminants (subsequently identified as six or more), which were sulfonamides, in the saccharin used by one laboratory where a few bladder tumors formed when saccharin was fed at the high level of 5% in the diet (P. Issenberg and D. N. Clayson, personal communication, 1973). These impurities at a level of 5,000 ppm in commercial saccharin prepared by the Remsen-Fahlberg process were implicated in the carcinogenesis. On the other hand, saccharin containing only 0.5 ppm of contaminant in a product produced by the Maumee process did not induce any bladder tumors.

It is axiomatic that the higher the exposure encountered, the higher the level of contaminant associated with the chemical agent being tested. Thus, the problem of overdosing, as noted by Issenberg and Clayson (1973) for saccharin, reflects not just the effect of the chemical but also the role of the contaminant. Thus, the alleged carcinogenic activity of the primary chemical may not be an issue when contaminants are removed.

Diluents or suspending mediums for injection or intubation of a test chemical also pose the problem of interactants. For example, in the study of detergents where oil and talc were in the suspending medium, the findings may be questioned because both oil and talc could play a role as cocarcinogens (A. D. Little, 1973).

Peacock and Spense (1967) found that lung tumors were increased in mice given a large dose of 500 ppm of sulfur dioxide, which parallels exposures in the work place. Laskin et al. (1970), however, found that sulfur dioxide at a level of 10 ppm did not induce cancer in rats. But when benzo-[a]pyrene at a level of 10 mg/m^2 was given in conjunction with sulfur dioxide at a level of 3.5 ppm for 494 days to rats, Laskin et al. did obtain some squamous cell carcinomas. It was not possible to induce lung tumors in rats by inhalation of benzo[a]pyrene alone.

Variation in Exposure

Exposure to an environmental chemical varies among individuals on a time basis. Susceptibilities also vary. As previously indicated, to compensate for this variability, maximum exposure levels are used in the calculation of risk. Such an approach, which is conservative as a predictive technique, may overstate the risk in an experimental endeavor. However, if the maximum experimental exposure is equated to the exposure for individuals in the work place, the estimate of risk and interpretations may have more toxicological significance and scientific acceptability.

It would thus seem appropriate that the risk for the total population be calculated for a given dose or exposure. This is, of course, a difficult task since human exposures are not always known. Nevertheless, where data exist or can be retrieved, one could multiply the calculated risk for a given dosage by the time for which such an exposure occurs; this could then be integrated over the distribution of dosages. This approach would provide some estimate of the average risk but not necessarily the high risk.

Epidemiological pursuits have been useful in building a data base on representative exposures in the human population. For pesticides, high-risk group-exposure measurements are feasible and some have been made. It is in the area of long-term, low-level exposure-response relationships that programs for assessment need to be devised, including methods for estimating, from animal experiments, the risk of cancer to human populations from exposure to chemicals. Such projects are now underway and will provide, hopefully, a data base for such assessments. It is regrettable that previous experimental studies on carcinogenic assessment have not given proper attention to this area.

CATEGORIZATION OF ENVIRONMENTAL CARCINOGENS

Attempts have been made to categorize carcinogens under such terms as *potent, weak, recognized, suspect,* or *potential* on the basis of toxicological studies. Some feel that a "carcinogen is a carcinogen," but such a rigid viewpoint provides no basis for risk assessment when considering the host of environmental agents that the individual encounters in his life.

Potent carcinogens, such as aflatoxin (Kraybill and Shimkin, 1964) and nitrosamine (Liijinsky and Epstein, 1970), produce a high incidence of cancers in experiments with small animal populations even at low levels in a diet or in the environment. The so-called weak carcinogens require a large population of experimental animals or the surveillance of a large group of humans (in the thousands) in epidemiological investigations, where there is a range in exposures, to define a carcinogenic response. Weak carcinogens pose a greater problem in detection than the more obvious or recognizable carcinogens.

As indicated from the standpoint of risk assessment in societal decisions and legislative and regulatory actions, the categorization into classes is essential when dealing with voluntary and involuntary types of human exposure. For proven carcinogens that are considered intentional additives in food, the Delaney amendment to the Federal Food, Drug and Cosmetic Act provides the legislative basis for banning and removing such chemicals from the marketplace. The greater problem is in dealing with inadvertent or unintentional additives in food, pollutants that are discharged into the air or water or appear in the food chain as a result of accidental discharge by industry and municipalities, and processes that contribute to environmental contamination (Kraybill, 1974a).

Involuntary exposure to carcinogenic environmental chemicals, a problem of increasing proportions, is a hidden health risk since inadequate intelligence systems for collection of data and information on their presence and level of occurrence may not be available. Too frequently the benefits of a chemical, later found to be carcinogenic, have been extolled without a comprehensive evaluation as to any potential hazard associated with a specific exposure to the chemical over a wide population group. When the persistence, degree of environmental transport, and biomagnification and residue accumulation in the food chain or the human body is revealed, then concern is aroused.

The cytotoxic agents that occur as natural carcinogens, such as aflatoxin, cycasin, and certain other plant materials, present some of the most serious problems because they are not recognized before extensive exposure has prevailed (Kraybill and Shapiro, 1969). Also, iatrogenic diseases have been evoked by the administration of drugs not recognized as carcinogens. The use for many years of thorotrast (thorium dioxide) in clinical practice to diagnose space-filling lesions, and later shown to induce angiosarcoma of the liver over a period of years, emphasized the need for assurance of the safety of drugs. Bergel (1974) has set in perspective the carcinogenic hazards in natural and man-made environments.

Maltoni (1973) describes the medical and legal terminology for the evaluation of risks of occupational carcinogens: (1) definite carcinogens where epidemiological evidence exists; (2) highly suspect carcinogens where strong experimental and/or some epidemiological evidence is present; and (3) potential carcinogens where experimental data give some indication of carcinogenic action of a compound on an experimental animal. Accordingly, he classifies certain agents according to these categories.

Roe (1968) in his excellent review, "Carcinogenesis and Sanity," emphasizes the need to distinguish between carcinogens and cocarcinogens. He considers it important to make this distinction before the list of compounds to be excluded from the environment becomes so long as to render the task utterly impossible, concluding that

> if cancer may be induced by an agent in a variety of species and following a variety of routes of administration, then the likelihood is that the agent is a true carcinogen. If cancer can only be induced in one species or under special circumstances, or if the effect observed is only an increase in the incidence of a type of tumor that arises commonly in the test species, or there is no clear relationship between dose and effect, then the likelihood is that where tumors appear the agent is acting only as a co-carcinogen.

Suggested Classification for Carcinogens

Recognized or proven carcinogens. An enumeration of carcinogens in the environment is, from an interpretative viewpoint, difficult. Some chemicals and materials are *recognized carcinogens* in animals or humans because they meet certain criteria, which are as follows: (1) epidemiological observations and surveys have established them as human carcinogens; (2) they appear on lists generally accepted by scientists as chemical or physical agents that have demonstrated a carcinogenic response in humans and experimental animals; (3) they are recognized as potent carcinogens because they evoke a response at low dose in one or more organ sites; (4) a dose response is confirmed in several or many species, strains, and several laboratories; and (5) the chemical or substance has been conclusively demonstrated to cause tumors, sometimes of a type frequently seen or sometimes appearing in an earlier time frame than otherwise expected. Implicit in such requirements is the statistical significance of tumor incidence, reproducibility of the tumorigenesis, and relevancy of route of exposure. Final confirmation is the observation that the tumors are transplantable.

Suspect carcinogens. Another classification assigned to certain chemicals tested experimentally for carcinogenesis is that of *suspect carcinogens*. In this case, no conclusive relationship to cancer production has been shown, but there is some inference based on (1) an association of increased tumor incidence with known exposures; (2) other biological indications such as malignant transformations in *in vitro* systems (cell cultures); and (3) a positive response, either in only one species or in a strain, but not a consistent response by both sexes or in accordance with a dose-response pattern that parallels nonoccupational and occupational exposure levels. However, with carcinogens categorized as suspect, there is no epidemiological evidence.

Potential carcinogens. A class of potential carcinogens can be separated out of the suspect carcinogen class. In this group are chemicals that have a structural similarity to proven carcinogens but have not yet been tested or on which there is suggestive evidence from mutagenicity data.

Inadequate data for classification. For many chemicals that may be inappropriately classified as carcinogens, there is either inadequate testing by prescribed protocols or there is insufficient data. Several kinds of deficiencies may be noted here, such as tests limited in time, inadequate dose schedule, insufficient test animals, nonrelevant exposure routes, improper species or strain, strong overlay of toxicity, and failure to recognize the role of a cocarcinogenic effect of contaminants.

It is essential to make all four of these classification distinctions, especially when public reaction or emotional response may upset the processes of legislative action or regulatory decision-making.

MULTIPLE STRESS AND MULTIPLE RISK

Quite frequently, scientific and regulatory decisions are made on the basis of exposure-response relationships relevant to a single stress agent or one route of exposure. In the environment, both humans and animals are exposed to multiple stresses via contaminants or additives in the air, water, and diet in addition to the insults received from drugs, biological agents (viruses, pathogens, parasites), and physical agents (radiation from gamma rays, X-rays, or ultraviolet rays). The multiple factors involved in human exposures may play either a synergistic or an inhibitory role. Test systems, on the other hand, are developed to detect the responses of specific agents. The role of combined factors in the induction of carcinogenic effects has been studied in too limited a number of cases.

Multiple Stress

Some examples of the synergistic or inhibitory effects of multiple stress are recounted in the following remarks.

Ascorbic acid blocks the nitrosation of aminopyrine, which forms the carcinogenic dimethylnitrosamine (Greenblatt, 1973). The nitrosation reaction, which involves secondary amines and nitrite to form nitroso compounds in the environment or in the gastric milieu, is dependent upon pH conditions. It is interesting to speculate whether orange juice will inhibit the appearance of the nitroso compounds during the ingestion of nitrite-preserved foods.

Montasano and Saffiotti (1968) have shown that the systemic treatment of hamsters with low doses of dimethylnitrosamine, which by itself induced few if any tumors of the respiratory tract, did induce some respiratory tumors by subsequent treatment with a polycyclic hydrocarbon that alone had a very low carcinogenic activity. The possible involvement of nitrosamines in human lung cancer in cigarette smokers is another case where nitrosamines in the smoke and perhaps in addition to polycyclic aromatic hydrocarbons may induce cancer in mammalian species (Magee, 1971).

Aflatoxin, a very potent hepatocarcinogen that produces liver tumors in a variety of species, showed an enhancement of liver tumorigenesis when a low level (0.4 ppb of aflatoxin B_1) was given to trout along with noncarcinogenic oils (sterculia) (Sinnhuber et al., 1968).

Many other examples of interactants could be cited. Some unpublished reports indicate that mixtures of 10 or 12 chemicals have been tested using a matrix system to detect the additive effect of various carcinogens. An interesting experiment would be to evaluate the carcinogenicity of a wide mixture of chemicals, 50 to 100, where the dose administered would simulate the exposure levels that the individual receives in his diet, inhaled air, and potable water. However, the matrix for such a large number of mixed agents or chemicals is rather complex and the cost of conducting such a study may be financially prohibitive.

Multiple Risk

Obviously, multiple stresses evoke some type of multiple risk, which may result in either a noncarcinogenic or carcinogenic response. The degree of risk is conditioned on the degree of susceptibility or hypersensitivity, which, in turn, may be related to genetic factors or immune competence. The magnitude of the risk is dependent upon the latent period for tumor induction and the residence time of the stress agent within the organ, tissue or cell. The intensity of the exposure is a reflection of the dose times the duration of the environmental stressor.

In many cases, there is a competitive risk from overt toxicity that may express itself in certain lesions or disease states. Such an overt toxicity may preclude the appearance of neoplastic lesions (by resulting in premature death) or may accelerate the onset of such cancers. Thus, one may observe multiple sites where the toxic agent or carcinogen has evoked a response, or some organ sites may be affected before others.

The human intake of a chemical may vary among individuals and frequently varies daily for a given individual. To provide for an adequate margin of safety in assessment of exposures and responses, it is often a practice experimentally to calculate risks for anticipated maximum exposure levels. One procedure advocated is to calculate the risk, mathematically, for the total population for a given dosage (a difficult task dependent on elaborate monitoring) and then multiply that risk by the time exposure occurs followed by integration over the distribution of doses. This approach would provide some estimate of average risk but does not consider those segments of the population that are at high risk.

Toxicological approaches, to date, have been rather simplistic since they are based on testing of single agents in isolation from the wide spectrum of chemicals to which the human population is exposed. Adding to this inadequacy is the fact that the techniques are relatively limited or insensitive to the detection of carcinogens individually or in combinations that really reflect the low or ambient levels of environmental exposure (Epstein, 1970, 1972; Kraybill, 1974b). One problem is that the experimental testing of small numbers of animals is based on the premise that a substance is or is not carcinogenic in the animals, and then extrapolations are made about a massive population presumed to be at risk. Such an experimental situation fails to consider the relative carcinogenic potential of different agents in risk assessment or the environmental and physiological levels of exposure likely to be encountered by the human population at risk. Therefore, the role of several carcinogens or carcinogens and non-carcinogen-promoting agents that could synergize carcinogenicity is not reflected in a typical bioassay study. Thus, one is confronted with possible false positives or false negatives, which do not help in the ultimate assessment of risk.

Another example of the problem of insensitivity of experimental methods is detailed in Epstein (1970). Assuming that the human is as sensitive as the rodent and that a chemical could carry a risk factor of 1 cancer in 10,000 humans exposed, this would mean about 22,000 cancers in the U.S. population. Obviously, 10,000 rodents would be required to demonstrate anything other than spontaneous occurrences of tumors. If one builds in a factor to allow for statistical significance, then about three to four times that number, or approximately 35,000 animals, would have to be used. Thus, when one uses groups of 50–100 animals to test a chemical at a low level of exposure, it is almost impossible to detect a response at such a low-dose challenge. This has led to the use of higher test doses, but the difficulties in using doses at, or in excess of, an MTD (maximum tolerated dose) have been described elsewhere (Burchfield et al., 1974).

Thus, the risk to animal and human populations should be evaluated wherever possible in terms of multiple stresses. One cannot assume that the effects of multiple stresses are necessarily additive; indeed, the influence can be inhibitory. When a weak response is observed, it is possible that the effect of contaminants in diet, water, or air may be cocarcinogenic. Some carriers and vehicles of pesticide chemicals may be carcinogenic or cocarcinogenic. There has been evidence reported in the literature that while there was synergistic action between the ingredients of particular pesticide preparations, there was no indication of additive carcinogenic potential among the pesticides investigated (Kay, 1974).

ASSESSMENT OF CARCINOGENICITY
IN ENVIRONMENTAL MEDIA

The preceding discussion has emphasized the significance of multiple stresses. The environment presents multiple exposures to the individual from carcinogenic insults in the air, water, diet, and medication. Exposure in the work place compounds the risk from environmental exposures. Therefore, experimental observations obtained in the assay of a single chemical or agent do not, in practice, reflect the carcinogenic risk from a series of microinsults in multiple exposures. Ultimately, assessments will have to be made on the combined effect of mixed environmental carcinogens as they are consumed in the diet, taken in through potable water, and inhaled in the air. Conceptually, there may be no disagreement as to this goal, but the design of studies to provide meaningful and interpretable data is most complex. However, the challenge may stimulate efforts to achieve this objective. Recent events as to environmental pollution and public concerns about the potential health hazard of carcinogens in the air, in municipal water supplies, and in the food chain will necessitate evaluations of the combined effects in these environmental media.

Aquatic Carcinogens

Some contaminants that occur naturally in waterways are largely of geologic origin. However, industrial technology, including chemical processing, has introduced a proliferation of chemical and biological agents into the aquatic environment around the world (Kraybill, 1974c). In large bodies of water, such as the ocean, there is a dilution effect. However, uncontrolled pollution has been detected through modern sophisticated analytical methods. The occurrence of aquatic carcinogens in one area of the globe and their transport to other areas has become a problem of international concern.

Some of the aquatic contaminants may be biodegradable and some may be removed by the treatment processes for potable water. However, many now are transferred into municipal water supplies as biorefractories. Tardiff and Deinzer (1973) and R. G. Tardiff (personal communication) have identified some 162 biorefractories that appear in U.S. municipal water supplies. Kraybill (1974c), in his classification of carcinogens in raw and treated water supplies, has identified six chemicals that are recognized carcinogens, about 4% of the total biorefractories of 162 chemicals. Similarly, there are 42 suspect carcinogens, or 25% of the total. The rest are either of unknown carcinogenic activity (67%) or negative for carcinogenicity (4%). About six cities and several watersheds have been involved in the identification of organic compounds in water supplies. Some recognized, suspect, and borderline carcinogens occurring in raw and treated water are listed in Table 4.

The primary interest of global aquatic pollution, other than esthetics and the destruction of marine animals, is the potential health hazard to humans, including neoplastic disease from swimming in such waters and the microcarcinogenic insult received from a mixture of chemicals in the drinking water. The adverse effects of pollution, including tumors, have been observed in finfish and shellfish for some time. These marine animals are thus suggestive evidence or early warning signals of the potential threat from aquatic carcinogens. Unknown is the carcinogenic effect of the interaction of chemicals in the water environment with respect to synergism and inhibition or their multiplicative effect on other carcinogens in the environment. The ingestion of contaminated fish would have to be considered in this context.

TABLE 4 Some Recognized and Suspect Carcinogens in Water Supplies[a, b]

Recognized	Suspect	
Arsenic	Benzene	Dieldrin
Benzidine	Chloroform	Heptachlor
Dibenz[a,h]anthracene	Aldrin	Chrysene
Vinyl chloride	Chlordane	1,2-Benzanthracene
Carbon tetrachloride	Heptachlor epoxide	Chromium (hexavalent)
Chloromethyl methyl ether	Cadmium	DDT
Asbestos compounds	DDE	Chlorodibromethane
3,4-Benzpyrene	BHC (Lindane)	Chloromethyl ethyl ether
1,2,7,8-Dibenzanthracene	Mirex	Benzene hexachloride
Ethylene thiourea	Polyurethane	
Bis(2-chloroethyl) ether		
Trichloroethylene		

[a]Data from Kraybill (1974c).
[b]In raw and potable waters.

An international program of systematic monitoring and surveillance on aquatic carcinogens, indicating qualitative and quantitative occurrence, is important. Epidemiologic and epizootic investigations should be correlated with these occurrences in an attempt to delineate any excesses of cancer in regions where point-source contamination or general pollution may be identified. In addition, experimental studies must be undertaken to evaluate the carcinogenic potency of aquatic biorefractory carcinogens in treated water, the mixtures of carcinogens in raw water, and the marine animals that retain these carcinogens as a body burden. Such studies are now under consideration. It is unfortunate that concern was expressed only after the public became aware of the fact that some chemicals, identified as recognized or suspect carcinogens, appeared in potable water as a result of chlorination but had not been previously identified in raw water supplies (Kraybill, 1974c; Kloepfer and Fairless, 1972). Since carcinogens appear in both raw and finished water, the overall problem is control and elimination of pollution. Thus, investigations on the marine or aquatic environment, including chemical identification, monitoring and surveillance, identification of finfish and shellfish tumors, and any demonstrated causal relationships between point-source contamination and cancer incidence, should play an important role in epidemiology of cancer. Leads from such studies should provide a basis for designing cancer control projects.

Carcinogens in the Air

The role of atmospheric contaminants in cancer mortality has been recognized for many years in research studies and through public health action programs. References to such studies are so extensive that only passing mention will be made to a few of them.

For the general population, there is a multiplicity of air contaminants that can act as carcinogens or cocarcinogens in cancer induction. Lung cancer is the leading cause of deaths associated with respiratory carcinogens. It was formerly responsible for the excess of male over female cancer deaths, but the increase in smoking among women has reduced the differential somewhat (Department of Health, Education, and Welfare, 1971a). Other primary sites involved in cancer deaths, for both sexes, in decreasing order of incidence, are the breast, colon, prostate, ovary, stomach, pancreas, cervix, bloodsystem, bladder, uterus, rectum, oral cavity, and esophagus (Wynder and Hoffman, 1972).

Nonoccupational groups receive, in addition to "personal" air pollution such as tobacco smoke, the effluents from industrial plants, automobile exhausts, and particulates and combustion products carried from combustion and incineration processes.

Cigarette smoke is an overriding factor in the evaluation of the effect of air pollutants on respiratory cancers. Thus, a direct causative association for a particular environmental exposure to air carcinogens must be made with standardization of data to nonsmokers. Wynder and Hoffman (1972) and Wynder and Hammond (1962) have indicated that lung cancer is affected by community air pollution and that the incidence in cities may be higher than in rural areas as a consequence of (1) higher degree of polluted air, (2) more industrial exposure, (3) more cigarettes smoked, (4) more cancers diagnosed, (5) different immigration and migration patterns, and (6) differences in socio-economic factors. Some investigators have made studies on a county basis in an attempt to correlate lung cancer incidence with air pollution indices. Such a study was reported by Buell et al. (1967) in California, but he found no correlation and concluded that the smog pollution existing in various counties had no effect on risk of lung cancer.

Polluted air concentrates contain a large number of polycyclic aromatic hydrocarbons (PAH compounds). These are formed as a result of the combustion of gasoline, industrial processes, and promiscuous burning of organic material by the population. Tobacco smoke contains PAH carcinogenic compounds but differs somewhat from community air pollutants in that there is a significant quantity of alkylated 4- and 5-ring aromatic hydrocarbons (Wynder and Hoffman, 1972). According to Wynder and Hoffman, the major difference between tobacco smoke and community air pollutants is the particle size and amount inhaled each day. A cigarette smoker who inhales takes in 5 billion particles per cubic centimeter of smoke. Some of these PAH compounds, well-established experimentally as carcinogens, are: (1) benz[a]anthracene, (2) benzo[a]pyrene, (3) dibenzo[a,h]pyrene, (4) benzo[b]fluoranthene, (5) benzo[j]fluoranthene, and (6) indeno[1,2,3-cd]pyrene.

There have been only inadequate surveys to demonstrate the degree of migration of industrial effluents that could impose a carcinogenic risk to the general population. In epidemiological studies on asbestos, Selikoff et al.

(1967) have shown that asbestos is not restricted to the work place but may occur in the household environment of an asbestos worker, in city air from disintegrated brake linings, in disintegrated floor tiles, and in a variety of asbestos products to which the general population may be exposed. On autopsy, asbestos fibers have been found in the lungs of urban dwellers.

Recent studies by the Environmental Protection Agency would indicate, from preliminary data, that vinyl chloride could migrate from a plant up to 3 miles away. Levels in the parts per million range were detected for this carcinogen up to 0.5 miles from a plant boundary. The highest level detected was 2 ppm adjacent to an industrial plant involved in manufacture of vinyl chloride monomer (Richardson, 1974). The drift of stack effluents to surrounding communities has been demonstrated in many cases, especially near smelter operations or, in the case of lead, as a dust fallout in urban areas (Schuck and Locke, 1970; Assaf and Biscaye, 1972; Sullivan, 1969).

Many pesticides (some of which have carcinogenic activity) used by the general population are airborne as particulates in various applications. In studying the epidemiology of DDT, Davies (1972) has shown that airborne levels of pesticides are responsible for higher body burdens of this pesticide where DDT is used continuously in Florida. Dust levels of pesticides in the home correlate well with plasma levels and are thus a useful index of exposure.

Table 5 lists some of the recognized and suspect carcinogens that might be considered as pollutants in the air and as insults to the general population.

TABLE 5 Some Recognized and Suspect Carcinogens Occurring in the Air as Exposures to the General Population

Chemical	Source
Benz[a]anthracene	Combustion products and cigarette smoke
Benzo[a]pyrene	Combustion products and cigarette smoke
Dibenzo[a,h]pyrene	Combustion products and cigarette smoke
Benzo[b]fluoranthene	Combustion products and cigarette smoke
Benzo[j]fluoranthene	Combustion products and cigarette smoke
Indeno[1,2,3-cd]pyrene	Combustion products and cigarette smoke
Arsenic	From pesticide use
Asbestos	Particles from asbestos products
Cadmium	Mining–smelting
Chromate (hexavalent)	Mining–smelting
DDT	Pesticide application
Aldrin	Pesticide application
Dieldrin	Pesticide application
Heptachlor	Pesticide application
Lindane	Pesticide application
Carbon tetrachloride	Industrial effluent
Vinyl chloride	Industrial effluent

Dietary Carcinogens

In the area of food, the provisions of the Delaney amendment to the Federal Food, Drug, and Cosmetic Act are rather rigorous in that any additive to food is prohibited if it is shown to be carcinogenic in any concentration under recognized toxicological procedures for testing. Thus, by legal definition, no food chemical or food additive intentionally added may be a carcinogen. Some additives used for years, such as food colors, flavorings, emulsifiers, stabilizers, antioxidants, sweeteners, and preservatives, have been considered GRAS compounds (Generally Regarded As Safe).

Despite all the rigorous control and precautionary measures and past history, some food chemicals have been found to be carcinogenic and consequently banned from use. Some compounds, however, occur naturally as degradation products or as toxic metabolites and are not commercial additives. They may be pyrolysis and radiolysis products or toxins such as aflatoxin and cycasin, etc. In these instances, the Food and Drug Administration maintains close surveillance to preclude the occurrence and distribution of such contaminated foods, sets tolerances and bans importation of food products such as copra (cocoanut oil), pistachio nuts, brazil nuts, and peanuts, that are shown to exceed the tolerances. An extensive review of the testing of food chemicals and the demonstrated carcinogenic activity of such chemicals that are now banned has been presented by Kraybill (1974d).

Some substances that were used as food chemicals and are now banned or limited on the basis of their carcinogenic properties are listed in Table 6.

Drugs and Medical Procedures and Carcinogenicity

Occupational exposure to chemicals has provided some of the best evidence of chemical carcinogenesis as determined in epidemiological studies on workers and confirmatory studies in experimental animals. Exposure to drugs is the next most important kind of exposure for accumulating data as a base for decision-making on carcinogenic risk. The population exposed to drugs may not be as large as that exposed to occupational hazards or food contaminants, but certainly the use of some drugs later proven to be carcinogenic in experimental animals warrants more extensive epidemiological studies where there is some suggestive experimental evidence.

This would entail prospective studies. However, some retrospective studies have revealed, for example, important findings in the use of DES (diethylstilbestrol) for threatened abortion during the first 17 wk of pregnancy. In studies since 1971, daughters of women treated with DES have been shown to have a demonstrably increased, but low, risk of cancer of the vagina and cervix. These clinical observations, buttressed by data in experimental animals where the carcinogenicity of DES has been recognized, led to legislative and regulatory activities on the use of DES as an animal feed additive.

TABLE 6 Some Chemicals and Natural Toxins in Foods Found To Be Carcinogenic[a]

Naturally occurring	Synthetic chemicals
Ergot	Dulcin
Luteoskyrin	Cyclamates[b]
Cyclochlorotine	Tween 60
Aflatoxins	Carboxymethylcellulose
Sterigmatocystin	Polyoxyethylenemonostearate
Ethionine	Oil orange E
Nitrosamines	Oil yellow HA
Polycyclic aromatic hydrocarbons	Oil orange TX
Pyrrolizodine alkaloids	Orange I
Safrole (from sassafras)	Yellow AB and OB
Oil of calamus	Light green SF
Cycasin	Brilliant blue FCF
Bracken fern	Fast green FCF
Thiourea	Butter yellow
Tannins (tannic acid)	8-Hydroxyquinoline
Carrageenan	FC&C red no. 32
Beryllium	Diethylpyrocarbonate (a tendency to form urethane)
Chromium (hexavalent)	Diethylstilbestrol
Cobalt	Ponceaux MX
Nickel	Citrus red no. 2

[a]Data from Kraybill (1974d) and Miller (1973).
[b]Carcinogenicity questioned.

The law now permits substances like DES, shown to be carcinogenic, to be used as feed additives provided no residues appear in any of the edible portion of the animal at time of slaughter. Medicated feed is used on the premise that cattle or sheep will grow more rapidly and thus consume less feed to obtain a marketable weight (Edwards, 1972; Wade, 1972).

Another case of physician-induced or iatrogenic disease is that resulting from the use of thorium dioxide or thorotrast as a radioactive contract medium for treating cancers of the cerebral vessel visualization system. Thorotrast was first used in 1925; but the first cases of liver angiosarcomas were not reported until 1947. Hundreds of cases of this liver cancer were produced, which is surprising since it was at first claimed that there was no danger from this alpha emitter. What was overlooked was the tendency for thorium dioxide to be stored in the liver. The standard dose of 75 mg gave a gamma radiation equal to 1.37 μg radium (Richardson, 1974). Since the half-life of thorium is 1.39×10 yr and radioactivity increases after 5 yr, the breakdown products are active and peak in 15 yr. Thus, the induction period is long and the end result tragic (MacMahan et al., 1947; Nettleship and Fink, 1961; Suckow et al., 1961; Hundeker et al., 1968; Kruckmeyer, 1963).

Many other drugs and agents could be cited here as inducers of cancer. Some of these drugs are listed in Table 7.

Energy Technologies and Carcinogenicity

Critical energy shortage has resulted in an atmosphere of urgency and so one may see the development of new technologies and processes to fulfill energy needs. These processes may lead to a proliferation of environmental pollutants as emissions into the atmosphere and effluents into streams and waterways. These additive pollutants may impose a stress that not only affects those occupationally involved but also those in the surrounding communities. The qualitative and quantitative aspects of these environmental insults and their relevance to environmental cancer must ultimately be evaluated.

Currently, there is a spectrum of technologies under consideration, some in the exploratory or pilot plant stage, others in the planning stage. A few of the technologies under consideration are as follows:

1. Increased energy efficiency, which includes recycling of materials, production of energy from waste, and improvements in, and increased use of, insulating materials. The latter implies extension and magnification of some released environmental carcinogens—plastics, asbestiform materials, etc.
2. Liquefaction and gasification of coal, which may introduce polycyclic aromatic hydrocarbons into the aquaphors and in the

TABLE 7 Some Drugs and Medical Procedures That Induce Cancer in Animals and Humans[a]

Chemical and/or procedure	Primary target organ	Animal	Human
Thorotrast	Liver		X
X-rays	Blood system (leukemia)		X
Arsenic	Liver, skin		X
Chlornaphazin	Bladder		X
Coal tar products	Skin	Mouse	X
INH (isonicotinic acid hydrazide)	Lung adenomas	Mouse	
Iron dextran	Soft-tissue sarcomas	Rat	?
Penicillin	Sarcomas on injection	Rodent	?
Griseofulvin	Liver and skin	Mouse	
Mitomycin C	Sarcomas at site of injection	Mouse	
Actinomycin D	Sarcomas and mesotheliomas on injection	Mouse	
Niridazole	Lung and stomach lymphomas	Mouse	
Flagyl	Lung lymphomas	Rat	
	Mammary fibroadenomas	Mouse	
Diethylstilbestrol	Vagina (offspring of treated patients)		X
L-Dopa	Malignant melanomas	Hamster	

[a]Data from Shubik (1972) and Miller (1973).

extraction process may release some carcinogenic contaminants into the air.

3. Improvement in current refinery or processing procedures on gas and oil, which, if not properly controlled, will introduce more contaminants into the environment.

4. Oil recovery from shale and tar sands. This process is now exploited in the Colorado plateau but not on a large scale. If fully developed, either by surface recovery or nuclear explosions, then an increased environmental pollution problem may be anticipated. Some environmental monitoring under a project by the National Science Foundation is underway in the Colorado region to establish the effect of this industry on contamination of the atmosphere and water.

5. Nuclear power and technology, which includes breeder and fusion technology, is so designed as to incorporate maximum safeguards in terms of human health protection. However, the possibilities remain that there will be a potential increase of plutonium and some fissionable materials, the long-term impact of which must be evaluated in terms of human cancer.

One of the first approaches in evaluating this problem would be a thorough review of what we do or do not know concerning these energy technologies. The second step would be to document the extent and conditions of human exposure to the pollutants released by these technologies in the past (if used), the present, and the foreseeable future. For example, in large-scale shale-processing operations, there are certain petroleum distillates or fractions obtained in retorting at 550–700° and above 700°F. In carbonaceous shale, coke, or spent shale waste, some polycondensed aromatic hydrocarbons in benzene extracts have been identified (Denver Research Institute, 1974). They are phenanthrene, benz[a]anthracene, dibenz[a,b]anthracene, 7,12-dimethyl benz[a]anthracene, fluoranthene, 3-methylcholanthrene pyrene, benzo[a]pyrene, dibenz[c,d]pyrene, perylene, and benzo[g,h,i]perylene. Some of these PAH compounds are carcinogenic.

Effluents of carcinogenic chemicals in the air and waterways will have to be monitored on a continuous basis to determine the concentration of the carcinogenic pollutant and the trends in the contamination (surveillance); samples from the air and condensed fractions from polluted waters will have to be biologically assayed to ascertain their carcinogenic activity and/or potency. In such an experimental evaluation of carcinogenicity of micropollutants, special procedures may be required beyond the traditional use of *in vivo* systems (where large quantities of material are available for bioassay in experimental animals).

Ultimately, the impact of such a large new energy development with its associated environmental and occupational health problems will have to be assessed through epidemiological studies to determine any excesses in human cancer and evaluate the benefits and hazards associated with these innovative processes required to meet national energy needs.

Interrelationships of Laboratory Information, Environmental Monitoring, Epizootics, and Epidemiology in a Systems Approach to Environmental Cancer

Traditionally, assessment of the carcinogenicity of a chemical is based on dose-response data in animal studies or on observations made in epidemiological studies. Human or mammalian systems may not evoke a carcinogenic or noncarcinogenic response from a singular environmental insult but may be conditioned by multiple exposures in the environment and the interaction of various chemicals or toxic agents. In the case of occupational exposure, the toxic stress may be so great and continuous that a cause-and-effect relationship from a single stress is quite evident.

Environmentally, the general population receives carcinogenic insults from the atmosphere, the water supply, and through additives or contaminants in the diet. The significance of these environmental factors has been discussed previously. In some instances, calculations have been made on the combined exposure to chemicals such as pesticides or heavy metals. Such information is useful in appraising integrated stress and potential risk (Kraybill, 1969; Committee on Biologic Effects of Atmospheric Pollutants, 1972b).

Frequently overlooked are observations on domestic animals, wildlife, and marine animals, especially, which may serve as indicators or monitors of the level of environmental exposure human beings are receiving. In addition, neoplasms are induced, such as those in marine animals, that reflect the degree of pollution in waterways. This effect is sometimes strikingly revealed in massive fish kills. Such presumptive evidence in epizootics may provide important clues to cancer among human populations in certain regions.

While bioassay data from experimental animals is useful, there are problems in extrapolation from experimental conditions of animal exposures to the more relevant situation in human exposure and carcinogenic response. An intelligence network that monitors and maintains a surveillance on the environmental exposures humans receive is an essential component in exploring exposure-response relationships in human population laboratories. Though the information from epizootics is another link in the human exposure-response chain, epidemiological studies, if they can be conducted, are the ultimate criterion in establishing cause-and-effect relationships relevant to neoplastic disease.

Integrating the information from all of the data bases should provide adequate evidence on carcinogenic risk (Fig. 4). Where environmental factors are involved and forecasts on hazards have been made, then, when human cancers appear at a significant rate or in excessive numbers in certain regions, that risk will be verified.

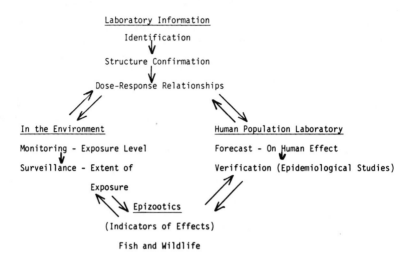

FIGURE 4 Laboratory information, environmental monitoring, epizootics, and epidemiology in a systems approach to environmental cancer (from Kraybill, 1974b).

EVALUATION AND SUMMARY

A description has been given of the methodological approaches employed in the assessment of carcinogenic risks for the general population, who receive nonoccupational environmental exposures to various chemicals and other agents. Such evaluations are facilitated either through studies on experimental animals (carcinogenesis bioassay) or by means of retrospective and prospective studies on specified human populations. The realization that a high percentage of human cancers may be induced by environmental agents has caused some concern; preventive medicine programs are indicated. Prevention of cancer should be one of the major efforts of our time, given the irreversibility of the neoplastic process in so many cases and the lack of success of therapeutic measures in arresting the course of this chronic and complex disease.

There have been advances and innovations in our methods of evaluating the carcinogenic potential of a wide array of environmental agents. But there are inherent problems in measuring the variability and predictability of carcinogenic activity when one is working with biological systems such as animal models or other systems such as cell cultures. Extrapolation of experimental findings to the human situation may be conditioned by many factors. The estimates and predictions on safety and/or hazard are not as precise as those used in the physical sciences. The biological response is conditioned on the validity of the test procedures; that is, how relevant the toxicological procedures are, how relevant the species and strain are, and how definitive the histopathology and the agreement on diagnosis made from histological observations are. Statistical analysis of the data on tumor incidence or comparative analysis of numbers of tumors in animals in control and test groups is insufficient to make a judgment on carcinogenic activity, particularly if the study is found to be lacking in numerous details. A premature release of information on the carcinogenicity of a chemical, without an adequate scrutiny of the validity of the data, will lead to regulatory and societal decisions that may be unwarranted and ultimately regretted. The decision-making process assumes that a very comprehensive and careful review of all data has been made and that the findings are unequivocally accepted by all scientific reviewers, representing many disciplines. Ideally, testing in laboratory animals should enable the prediction of those agents responsible for human cancer, their effect on the human being, and the dose range that might produce that effect.

Frequently, experimental data fall short of this ideal. Often, estimates of carcinogenic risk are made directly from epidemiological studies and observations on human beings and only later confirmed in experimental animals. It is, of course, unfortunate that in these cases the human turns out to be the test animal, so to speak. In the future, it is hoped that the animal model will be the early-warning indicator for what may lie ahead for the human population.

There are also situations where the indicators of carcinogenesis in the experimental systems are not verified by observations on the human population. This raises several questions: (1) Is the compound noncarcinogenic to humans (that is, is there a species variability)? (2) Has the induction period for the development of human tumors not yet been attained or is the latency period greater than the human life span? (3) Is the proper epidemiological study yet to be accomplished? (4) Are the available data being misinterpreted?

Animal studies suggesting tumorigenesis are frequently of insufficient quality and, as with any living system, may yield some false negatives and false positives. Also, the animal test system may not be predictive of the exact dose that produces cancer in humans. Many studies provide insufficient data in that dose-response analyses, which would be of great value in characterizing the carcinogenic potential of the test chemical, have not been done. The reliability of prediction from animals to humans is, of course, enhanced when tumors are produced at a significant level in several animal species and strains, including rodents and nonrodents, and are repeatedly confirmed in several laboratories. Unfortunately, these criteria are not always met.

One can never be certain that even the best animal data are not reflecting false positives or false negatives. The final verification, unfortunately, usually comes from observations made on human populations if a cause-and-effect relationship does indeed exist between a certain environmental exposure and cancer. To achieve maximum predictability, it is most important that our testing programs for carcinogenesis, using various bioassay procedures, be the best that can be developed. This requires that our evaluation studies include adequate data on dosing, time-to-tumor formation, metabolic fate, sufficient numbers of animals, and other features of a good design.

Certainly what is also needed are criteria for evaluating the predictive value of animal data for human cancer. Some efforts are being made in this direction through national and international advisory bodies. This reduces the tendency toward unilateral decisions made by scientists motivated to take on this awesome decision-making power.

Virtually all information other than direct human studies comes from assessment of the potency of a chemical carcinogen in experiments on mice, rats, and other conventional test animals. These animals may be subjected to doses much higher than those usually experienced by humans. The reasons for adopting such procedures are described earlier in this chapter. Higher test doses are not used to obtain quicker results with fewer animals at lower cost, but they are an expedient compromise to the alternative of a million-mouse experiment designed to match the population size for human exposures. There is, of course, the problem of dose-response relationships seen at these higher levels being extrapolated downward to levels comparable to human exposure.

The types of exposures received by the individual from his environment are multiple and thus present a multiple risk. Although some experimental studies have been designed to evaluate the effect of mixed agents and to test their synergistic and/or inhibitory role as interactants, more studies of this type should be undertaken. The design is difficult, but certain matrixes, providing for the simultaneous testing of at least 12 chemicals, have been made available. The biological assay of single chemical agents is not reflective of environmental situations for humans; that is, the assessment of a single-agent response is not reflective, from a pragmatic viewpoint, of the potential for synergistic and/or inhibitory effects.

An alternative approach to evaluation of carcinogenic risk would be to consider the combined effect of the environmental chemicals to which humans are exposed. This approach to environmental cancer could first be explored by determining, in a suitable test system, the biological response of total extracts and subfractions of extracts of polluted water, polluted air, and contaminated diets. Such an approach is now under consideration for evaluating the mutagenicity and carcinogenicity of the biorefractories in municipal water supplies.

Finally, in a comprehensive evaluation of the problem of environmental cancer, one must utilize all of the data bases available from experimental oncology, the environmental monitoring and surveillance networks, and the observations on neoplasia in marine and terrestrial animals and then correlate these data with observations in human population laboratories. The importance of establishing a "crosswalk" between such areas for the development of clues and evidence of human cancer has not been fully realized. The limiting objectives of categorical disease programs do not easily lend themselves to the exploitation of such interfacing and thus do not maximize the utilization of these resources in problem identification and resolution directed toward the conquest of cancer.

REFERENCES

A. D. Little, Inc. 1973. Current status of human safety and environmental aspects of fluorescent whitening agents used in detergents. Report issued to Minor Additives Committee, Soap and Detergent Assoc.

Agricultural Research Council. 1960. Radiobiological Laboratory, report no. 3. London: Her Majesty's Stationery Office.

American Cancer Society. 1974. *Cancer facts and figures*, p. 3. New York.

Assaf, G. and Biscaye, P. E. 1972. *Science* 175:890–884.

Baird, V. C. 1967. *J.Occup.Med.* 8:415–420.

Barnes, J. M. and Denz, F. A. 1954. *Pharmacol. Rev.* 6:191–242.

Berg, J. W. and Burbank, F. 1972. In *Geochemical environment in relation to health and disease*, ed. H. C. Hopps and H. L. Cannon, vol. 199, pp. 249–265. New York: New York Academy of Sciences.

Bergel, F. 1974. *Proc. Roy. Soc., London Ser. B* 185:165–181.

Boyland, F. 1969. *Exp. Tumor Res.* 11:222–234.

Buell, P., Dunn, J. E. and Breslow, L. 1967. *Cancer* 20:2139–2147.

Burchfield, H. P., Storrs, E. E. and Kraybill, H. F. 1974. In *Pesticides, environmental quality and safety supplement*, ed. F. Coulston and F. Korfe, vols. 3 and 4. Stuttgart: Georg Thieme. In press.

Comar, C. L. and Georgi, J. R. 1961. *Nature* 191:390–391.

Committee on Biologic Effects of Atmospheric Pollutants. 1972a. In *Particulate polycyclic organic matter*, ed. Committee on Biologic Effects of Atmospheric Pollutants, chap. 3, pp. 13–37. Washington, D.C.: National Academy of Sciences.

Committee on Biologic Effects of Atmospheric Pollutants. 1972b. *Airborne lead in perspective*, pp. 132–192. Washington, D.C.: National Academy of Sciences.

Creech, J. L., Jr. and Makk, L. 1975. *Ann. N.Y. Acad. Sci.* 246:88–99.

Davies, J. E. 1972. In *Epidemiology of DDT*, ed. J. E. Davies and W. F. Edmonson, pp. 39–48. Mount Kisco, N.Y.: Futura.

Davies, J. E. and Edmundson, W. E. 1972. In *Epidemiology of DDT*, ed. J. E. Davies and W. E. Edmundson, pp. 27–125. Mount Kisco, N.W.: Futura.

Denver Research Institute. 1974. The disposal and environmental effects of carbonaceous solid wastes from commercial oil shale operations, App. B, First Annual Report.

Department of Health, Education and Welfare. 1960. *Radiological health data.* vol. 1, no. 7, p. 37.

Department of Health, Education and Welfare. 1971a. *Health consequence of smoking: Report to the surgeon general*, pp. 251–252. Washington, D.C.: Government Printing Office.

Department of Health, Education and Welfare. 1971b. *Radiological health data*, vol. 2, no. 5, pp. 16–17.

Department of Health, Education and Welfare. 1973. *The strategic plan.* National Cancer Program, DHEW publication no. (NIH)–74–569.

Dunham, W. F., Armstrong, J. F. and Quinby, G. E. 1965. *Arch. Environ. Health* 11:641.

Edwards, C. C. 1972. Statement before the Subcommittee on Health, Senate Committee on Labor and Public Welfare, July 20.

Egbert, D. S. and Geiger, A. 1936. *Amer. Rev. Tuberc.* 34:143–150.
Epstein, S. S. 1970. *Nature* 228:816–819.
Epstein, S. S. 1972. *Amer. J. Pathol.* 66:352–374.
Epstein, S. S. 1974. *Cancer Res.* 34:2425–2435.
Goldblatt, M. W. 1947. *Brit. Med. Bull.* 4:405–417.
Goldblatt, M. W. 1958. *Brit. Med. Bull.* 14:136–140.
Greenblatt, M. 1973. *J. Natl. Cancer Inst.* 50(4):1055–1056.
Heller, J. and Henry, S. A. 1930. *J. Indust. Hyg. Toxicol.* 12:169–197.
Higginson, H. 1969. *Can. Cancer Conf.* 8:40–75.
Hueper, W. C. 1969. In *Occupational and environmental cancers of the urinary system*, ed. W. C. Hueper, chap. 3, pp. 118–180. New Haven: Yale University Press.
Hundeker, M., Berger, H. and Petres, J. 1968. *Ark. Klin. Exp. Dermatol.* 232:56–65.
Innes, J. R. M. et al. 1969. *J. Natl. Cancer Inst.* 12:1101–1114.
Jones, H. B. 1974. Estimation of environmental factors in the origin of cancer and the hazard of carcinogenesis, pp. 1–10. Presented at Amer. Assoc. Adv. Sci. Symposium, February 25–March 2. Washington, D.C.
Kay, K. 1974. *Environ. Res.* 7:243–271.
Kloepfer, R. D. and Fairless, B. J. 1972. *Environ. Sci. Technol.* 6(12):1036–1037.
Kraybill, H. F. 1969. *Can. Med. Assoc. J.* 100:204–215.
Kraybill, H. F. 1973. Reappraisals in carcinogenesis: A primer. Presented at Food and Drug Law Institute Seminar, May 21–22. Washington, D.C.
Kraybill, H. F. 1974a. In *Environmental quality and food supply*, ed. P. L. White and D. Robbins, pp. 173–184. Mount Kisco, N.Y.: Futura.
Kraybill, H. F. 1974b. In *Symposium for chemicals and cancer.* In press.
Kraybill, H. F. 1974c. In *Progress in experimental tumor research*, vol. 21, *Tumors in aquatic animals*, ed. F. Homburger. Basel: Karger. In press.
Kraybill, H. F. 1974d. In *Handbook of trace substances in health*, ed. P. M. Newberne. New York: Marcel Dekker. In press.
Kraybill, H. F. and Shapiro, R. E. 1969. In *Aflatoxin*, ed. L. A. Goldblatt, chap. 15, pp. 425–428. New York: Academic Press.
Kraybill, H. F. and Shimkin, M. B. 1964. *Adv. Cancer Res.* 8:191–248.
Kraybill, H. F., Calvert, C., Decker, W. M. and Terrill, J. G. 1962. *Health Phys.* 8:27–33.
Kulp, J. L., Schulert, A. R. and Hodges, E. J. 1960. *Science* 132:448–454.
Kruckmeyer, K. 1963. *Urologie* 2:73–76.
Laskin, S., Kushner, N. and Drew, R. T. 1970. Studies in pulmonary carcinogenesis. In *AEC symposium series no. 18*, ed. M. G. Hanna, P. Nettesheim, and J. R. Gilbert, pp. 321–351. Washington, D.C.: Government Printing Office.
Lewin, R. 1974. *SR/World*, Science Section, pp. 50–51. April 20.
Liijinsky, W. and Epstein, S. S. 1970. *Nature* 225:21–23.
Loomis, T. A. 1969. Statement on carcinogenic activity of DDT. Presented at hearings of Washington State Department of Agriculture, October 16.
Lorenz, E. 1944. *J. Natl. Cancer Inst.* 5:15.
Lundin, F. E. 1969. *Health Phys.* 16:571.
MacMahan, H. E., Murphy, A. S. and Bates, M. I. 1947. *Amer. J. Pathol.* 23:585–611.
Magee, P. N. 1971. *Food Cosmet. Toxicol.* 9:207–218.
Maltoni, C. 1973. In *Advances in tumor prevention, detection and characterization*, vol. 2, *Cancer detection and prevention*, ed. C. Maltoni, p. 6. Int. Congress Series no. 322. New York: American Elsevier.

Maltoni, C. and Lefemine, G. 1974. *Environ. Res.* 7(3):387–405.

Merten, D. and Knoop, L. 1960. Report for the UN Scientific Committee on the Effects of Atomic Radiation, Report IIC-6930-1, pp. 1–18. Bad Godesberg, Germany.

Miller, J. A. 1973. In *Toxicants occurring naturally in foods*, 2nd ed., ed. Committee on Food Protection, pp. 508–550. Washington, D.C.: National Academy of Sciences.

Montesano, R. and Saffiotti, U. 1968. *Cancer Res.* 28:2197.

Nettleship, A. and Fink, W. J. 1961. *Amer. J. Clin. Pathol.* 35:422–426.

Peacock, P. R. and Spence, J. B. 1967. *Brit. J. Cancer* 21:606–618.

Pott, P. 1775. *Chirurgical works*, vol. 5, p. 63. London.

Richardson, H. L. 1974. Report on vinyl chloride exposure and neoplastic and nonneoplastic disease. Interagency Collaborative Group on Environmental Carcinogenesis, National Cancer Institute, April.

Roe, F. 1968. *Food Cosmet. Toxicol.* 6:485.

Rose, D. J. 1971. *Science* 172:797–800.

Sadarangani, S. H., Sahasrabudha, S. G. and Soman, S. D. 1973. In *Tritium*, ed. A. D. Moghissi and M. W. Carter, pp. 327–333. Phoenix, Ariz.: Messenger Graphics.

Schuck, E. A. and Locke, J. K. 1970. *Environ. Sci. Technol.* 4(4):324–330.

Selikoff, I. J., Bader, R. A., Bader, M. E., Churg, J. and Hammond, E. C. 1967. *Amer. J. Med.* 42(4):487–496.

Selikoff, I. J., Hammond, E. C. and Churg, J. 1968. *J. Am. Med. Assoc.* 204:106–112.

Shimkin, M. B. 1969. *Science and cancer*, p. 66. Dept. of Health, Education and Welfare Publ. No. PHS 1162. Washington, D.C.: Government Printing Office.

Shubik, P. 1972. In *Environment and cancer*, pp. 142–156. (A collection of papers presented at the University of Texas at Houston, M.D. Anderson Hospital and Tumor Institute, 24th Annual Symposium on Fundamental Cancer Research, 1971.) Baltimore: Williams & Wilkins.

Sinnhuber, R. O., Wales, J. H., Ayres, J. H., Engebrecht, J. and Amend, D. L. 1968. *J. Natl. Cancer Inst.* 41:711–718.

Smoron, C. L. and Battifora, H. A. 1972. *Cancer* 30:1252–1259.

Suckow, E. G., Henegar, G. G. and Baserza, R. 1961. *Amer. J. Pathol.* 38:663–677.

Sullivan, R. J. 1969. *Preliminary air pollution survey of arsenic and its compounds: A literature review*. Prepared for Department of Health, Education and Welfare, Raleigh, N.C., October.

Tardiff, R. G. and Deinzer, M. 1973. Toxicity of organic compounds in drinking water. Paper presented at 15th Water Quality Conference, February 7–8, University of Illinois, Urbana, Ill.

Vigliani, E. C. and Barsotti, M. 1962. *Acta Univ.* 18:670–675.

Wade, N. 1972. *Science* 177:335–337.

Walker, K. C., Goette, M. B. and Batchelor, G. S. 1954. *J. Agr. Food Chem.* 2:1034.

Walpole, A. L. and Williams, M. H. C. 1958. *Brit. Med. Bull.* 14:141–145.

World Health Organization 1964. *Prevention of cancer, technical report services*, pp. 1–53. Geneva.

Wynder, E. and Hammond, E. C. 1962. *Cancer* 15:79–92.

Wynder, E. and Hoffman, D. 1972. In *Environment and cancer*, pp. 119–141. (A collection of papers presented at the University of Texas at Houston, M. D. Anderson Hospital and Tumor Institute, 24th Annual Symposium on Fundamental Cancer Research, 1971.) Baltimore: Williams & Wilkins.
Zbinden, G. 1973. In *Progress in toxicology*, vol. 1, chap. 2, pp. 17–19. New York: Springer-Verlag.

Chapter 3

OCCUPATIONAL CARCINOGENESIS

Donald V. Lassiter

Center for Occupational and Environmental Safety and Health
Stanford Research Institute
Menlo Park, California

INTRODUCTION

Scope

An update or state-of-the-art assessment of the field and activities associated with environmental cancer must, necessarily, include a chapter devoted to the contribution of occupational exposures to the overall understanding of this subject.

The role of occupation in induction of cancer has taken on increasingly greater significance during the 1970s with the realization that workers exposed in previous years to substances such as asbestos or vinyl chloride have developed malignant neoplasms as a result of such exposures. These discoveries have signaled a new era for cancer research and prevention activities as the proportional contribution of occupational exposure to environmental carcinogenesis has become increasingly manifested.

At the outset it is necessary to mention several extensive works in the field of occupational cancer. In 1964, Hueper and Conway published a text that has become a standard reference in the field of chemical carcinogenesis and that included an in-depth treatise on the determinant role of occupation. Both Eckardt (1959) and Dinman (1974) have published excellent monographs concerning the nature of occupational cancer, including recommendations for classification of carcinogenic substances and exposure control methodologies. In addition, the published proceedings (Saffiotti and Wagoner, 1976) of a conference on occupational carcinogenesis held by the New York Academy of Sciences in 1975 provides an excellent update of the field. It would be superfluous to attempt to enlarge on these works in this chapter, and the reader is referred to them for a more comprehensive treatment of this subject. That which is needed for inclusion in this present work on environmental cancer is the role of occupation, as it is presently perceived, in assessing overall risk of cancer in conjunction with other environmental factors and within the framework of existing legislation. It is not the purpose of this chapter, therefore, to reiterate information contained in other works on this subject, but rather to dwell on such material only to the extent necessary to attain perspective on problems as they are viewed in the light of present knowledge. In this chapter then we shall consider the importance of the occupational environment in relation to its impact on the induction of cancer and the role of federal regulatory authority-mandated responsibility for prevention and control of occupational cancer.

Estimates of the influence of environmental factors on expression or induction of cancer have ranged as high as 70% (Higginson, 1968) to 90% (Boyland, 1969). Because precise quantitation of environmental "connections" must await advances in determination of mechanisms of tumor induction, subjective estimations of proportionate etiology are of interest primarily from the standpoint of recognition that extraneous factors probably play a dominant role in development of the second leading cause of death from disease in the United States. For the biomedical community and for those legally responsible for protection of the nation's health, acceptance of this premise logically leads to the conclusion that real advances in reduction in cancer incidence can be assured as environmental factors are identified and controlled. However, the practical application of scientific knowledge in this area may very often meet not with social acceptance but with reluctance of society to undertake necessary ameliorative adjustments.

The Occupational Safety and Health Act of 1970 (PL 91-596)

This update of the field of occupational cancer is particularly relevant at this time because of the influence on the course of prevention and control of these diseases through activities and programs developed in response to the Occupational Safety and Health Act of 1970 (PL 91-596). This landmark legislation has been hailed as a panacea to occupational health problems by some and criticized as one of the most oppressing acts ever passed by the Congress by others. Certainly this act has sparked a great deal of controversy in the labor–management area, if not in the public health community itself. The extremely broad mandate contained in this legislation and the rulings of the judiciary on promulgated standards have created a wide policy range for consideration of regulatory actions to deal with actual and potential occupational safety and health problems.

Prior to passage of the Occupational Safety and Health Act it was considered by many that the extremely broad legislative authority mandated to the Secretary of Labor would result in great controversy concerning the degree to which mandatory controls to protect the health of workers could be exercised under the act. No small part of this controversy was the degree to which the Secretary, acting through the Occupational Safety and Health Administration (OSHA), could promulgate standards to protect workers from exposure to carcinogenic substances encountered in their working environ ment. Questions previously academic to the area of cancer induction began to take on new significance as it became apparent that regulatory control of chemical substances based on their demonstrated potential to induce tumors would rapidly become a central feature of OSHA's program to protect employee health. The fact that many such questions have been the subject of considerable debate among experts representing various disciplines of the scientific community has served to assure that regulatory decisions citing one side or the other of such controversial issues as supportive rationale would be appealed to the highest courts for final, judicial resolution.

It has become clear that the scientific community, in general, is reluctant to become further embroiled in this controversy and equally clear that definitive answers to many of these questions must await results of future animal research and epidemiologic investigations. In the meantime, however, OSHA cannot relent in efforts to fulfill its legislative mandate to protect the health of employees whose work may bring them into daily contact with potentially carcinogenic substances. The dilemma created by these circumstances resists facile resolution and requires the involvement of those individuals most capable of exercising balanced scientific judgment in this area to assist both regulatory and research agencies, as well as the courts, in reaching decisions concerning the social consequences of permitting long-term exposures to recognized carcinogenic substances with resultant health hazards for the exposed worker.

REGULATORY APPROACHES TO CONTROL
OF OCCUPATIONAL CANCER

Contemporary impetus for control of occupational cancer in the United States on the part of employers has been stirred principally through passage in 1970 of the Occupational Safety and Health Act. Prior to that time there were few mandatory constraints to production or use of chemical substances based on knowledge of potential toxicity or carcinogenicity. Constraints that did exist were, for the most part, those voluntarily adhered to as set forth by private standards setting organizations such as the American Conference of Governmental Industrial Hygienists (ACGIH), the American National Standards Institute (ANSI), and the American Industrial Hygiene Association (AIHA). The foremost of these organizations in developing recommended exposure standards has been the ACGIH. This nongovernmental organization began development in 1946 of a growing list of recommended threshold limit values (TLVs) designed, in general, to limit worker exposure to airborne concentrations of chemical substances in common production or use by industry to less than harmful quantities (ACGIH, 1946). In 1962 the list (ACGIH, 1962) included, in a separate appendix, three carcinogenic chemicals for which extremely stringent controls were recommended. By 1968 the list (ACGIH, 1968) had been expanded to contain nine carcinogenic substances.

Specifically, the ACGIH recommendation was that no exposure to these substances should be permitted by any route. This philosophy, voluntarily expressed by the industrial health community itself, served as a consensus on the degree to which occupational exposure to recognized carcinogenic chemical substances should be controlled. This philosophy was developed prior to enactment of legilsation providing for mandatory exposure controls and represents the clear understanding and appreciation by the industrial health community of the health risk posed by exposure to carcinogens. The philosophy embodies the principle that exposure to even minimum concentrations of a carcinogenic substance may pose increased risk of cancer induction and, possibly, that absolutely safe exposures may not exist for such a substance. The modifying influence of the Occupational Safety and Health Act of 1970 on this general philosophy has been evidenced by subsequent recommendations of the ACGIH concerning control of specified carcinogens. In 1972 the annual list (ACGIH, 1972) of threshold limit values arbitrarily divided the carcinogens contained in Appendix A into two groups according to whether they were considered to be primarily animal or human carcinogens. In 1973 the classification scheme (ACGIH, 1973) for Appendix A was altered to include exposure values for several of the substances.

The strong influence of the ACGIH on the course of the Occupational Safety and Health Act should not be underestimated. The approximately 400 health standards (*Federal Register*, 1971) initially promulgated by the Occupational Safety and Health Administration (OSHA) in 1971 derived predominately from the 1968 TLV list of the ACGIH. The 1968 edition (ACGIH, 1968) of Appendix A, however, failed to be promulgated by OSHA along with the main body of environmental exposure standards. But in 1972 Appendix A served as the principal guideline for a recommendation by the National Institute for Occupational Safety and Health (NIOSH) to OSHA that occupational exposure to 15 carcinogenic substances should be controlled. These substances included (1) 4-aminobiphenyl, (2) 4-nitrobiphenyl, (3) bis-(chloromethyl) ether, (4) chloromethyl methyl ether, (5) 4-dimethylaminoazobenzene, (6) N-nitrosodimethylamine, (7) 2-acetylaminofluorene, (8) β-naphthylamine, (9) α-naphthylamine, (10) benzidine and salts, (11) 3,3′-dichlorobenzidine and salts, (12) ethyleneimine, (13) 4,4′-methylene-bis(2-chloroaniline), (14) β-propiolactone, and (15) dimethyl sulfate.

Of the 15 substances dimethyl sulfate was deleted later by OSHA with NIOSH concurrence. In addition, α-naphthylamine was not recognized by the ACGIH as carcinogenic, although it was so considered by NIOSH in their recommendations to OSHA. Final regulatory standards for the 14 substances were promulgated by OSHA on January 29, 1974, in the *Federal Register* (1974).

Other, voluntary constraints to production/use of certain carcinogenic chemicals prior to 1971 were occasioned by the available information published in the open scientific literature clearly documenting a probable risk of cancer for exposed employees. How frequently and widespread the principle of "looking prior to leaping" has been practiced by employers probably never will be known. It can only be recorded that by the 1970s a large body of scientific evidence existed detailing the possible carcinogenic nature of hundreds of chemical substances in use by industry. Certainly the knowledge that scores of these substances clearly posed substantial risk of cancer for exposed employees could not have been overlooked by the professional, industrial biomedical community.

The major impact of the Occupational Safety and Health Act in this area has been the demonstration that stringent control of employee exposure to a chemical substance could be required by OSHA based on the judgment that because the substance was carcinogenic in experimental animals it posed an unacceptable carcinogenic risk to employees. The dilemma this situation has created for industry is a matter of public record. The technologic and economic problems associated with mandatory, drastic reductions in levels of employee exposures to asbestos, benzidine, bis(chloromethyl) ether, vinyl chloride, coke oven emissions, etc. have been detailed in the records of public hearings on proposed OSHA regulations. These records are replete with inferences as to why substance X is not carcinogenic; or if it is admittedly carcinogenic in animals, why it does not pose carcinogenic risk for workers; or if it is carcinogenic to workers in excess of a certain concentration or dose, why it is not carcinogenic at a much lower concentration or dose; or if it is carcinogenic even at extremely low concentrations (dosages), why it does not pose a substantial risk to workers because of a presumably extremely long latency period (i.e., longer than normal life expectancy); or barring all considerations of possible health consequences, why the stringent regulation of substance X poses extreme economic hardship and is therefore not in the nation's "best" interests.

It is this latter consideration that presents the real dilemma for a regulatory agency. If little economic effect could be anticipated as a result of an extremely stringent regulatory action, few would argue the merits of taking such action in the face of perceived significant health risk to workers. Under such circumstances it would also be anticipated that the scientific community as a whole would more generally agree on drastic courses of regulatory action.

Often, however, because of the magnitude of possible economic consequences of proposed regulatory controls, the scientific community may discover itself fragmented into special interest groups, each group believing it has correctly reviewed and evaluated the pertinent scientific evidence in reaching its position. Because of the dearth of critical, reliable scientific information available in many of the more important subject areas, though, it is not unusual for conjecture and opinion to lead to such differing points of view. This situation coupled with differing philosophies concerning national interests and the role of science and the scientist in society can lead to honest differences of opinion on the relative merits and evaluation of a given scientific work, or body of works, used by an agency in support of a particular regulatory decision. When factual scientific evidence is insufficient, resultant regulatory actions may reflect either decisions based almost entirely on policy judgments or, if established, on policy judgments modified by policy guidelines. Such guidelines, although limiting the range of possible policy alternatives, serve to clarify and facilitate policy judgments within a framework of established principles. Thus, the Delaney amendment (PL 85-929) to the Federal Food, Drug and Cosmetics Act has provided legislative guidelines for the U.S. Food and Drug Administration (FDA) in the form of a mandate to exclude food additives that have a demonstrated carcinogenic potential for humans or for animals whose exposure routes were comparable to those for humans. The Occupational Safety and Health Act, although not specifically addressing the question of occupational exposure to carcinogens, does provide that criteria for standards must assure, insofar as practicable, that no worker shall suffer diminished health, loss of functional capacity, or decreased life span as a result of his work experience. Obviously, occupationally induced cancer touches on all three of these areas. It was largely with this very general mandate, and with no established policy guidelines, that OSHA entered into the area of promulgating regulations requiring mandatory control of occupational exposure to the 14 carcinogenic substances listed earlier.

Regulatory approaches to control of occupational carcinogenesis may take a myriad of directions depending on scope and limits of authority of the responsible agency, criteria for determination of carcinogenicity and of carcinogenic risk to employees, and extent to which considerations of feasibility of controls may modify original determinations of risk. Regulatory control of carcinogenic chemicals in the workplace may include an outright ban of production and/or use, mandatory substitution, whenever possible, or limiting exposure to within prescribed limits. Variations on these control measures may include reduction of concentrations to ambient, or background levels, establishment of a licensing authority or use permit system, and development of special work practices based on best available technology. Where the authority of a regulatory agency does not include the power to ban production and/or use of a particular substance considered to be carcinogenic, the agency must establish regulatory controls consistent with the maximum degree of health protection absolutely possible. Although the degree of health protection that is absolutely possible may not necessarily be either technically or economically possible in the immediate sense, the objective of the regulatory agency under these circumstances should be to achieve what is immediately both technically and economically feasible, with the goal of attaining what is absolutely necessary as it becomes technically and economically possible. Because this final goal for control may impose severe economic hardship, employers must carefully consider the costs of continued production or use of the substance or of the process in question. Economic considerations by the employer must include not only the short-term, possibly minimal, costs associated with attaining immediate compliance with preliminary control measures but also the projection of future economic obligations as more stringent control measures become technically feasible. Long-term considerations may include the necessity for complete modification of existing production or use facilities or the building of new facilities design engineered to provide as closed a production system as is technically possible. In design of engineering controls and of systems for incremental or continuous environmental sampling, the employer should be cognizant that advance designs or breakthroughs by one portion of the industry may very well set the stage for mandating the implementation of such controls or systems throughout the affected industry.

For the multinational corporation longer-term planning undoubtedly will include considerations of the economic desirability of producing carcinogenic substances in nations with few, or far less stringent, control measures. In the case of substances such as asbestos and vinyl chloride, although industrial processes associated with the milling and processing of the former and of the synthesis or polymerization of the latter pose greatly increased risks of cancer to employees, other "downstream" processes may present little, if any, such excess risks. Transfer of these "dirty" processes to nations that fail to provide effective regulatory exposure controls, thereby rendering the operation more economically feasible, also results in exposing a completely new workforce to concentrations of a carcinogenic substance that are very likely far in excess of concentrations sustained by employees in the parent nation.

The primary consideration when dealing with toxic or potentially carcinogenic substances in the occupational environment is control of employee exposure to such substances by reducing ambient concentrations to safe levels. The degree of safety that is assured where exposure to a carcinogen is concerned is a matter of considerable debate, as discussed elsewhere in this chapter. The simple, traditional approach to accomplish exposure control is through implementation of local exhaust or general dilution ventilation schemes. Design of effective general dilution ventilation schemes, however, can become extremely complex when dealing with point source emissions, including leaks, in a large enclosed facility. With either type of ventilation scheme (or combinations thereof) contaminated air is normally exhausted into the outside environment. Some type of emission control or "scrubbing" device may be employed to entrap or absorb particular contaminants. However, unless the emission includes a readily detectable irritant gas, nuisance odor, or particulate or unless otherwise required by regulation, emission control devices in all likelihood will not be used. The employer considers his ventilation system successful if the employee is protected from exposure to concentrations of the contaminant(s) believed to be harmful. In the case of industrial processes involving emissions of confirmed or suspected chemical carcinogenic substances, the primary concern of employers is effective removal of "harmful" quantities of the carcinogen away from the working environment prompted either by their own initiative or when required to do so by regulation. In most such situations the concentration or fate of the carcinogen outside the working environment is of little concern to the employer, unless otherwise regulated, because of the belief that the great dilutatory effect of the general environment will reduce concentrations of the substance to less than harmful quantities. It may not be readily appreciated that safe levels of exposure to the particular carcinogenic substance in question may not have been demonstrated. From the standpoint of the employer, industrial facilities, especially those in warmer climates, not enclosed present an ideal, as well as an economical, solution to this problem by using natural ventilation to accomplish removal of the carcinogen from the immediate workplace. In such situations the potential conflict between regulatory agencies responsible for protecting different portions of the population/environment is obvious. One cannot simply remove a harmful substance from one portion of the environment to another without subsequent contamination of the latter.

EVALUATION OF OCCUPATIONAL CARCINOGENESIS HAZARD AND RISK

Prior to determination of the extent to which exposure to occupational carcinogens should be controlled, it is essential that criteria or policy guidelines be developed to assist in evaluating scientific literature and other information concerning carcinogenic hazard posed by exposure. Both human epidemiologic and experimental animal exposure data must be considered and evaluated in making these determinations. Recent findings (McCann and Ames, 1976) demonstrating that a high proportion of carcinogenic chemicals tested are also mutagenic will, no doubt, force a reconsideration by employers in situations where those chemicals discovered to elicit a mutagenic response are present.

Regulation of occupational exposure to chemicals based on perceived carcinogenic hazard must, therefore, include an exhaustive literature search followed by in-depth review and evaluation to determine relevancy to the occupational environment. The search itself must focus not only on those domestic sources readily obtainable in the open, published scientific literature but also on efforts to obtain previously unpublished data and updated reports of research in progress. Much greater efforts are required to obtain similar scientific literature and published research reports from foreign sources, but if the search is to be truly complete and updated to a specified point in time, the additional effort required to gather literature from other than readily available domestic sources must be undertaken. In most cases this additional effort will require translation services, which will greatly increase cost of the overall literature retrieval effort. The use of automated information storage and retrieval services such as those available from the National Library of Medicine and the National Academy of Sciences has greatly decreased the amount of time required to accomplish a preliminary scan of the scientific literature for pertinent articles.

Retrieval of "hard copy" reproductions or originals of papers considered pertinent during the scan phase of the search is required to permit in-depth evaluation of the complete paper. Abstracts of published works alone rarely permit an analysis with any greater value than assisting in defining the scope of the initial scan. Reliance on translated abstracts for analysis of foreign works introduces the possibility of at least two major errors. Persons performing the translation may be technically unfamiliar with the work and, therefore, may misinterpret the data, and if a different individual performs the abstraction, additional error may be introduced.

Evaluation of information should be accomplished on two levels. The first level involves assessing the carcinogenicity or carcinogenic potential of specific chemical substances, physical agents (e.g., ionizing radiation, ultraviolet light, and X-irradiation), or undefined mixtures (e.g., wood dusts, coke oven emissions). The second level of evaluation involves assessing the particular carcinogenic hazard posed by exposure to the substance or agent in the occupational environment. Carcinogenic potential may bear little relationship to exposure hazard when the latter is properly contained. It is a major tenet of industrial hygiene that toxicity and hazard are not synonymous terms and that extremely toxic substances may pose a minimum of hazard if workplace exposure is adequately controlled. The same undoubtedly holds true for most carcinogenic substances used in the workplace. That is, risk of cancer induction is probably closely correlated with effective dose, and both may be reduced through methods of exposure control.

Absolute exposure control, accomplished by means of a complete ban on production and/or use, will eliminate the hazard and, therefore, the attendant risk. However, if this ultimate recourse is not possible (e.g., not within the legal mandate of a regulatory agency), then some exposure, regardless of how minimal, will undoubtedly occur, and some attendant risk of cancer, although possibly extremely minimal, will exist. To presume otherwise is to completely ignore the fact that so-called no-effect levels of exposure to carcinogenic substances are extremely difficult, if not practically impossible, to conclusively demonstrate. Under such circumstances and legal constraints then the control objective must be hazard reduction with concomitant minimization of risk. The immediate problem becomes one of hazard assessment under various conditions of workplace exposure. Because dose–response relationships for even the most intensively investigated carcinogens fail to provide definite answers for very low levels of exposures, assumption of some minimum, though possibly undefined, risk must be accepted even for those exposure concentrations less than the lowest concentration clearly demonstrating carcinogenic effect.

Recognition of occupational exposure as a determinant of cancer induction usually has required either that large numbers of workers be exposed to carcinogenic substances over long periods of time sufficient to reveal substantive differences in tumor induction with unexposed cohorts or that the incidence of a certain type of tumor normally considered rare in the general population occurs with greater frequency among exposed workers. The recognition of scrotal cancer in chimney sweeps, as documented by Sir Percival Pott (1775), and of cancer of the urinary bladder, as first described by Rehn (1895), represent classic examples of this requirement. More recently the health consequences of previous exposures to asbestos, vinyl chloride, or bis(chloromethyl) ether have been realized as workers at risk developed tumors of definitive etiology.

Although both epidemiologic investigations and animal experimentation have been recognized as the two primary sources of evidence necessary to establish etiology of occupational cancers, the impact of information from these sources on development of control measures often has been less than substantial. In addition, recognition of risk of cancer by public health authorities has usually differed from similar recognition by industrial management. Under circumstances where absolute proof of cancer induction elicited by exposures to specific substances is hardly possible, overall assessment of risk of cancer based on available epidemiologic and experimental animal investigations is subject to a wide range of scientific opinion. Workers, with a very limited appreciation of either the biology of cancer or of the special risks associated with their particular employment, are, of course, placed in the middle of this predicament.

Several problems immediately confront a regulatory agency in attempting to control occupational exposure to carcinogenic substances. First, as previously discussed, unless authority to ban substances based on toxicity, including irreversible delayed toxicity associated with tumor induction, is included in its mandate, a regulatory authority must evaluate the health consequences of continued exposure to hazardous substances at some average or ceiling concentration that is both compatible with available sampling and analytical methodology and that is considered technologically attainable by industry, even if practical considerations would preclude its immediate attainment. Such considerations may include the admission that the state of presently available technology does not yet include development of the engineering methodology necessary to achieve compliance with the exposure standard believed to be ultimately necessary.

The same can be said of sampling and analytical methodology. Unless compliance with the ultimate standard can be satisfactorily determined with known accuracy, a less precise standard represents the only practical solution. This is not to say that advances in sampling and analytical technology, in a manner similar to technology concerned with development of engineering controls, cannot be the subject of reasonable speculation and that regulatory controls cannot include future "benchmark" dates to spur on the development of necessary technology.

Because even the most effective methodology for control of carcinogenic substances in the workplace will never completely eliminate risk of cancer associated with exposure to a regulated substance, the absolute best that can be achieved is substantive minimization of risk. A society that accepts this consequence as a condition of worker exposure likewise accepts the responsibility of assuring that the worker employed in the risk-associated occupation clearly understands the possible health consequences of this employment and is provided the greatest exposure protection possible. The worker must sufficiently understand the particular risks associated with the employment in order to be able to choose intelligently not to accept such risks—even when this may entail loss of employment. However, for a subject as complex as the biology of tumor induction and development of cancer, on which even the scientific community is often divided, it is not certain that workers perhaps even without the benefit of secondary school biology, can comprehend sufficiently this scientifically sophisticated knowledge to assure that they are capable of intelligently evaluating their particular risks. Therefore, an essential element of occupational cancer control, including development of regulatory standards, must be a comprehensive program for education and training of potentially exposed employees to include explanation of risk and instruction in environmental control methods and procedures. Such programs must not be limited only to employees but must include their supervisors, management, and the families of the workers as well.

EMPLOYER CONCERNS FOR OCCUPATIONAL EXPOSURE STANDARDS FOR CARCINOGENIC SUBSTANCES

Many employers now realize that hundreds of chemicals have been demonstrated to induce cancer in animals and that employees exposed to these and related chemicals probably incur increased risk of cancer. Such employers also may have observed that several decisions by U.S. Circuit Courts of Appeal (1974) have vigorously upheld stringent regulatory controls for chemical substances considered to be carcinogenic by regulatory authorities, including such control measures as drastic reduction in permissible exposure concentrations, specification of detailed work practices, and requirement of specified medical examinations and tests. The recent toxic substance control legislation with requirements for testing new, as well as certain "old," chemical substances based on assumptions of possible carcinogenicity, places the manufacturer in a situation of proving safety prior to marketing.

It is entirely possible that new questions of employer responsibility will be raised concerning legal liability for exposing employees even to unregulated substances when the employer has sufficient reason to believe that such exposure may entail substantial carcinogenic hazard. Questions concerning employer responsibility for reporting of results of in-house experimental animal testing and epidemiologic studies of employee populations are unresolved. Unless such results are published in the open scientific literature, it is possible that knowledge of such studies will never come to light. Yet it seems reasonable to assume that most employers introducing a new chemical into large-scale production would make at least an initial attempt to discover acute toxicologic properties of the substance. It also seems plausible that similar tests, however rudimentary in design and scope, have been performed in the past by employers to analyze the more chronic effects of exposure, possibly including induction of tumors. If this is the actual case, it can be concluded that absence of sufficient incentive precludes the employer from sharing such vital knowledge with competitors or with the scientific community as a whole.

The seeming reluctance of employers to provide adequate, realistic exposure protection for employees has been demonstrated repeatedly in testimony presented during the course of public hearings on proposed OSHA rule making for control of carcinogens in the workplace. Time and again these hearing records reveal that employers have provided testimony strongly advocating positions apparently based more on desire than on evaluation of scientific data. One such position can be generally stated as, "Chemical X has been in production for Y years and has never resulted in a case of tumor Z." In such situations, however, the size of the exposed worker population often has been insufficient to render the results statistically conclusive. In most such circumstances there is only a miniscule amount of data pertaining to exposure concentrations, especially over long periods of time. Too often only currently employed workers, or those who have left within a few years of the study, are included as the population at risk. Workers who were employed very early in the operation in question and who, therefore, probably incurred much greater exposures to the carcinogen are often extremely difficult to trace, especially those who worked for only a year or so. Even if this early worker population is not large, it represents a group of employees with proportionately longer latency periods since initiation of exposure who are, therefore, presumably at greater risk of cancer. In the case of experimental animal studies sponsored or performed by industry results have sometimes been equivocal.

CLASSIFICATION AND PRIORITIZATION OF OCCUPATIONAL CARCINOGENS

An initial step for a regulatory agency in developing standards for occupational carcinogens concerns priority classification for evaluation of the large number of chemical substances that have been demonstrated to possess at least some degree of carcinogenic potential. Various schemes have been proposed for classifying carcinogenic chemical substances used in the occupational environment. Examples of such plans are those developed by Hueper and Conway (1964), Eckardt (1959), Dinman (1974), Cole and Goldman

(1975), Rose (1976), and the ACGIH (1973). Such schemes invariably involve attempts to categorize chemical substances based on estimates of degree of carcinogenic potency from experimental animal and/or human epidemiologic evidence. Although evaluation of such parameters is largely subjective, approximations of carcinogenic potency are worthy of consideration for the same reason that chronic toxicity is considered when evaluating potential occupational exposure hazards posed by toxic substances.

Classification schemes, in addition, can serve important functions. For example, a categorization of chemical substances on the basis of perceived carcinogenic potency represents at the minimum a contemporary evaluation of existing information in this field. Such a scheme can serve to inform the general public and especially industry of the relative carcinogenic importance being assigned by the scientific community or regulatory authority to certain of the chemicals being used by industry. If parameters are chosen that include those of major importance concerning carcinogenicity, it may be possible to approximate the relative carcinogenic potency among chemical substances. However, it must be emphasized that such schemes, although organizing information concerning carcinogenic potency in a relative sense, do not indicate such potency in an absolute sense. This idea supposes, of course, that sufficient information concerning the chosen parameters is available for each substance.

It also should be realized that chemicals exhibiting only weakly carcinogenic properties may be extremely important from the standpoint that greater numbers of workers eventually may be exposed over a greater time interval such that the final outcome in terms of the number of workers eventually developing cancer may be highly significant. The increased incidence of lung cancer among cigarette smokers is an example of a large population exposed to a weakly carcinogenic stimulus with the resultant toll in human lives. Although this distinction between strong and weak carcinogenic substances is more than academic, from the practical standpoint substances with more readily recognizable carcinogenic potentials (i.e., extremely potent carcinogens) usually provide the social visibility that assures their priority consideration. Also, regulation of substances with recognized carcinogenic potency based on sound scientific evidence presents far fewer difficulties than attempting to regulate weaker, though possibly widely dispersed, carcinogens. The real value to research and regulatory organizations of developing a priority ranking system for consideration of carcinogens is to assure the optional allocation of the agencies' resources available to develop control measures to minimize risk associated with exposure.

The classification scheme presented in Table 1 was developed from information provided in a series of monographs produced by the International Agency for Research on Cancer (IARC, 1972-1975). This information concerning evaluation of carcinogenic risk of chemicals to humans was developed into a classification scheme subject to the following criteria:

Category	Criteria
I	Definitive epidemiologic and/or case studies
II	Some epidemiologic and/or case studies and/or definitive experimental animal investigations
III	Suggestive experimental animal investigations; epidemiologic and/or case studies, if available, inconclusive
IV	Available data inconclusive or equivocal

Certainly, of all disease conditions associated with workplace exposure, occupational cancer has been the most intensively investigated during the recent past. The insidious nature of these diseases with latency periods between initiation of exposure and clinical recognition of symptoms of 10, 20, or 30 or more years means that large numbers of workers may accrue significant exposure to carcinogenic substances prior to the recognition of exposure hazard. It is, then, in those activities concerned with hazard recognition that much of the resources of research and regulatory organizations should be concentrated. Such hazard recognition activities should include surveillance of the workplace to determine conditions of exposure, recognition of etiologic agents, and detection of tumors.

In developing a prioritization model to allocate program resources for prevention and control of occupational cancer, it would be desirable to determine the number of "excess" cancers that could be expected in a worker population exposed to defined chemical substances or mixtures of such substances. If this information could be determined within known confidence limits, it would be possible to view the prioritization problem in greater perspective. That is, if it were possible to predict yearly excesses of cancers associated with recognized occupational exposures, then this information could be used by both research and regulatory agencies alike in developing programs whose goals involve prevention of such excesses. Although data and information are not available at present to the extent required to accomplish this task with great accuracy and reliability, it is interesting to speculate on how this goal could be approximated through the use of presently available information. The essential elements of information required to reach the desired ultimate goal include accurate knowledge of the health experience of large numbers of workers classified according to age, sex, race, and, if possible, smoking and drinking histories. Other parameters, including genetic and nutritional factors, reasonably could not be expected to be included in a scheme of national magnitude. Of course, it would be necessary to have accurate information concerning workplace exposures obtained through detailed, comprehensive occupational histories. Finally, it would be necessary to know the health significance of discrete and multiple exposures detailed in the occupational histories. Knowledge of the health experience of workers by

TABLE 1 Classification of Certain Occupational Carcinogens with Respect to Perceived Risk and Relative Potency

Chemical substance	Priority ranking[a]	Epidemiologic and/or case studies	No. animal species positive[a]	Route tested (positive)		Tumor site		Latency (lifespan)		Incidence		Regulatory status[b]
				Inhalation	Other[a]	Local	Systemic[a]	1st half	2nd half[a]	<50%[a]	>50%[a]	
Category I—Confirmed Human Carcinogen; definitive epidemiologic and/or case studies												
Benzidine	26	Both	4	X	2		X		X		X	C
bis(Chloromethyl) ether	25	Both	2	X	1		X	X			X	C
Chloromethyl methyl ether	24	Cases	1	X	1	X	X	X			X	C
Vinyl chloride	24	Cases	2	X	1	X	X	X			X	C
Asbestos (crocidolite)	22	Both	1	X	1		X		X		X	T
Asbestos (chrysotile)	21	Both	4	X	2		X		X	X		T
β-Naphthylamine	19	Cases	6		1		X	X			X	C
Asbestos (amosite)	17	Both	1	X	1		X	X		X		T
Auramine	15	Both	2		1		X	X			X	
4-Aminobiphenyl	15	Epid.	4		1		X		X	X		
Arsenic and compounds	–	Both	(Animal studies are inconclusive to date)									C
Category II—Probable Human Carcinogen; some epidemiologic and case studies and/or definitive experimental animal investigations												
3,4-Benzo[a]pyrene	36	–	9	X	5		X	X	X		X	T
Beryllium and compounds	28	Cases	4	X	2		X	X			X	T
Diazomethane	25		2	X	1	X	X	X			X	
Dimethyl sulfate	23	Cases	1	X	2	X	X		X		X	T
Carbon tetrachloride	22	Cases	4	X	3	X	X		X	X		T
N-methyl-N'-nitro-N-nitroso-guanidine	22		5	X	5	X	X	X			X	
Nitrosoethyl urea	20		4	X	4	X	X	X			X	
o-Aminoazotoluene	18		4	X	2	X	X	X			X	
p-Dimethylaminoazo-benzene	18		3	X	3	X	X	X			X	

TABLE 1 Classification of Certain Occupational Carcinogens with Respect to Perceived Risk and Relative Potency (*Continued*)

Chemical substance	Priority ranking[a]	Epidemiologic and/or case studies	No. animal species positive[a]	Route tested (positive) Inhalation	Route tested (positive) Other[a]	Tumor site Local	Tumor site Systemic[a]	Latency (lifespan) 1st half	Latency (lifespan) 2nd half[a]	Incidence <50%	Incidence >50%[a]	Regulatory status[b]
β-Propiolactone	18		4		4	X	X		X		X	C
Asbestos (anthrophyllite)	17	Both	1	X	2		X		X	X		T
Propyl thiouracil	17	Both	4		1		X	X			X	
Nickel (insoluble) compounds	16	Cases	3	X	1	X		X		X		
Amitrole	15	Epid.	3	X	2	X	X		X		X	
1,3-Propanesultone	15		2		3	X	X	X			X	
Nickel carbonyl	13	Cases	1	X		X		X		X		T
Estradiol-17β	11		4		2	X			X	X		
Calcium chromate	10	Cases	2		1	X	X	X		X		
Benzene	9	Both	1		1		X	X		X		T
Nickel (soluble) compounds	5	Cases	2		1	X		X		X		T
Chromate (insoluble) compounds	3	Cases	1	X	2	X			X	X		T
Cadmium oxide (fume)	—	Cases	(Animal studies negative in only route and species tested)			X	X		X	X		T
Coal tar pitch (volatiles)	—	Epid.	(No significant animal studies)									T
Hematite	—	Epid.	(No significant animal studies)									
Iron oxide	—	Epid.	(Animal studies negative in three species tested by inhalation route)									T
Lead arsenate	—	Both	(Animal studies negative in only route and species tested)									T

Category III—Suggestive Experimental Animal Investigations; epidemiologic and/or case studies, if available, inconclusive (possible human carcinogens)

Urethane	28		3	X	3	X	X	X			X	
Estrone	19		3		3		X	X			X	
Thiourea	18		3		3		X	X			X	

78

Chemical								Class
Isonicotinic acid hydrazine	17	2				X	X	
Dibenz[ah]acridine	16	1	X			X	X	C
Dibenz[ah]anthracene	16	1	X		X	X	X	C
3,3'-Dichlorobenzidine	16	2	X		X	X	X	
Ethylenimine	16	2				X	X	
Isosutrole	16	2				X	X	
Lead phosphate	16	1				X	X	
Aramite	15	2				X	X	
Lead acetate	15	2				X	X	
Safrole	15	2				X	X	
BCH (alpha, beta, gamma)	14	1				X	X	
Chrysodine	19	1	X			X	X	
1,2-Diethylhydrazine	14	1	X			X	X	
1,1-Dimethylhydrazine	14	1	X			X	X	
Hydrazine	14	2	X		X	X	X	T
Lead sybacetate	14	1	X			X	X	
4-Nitrobiphenyl	14	1	X			X	X	C
Ethylene thiourea	13	2			X	X	X	
Thioacetamide	13	2			X	X	X	
Chloroform	12	1			X	X	X	T
TDE and DDE	12	1			X	X	X	
1,1-Dimethylhydrazine	12	1			X	X	X	T
4,4-Methylenebis-(2-methylaniline)	12	1			X	X	X	
1,4-Butanediol di-methanesulfonate	10	2			X	X		
3,3-Dimethoxybenzidine	10	2		X	X	X		C
Acetamide	9	1		X	X	X		
Citrus red no. 2	9	2		X	X	X		
Dihydrosulfrole	9	1		X		X		
4,4-Methylenebis-(2-chloroaniline)	9	2		X	X	X		C

TABLE 1 Classification of Certain Occupational Carcinogens with Respect to Perceived Risk and Relative Potency (*Continued*)

Chemical substance	Priority ranking[a]	Epidemiologic and/or case studies	No. animal species positive[a]	Route tested (positive)		Tumor site		Latency (lifespan)		Incidence		Regulatory status[b]
				Inhalation	Other[a]	Local	Systemic[a]	1st half	2nd half[a]	<50%	>50%[a]	
α-Naphthylamine	9		2		2		X		X	X		C
PCB-Arochlor 1259	9		1		1		X	X		X		T
PCB-Kanechlor 500	9		1		1		X	X		X		T
Cadmium chloride	8		2		1	X	X		X	X		
Mestranol	8		2		1		X		X	X		
Ponceau MX	8		2		1		X		X	X		
Streptozotocin	8		2		1		X		X	X		
Cadmium (metal)	7		1		1	X	X		X		X	T
Mirex	7		1		1	X			X	X		
4,5-Benzo[e]pyrene	4		1		1	X		X		X		
Cadmium sulfate	4		1		1	X		X		X		

Category IV—Available data inconclusive or equivocal

Chemical substance			No. animal species positive[a]	Route tested (positive)								Regulatory status[b]
				Inhalation	Other[a]							
Aldrin			2		1							T
Amaranth			3		2							
Aniline			2		2							T
Azobenzene			1		1							
Carmoisine			1		1							
Chlorobenzilate			1		1							
Chromium (metal)			3		1							T
C.I. disperse yellow			1		1							
Damd C red 9			1		1							
2,6-Diamino-3-phenylazo-pyridine hydrochloride			1		1							

Chemical			Regulatory status
Dieldrin	4		T
Diethyl sulfate	1	1	
3,3-Dimethylbenzidine	2	1	T
Endrin	1	1	T
Heptachlor	2	1	
Lead carbonate	1	1	
Magenta	2	3	
Maleic hydrazine	1	2	
Methoxychlor	1	2	
PCB-Kanechlor 300 and 400	1		T
Orange G	3	2	
Ponceau SX	3	2	
Scarlet red	2	2	
Sudan I and II	1	1	
Sudan III	2	2	
Sunset yellow FCF	2	2	

[a]Priority ranking determination based on parameters of experimental animal evidence:

Parameter	Numerically weighted factor	Parameter	Numerically weighted factor
A. Route of administration		2. Tumors observed only during second half of animal life span	0
1. Inhalation	10	D. Tumor incidence	
2. Each other route (positive)	1	1. Greater than 50%	5
B. Tumor site		2. Less than 50%	0
1. Local (e.g., injection site)	0	E. Each species tested with positive findings of tumor induction	1
2. Systemic (i.e., distant site and/or metastasis)	5		
C. Tumor latency			
1. Tumors observed during first half of animal life span	2		

[b]Regulatory status of the chemical substance: C, regulated as a carcinogen by OSHA. T, regulated as a toxic substance by OSHA.

Note: The author expresses his appreciation to Grover V. Foster, Jr., Ph.D., and acknowledges his professional assistance in preparation of this table.

occupational exposure history could be used to generate reliable statistical conclusions concerning increased risk of many chronic diseases, including cancer. Information concerning various components of exposures could then be used to assist further in planning more definitive investigations into etiology and determination of mechanism of disease induction.

That this ideal situation was only a distant realization in the United States even a decade ago is attested to in a statement (DHEW, 1966) to the Surgeon General of the U.S. Public Health Service in 1966:

> It is almost inconceivable that this nation with its vast resources and technical skills, has never developed a comprehensive picture of the work environment to determine the relationship with the health status of its productive work force. Nor are all the health hazards to which its workers today are exposed identified clearly to determine the presence and trends of disease observed. . . .

Certain parcels of data and information, however, are becoming available, which, when all are considered together, may be sufficient to permit reliable estimates of cancer excesses in certain industries and perhaps even provide for differentiation among occupations within an industry. Of course, where reliable studies have been published concerning excess risk of cancer in groups of workers exposed to particular chemical substances, the task of eliminating or minimizing such risks through substitution of less hazardous materials, or, where this is not possible, through stringent exposure controls becomes the obvious course of action.

Information concerning populations employed in broad occupational and industrial categories by geographic areas is collected by the U.S. Bureau of the Census. Crude estimates of numbers of workers occupationally exposed to approximately 450 of the most common chemical substances and physical agents have been developed by the National Institute for Occupational Safety and Health (NIOSH). Further refinement of the NIOSH estimates to provide more reliable information is expected to be available in 1977 from data obtained through a National Occupation Hazard Survey (NOHS) performed by NIOSH. The information to be obtained from the NOHS activity will be all the more important because occupational exposures to specific chemical substances will be keyed to the U.S. Bureau of Census occupation/industry classification system.

It should be noted that the U.S. Bureau of Labor Statistics (BLS), in the U.S. Department of Labor, conducts a yearly national statistical sampling survey for determination of incidence of occupationally related illnesses and injuries in the U.S. work force. Although these estimates are subject to considerable controversy concerning their significance and reliability, the Standard Industrial Classification (SIC) used by BLS to place individual worker reports of illness/injury into industrial categories is more extensive than the corresponding U.S. Bureau of Census Classification System for industry. The SIC system does not, however, include occupation, as does the

U.S. Bureau of Census Classification System. It may be possible, however, to roughly combine the industrial categories of the two systems.

It is possible, therefore, to estimate on a national basis numbers of workers employed in broad industrial/occupational classes and perhaps by 1977 also to include estimates of occupational exposure to particular chemical substances. The latter information is presently unobtainable except for vertical in-depth, comprehensive surveys of particular industries, which are both difficult and expensive.

Information available from the Third National Cancer Survey (DHEW, 1975) conducted during 1969-1971 may be a most valuable resource in providing key links to attaining the goal of estimating cancer excesses by occupation. An approximate 10% sample of all cancer cases identified during the 3-yr survey was selected for purposes of obtaining supplementary information concerning treatment, duration of hospitalization, cost of medical care, and economic impact of cancer treatment on the family. In addition, this 10% sample of supplementary information included the occupation of the cancer patient at the time of tumor diagnosis, the occupation following diagnosis, and the occupation at which the patient had been employed for the longest period of time. Because of the large sample size of the National Cancer Survey itself (i.e., 10% of the U.S. population) and the exhaustive efforts to obtain practically all cases of cancer occurring during the 3-yr survey in the six Standard Metropolitan Statistical Areas and two states where the survey was conducted, the results obtained in the survey should be closely representative of the cancer experience of the U.S. population as a whole. In the eight areas where the smaller 10% sample was obtained, the relation of cancer incidence by histologic type and primary site during 1969-1971 to usual occupation of the patient can be determined. It also is possible to estimate cancer risk for each major organ site by occupation and industry (U.S. Bureau of Census Classification). Thus, it should be possible to estimate excess numbers of specific cancers occurring yearly in a particular occupation/industry in the eight areas in the 10% sample. The extrapolation of these estimates to the entire U.S. work force will require standardization of pertinent variables including occupational/industrial differences in the U.S. work force with those in the eight areas. This could be accomplished by comparing detailed U.S. Bureau of Census data for the eight areas in question with that for the U.S. as a whole. By coupling these data concerning tumor incidence by occupation/industry with data obtained from the NIOSH NOHS activity, both suspected agents of etiology and occupations associated with high incidences of specific tumors can be identified and accorded priority consideration. It should be recognized that this approach would seldom establish definitive tumor etiology. Both bioassay testing and epidemiologic investigations are required to establish tumor etiology with certainty. The approach proposed, however, would assist in determining which chemicals should receive priority consideration for bioassay testing and, similarly, which worker populations should receive consideration for epidemiologic investigations.

TABLE 2 Excess Cancers Attributable to Occupational

Chemical substance	Target organ	NIOSH estimate of worker population[a]	Incidence per 100,000 U.S. males[b]	Incidence per 100,000 U.S. males >40 yr old[c]	Risk factor[d]	Risk factor (100-fold decrease)
Asbestos	Lung, pleural and peritoneal mesothelium	5,000,000	72.1	194.3	12	1.12
Arsenic	Lung	1,500,000	72.1	194.3	8	1.08
Benzene	Blood	2,000,000	12.7	27.7	3	1.03
Chromium	Lung	160,000	72.1	194.3	40	1.4
Coal tar pitch volatiles and coke oven emissions	Lung	60,000	72.1	194.3	6	1.06
Iron oxide	Lung	100,000	72.1	194.3	5	1.05
Nickel	Lung	50,000	72.1	194.3	10	1.10
Vinyl chloride	Liver	20,000	0.02	0.02	400	4

[a]DHEW (1974).

[b]Average annual age-adjusted (1970 U.S. census) incidence rate per 100,000 U.S. males (DHEW, 1975).

Yet another approach, suggested in a presentation by Bridbord (1975), and one of more immediate practical application involves an estimation of the number of male workers potentially exposed to specific chemical substances (e.g., estimates developed by NIOSH) and the yearly incidence of specific cancers or of cancer deaths in the total U.S. work force. An application of this approach is presented in Table 2, which was developed to demonstrate the conceptual utility of a particular approach in estimating the influence on cancer incidence of occupational exposure to a particular carcinogenic chemical substance. In this instance, the desired information is the number of excess deaths per 100,000 each year in a worker population at risk. The incidence rate used to derive this information was for workers (U.S. males) over 40 yr of age. This particular rate was used to provide an approximate 20-yr latency estimation for this population. The risk factors used in Table 2 are those presented by Cole and Goldman (1975) in a review of the literature pertaining to the range of published risk information. Finally, the predicted number of excess cases of cancer per year per 100,000 population at risk are presented both for the highest published risk data and for a 100-fold reduction in this data. As already mentioned this approach is one involving application of presently available information for the chosen parameters. As the statistical validity of a particular parameter increases through greater knowledge, the

Exposures to Certain Chemical Substances at Different Levels of Risk

Expected no. cases of cancer per year in workers >40 yr old	Predicted no. cases of cancer per year if all workers (>40 yr old) at highest risk	Predicted no. cases of cancer per year if all workers (>40 yr old) at reduced risk (i.e., 100-fold decrease)	Predicted no. excess cases of cancer per year in workers >40 yr old at highest risk	Predicted no. excess cases of cancer per year in workers >40 yr old at reduced risk (i.e., 100-fold decrease)
3530.9	42,370.8	3,954.6	38,839.9	423.7
1059.3	8,474.1	1,144	7,414.8	84.7
201.3	603.9	207.3	406.6	6
113	4,520	158.2	4,407	45.2
42.4	254.4	44.9	212	2.5
70.6	353	74.1	282.4	3.5
35.3	353	38.8	317.7	3.5
Negligible	1.5	Negligible	1.5	Negligible

[c]Average annual age-adjusted (1970 U.S. census) incidence rate per 100,000 U.S. males (>40 yr of age) (DHEW, 1975).

[d]Highest published risk data (Cole and Goldman, 1975).

reliability of the predicted yearly excesses of cancer increases. The value of the approach used in Table 2 is not related as much to defining etiology as to identification of populations at increased risk of cancer. Such information should have wide application in development of priorities for epidemiologic research and bioassay testing.

If predictions of the amount of cancer extrinsically related are correct, then many of the substances to which each of us is daily exposed must be of suspected tumorigenic influence at some level of initiation, promotion, or exacerbation. Certainly hundreds of chemical substances have been demonstrated to induce tumors in animals under a wide variety of exposure regimens. It is the extrapolation of this information to humans, exposed to such substances during the course of normal employment and under exposure conditions that may be radically different from those in animal experimentation, that most frequently is the cause of considerable scientific deliberation. Such obvious considerations, however, should not be used to mitigate the importance of animal models in the bioassay of chemical substances. The important factor is that exposure protocols of a particular investigation be clearly defined in order that the importance of the results of the study and their possible relation to the occupational environment may be properly evaluated. Although it is not necessary that animal studies closely duplicate the occupational environment in development of exposure protocols, those studies in which exposure conditions closely approximate the occupational exposure situation must be adjudged more pertinent in terms of positive findings of tumor induction.

REFERENCES

American Conference of Governmental Industrial Hygienists. 1946. *Threshold limit values for 1946.*
American Conference of Governmental Industrial Hygienists. 1962. *Threshold limit values for 1962.*
American Conference of Governmental Industrial Hygienists. 1968. *Threshold limit values for 1968.*
American Conference of Governmental Industrial Hygienists. 1972. *Threshold limit values for 1972.*
American Conference of Governmental Industrial Hygienists. 1973. *Threshold limit values for 1973.*
Boyland, E. 1969. *Progr. Exp. Tumor Res.* 11:222.
Bridbord, K. 1975. In *Proceedings of nineteenth meeting: Interagency collaborative group on environmental carcinogenesis*, ed. H. F. Kraybill, pp. 57–59. Bethesda, Md.: National Cancer Institute.
Cole, P. and Goldman, M. B. 1975. In *Persons at high risk of cancer—An approach to cancer etiology and control*, ed. J. F. Fraumeni, Jr., pp. 167–183. New York: Academic Press.
Dinman, B. D. 1974. *The nature of occupational cancer.* Springfield, Ill.: Thomas.
Eckardt, R. E. 1959. *Industrial carcinogens.* New York: Grune and Stratton.
Federal Register. 1971. 36:10466.
Federal Register. 1974. 39:3756.
Higginson, J. 1968. *Proceedings of the 8th Canadian cancer conference, Honey Harbour, 1968*, p. 40. New York: Pergamon Press.
Hueper, W. C. and Conway, W. D. 1964. *Chemical carcinogenesis and cancers.* Springfield, Ill.: Thomas.
International Agency for Research on Cancer (IARC). 1972–1975. *Monographs on the evaluation of carcinogenic risk of chemicals to man*, vols. 1–8. Lyon, France.
McCann, J. and Ames, B. N. 1976. *Ann. N.Y. Acad. Sci.* 271:5.
Pott, P. 1775. *Chirurgical observations.* London: Hawes, Clarke, and Collings.
Rehn, L. 1895. *Arch. Klin. Chirurg.* 50:588.
Rose, V. E. 1976. *J. Occup. Med.* 18:81.
Saffiotti, U. and Wagoner, J. K., eds. 1976. *Ann. N.Y. Acad. Sci.* 271.
U.S. Circuit Courts of Appeal. 1974. *Synthetic Organic Chem. Mfr. Assn. v. Brennan* (C.A. 3, Nos. 74-1129, 74-1149, 74-1268 decided Dec. 17, 1974).
U.S. Department of Health, Education and Welfare (DHEW), Division of Occupational Health. 1966. *Protecting the health of eighty million Americans—A national goal for occupational health.* Washington, D.C.
U.S. Department of Health, Education and Welfare (DHEW), National Institute for Occupational Safety and Health (NIOSH). 1974. *NIOSH priority list for criteria document development for toxic substances and physical agents.* Rockville, Md.
U.S. Department of Health, Education and Welfare (DHEW), National Cancer Institute. 1975. *Third national cancer survey—Incidence data.* National Cancer Institute Monograph 41. Bethesda, Md.

Chapter 4

CONCEPTS OF A BIOASSAY PROGRAM IN ENVIRONMENTAL CARCINOGENESIS

Norbert P. Page

National Cancer Institute
National Institutes of Health
Bethesda, Maryland

INTRODUCTION

As pointed out in other chapters, the English surgeon Percivall Pott is generally acknowledged to have been the first person to implicate an environmental agent as a causative factor in cancer. Pott reported in 1775 his observations of scrotal cancers among chimney sweeps, claiming that chronic exposure to soot was the probable cause. A century later, in 1895, the German clinician Ludwig Rehn provided further support for the concept of chemical carcinogensis when he linked cancer of the bladder with occupational exposure to chemicals in the aniline dye industry. As discussed in the excellent review by Shimkin (1975), other chemicals or environmental agents were to be associated with cancer as the clinicians and epidemiologists examined trends of cancer incidence in people.

Not until well into the twentieth century was experimental induction of cancer in animals to be achieved. Yamagiwa and Ichikawa (1915) reached this milestone by inducing cancers by repeatedly painting the ears of rabbits with

Dr. Page was Director of the National Cancer Institute's Carcinogenesis Bioassay Program from April 1973 to June 1976. Before that period Drs. Elizabeth and John Weisburger shared that responsibility. Acknowledgement is extended to those of the National Cancer Institute who contributed to the management of the Carcinogenesis Bioassay Program. Concepts presented were developed largely through the experiences gained in earlier bioassay studies with the assistance of expert scientific panels. These concepts reflect procedures in use at the time of this writing (May 1976). I am particularly grateful to Drs. Umberto Saffiotti, James M. Sontag, Cipriano Cueto, Jr., and Elizabeth Weisburger for their assistance and guidance. The contributions of Ms. P. Steinour were extensive, not only in coordinating program activities but in preparing and editing this chapter.

Dr. Page's present address is National Institute for Occupational Safety and Health, Park Building, Room 3-18, 5600 Fishers Lane, Rockville, Maryland 20852.

coal tar. In 1922, Passey confirmed the carcinogenicity of soot in similar studies. Years later Kennaway and his group, in the early 1930s, performed studies with benzpyrene that provided the impetus for experimental animal carcinogenesis (Kennaway, 1955). From those scant undertakings only 40 years ago, the field of carcinogenesis research has blossomed with exciting studies and results.

Much has been accomplished in these last two decades, not only in detecting carcinogenic chemicals by animal tests but in learning about basic mechanisms of cancer induction and host modifying factors. While the prediction of human health hazards from results obtained from animal tests is admittedly imprecise, the long-term animal bioassay is still acknowledged to be the most reliable prognosticator of a chemical's carcinogenic potential.

With today's test procedures and emphasis on carcinogenicity testing, more human carcinogens will probably be detected first by experimental tests rather than by epidemiologic studies, as in past years. More than ever, experimentalists and epidemiologists can interact to provide direction and leads to the enormous task of exploring the complex problems associated with chemicals and cancer in our society.

While there can be little doubt that properly conducted epidemiologic studies provide the best evidence of a chemical's potential to cause cancer in humans, such studies are of limited use for new chemicals entering the environment. With the long latent period of 15–20 yr for many chemically induced cancers, it is likely that only strong carcinogenic chemicals to which a well-defined population has been exposed for several years will be detected by epidemiologic means alone. On the basis of a thorough review of geographic variations, Higginson and Muir (1973) supported the World Health Organization estimates of 1964 and those of Boyland (1969) that over three-fourths of the world's cancer incidence was environmentally related and thus preventable. Regardless of the actual figure, scientists are in general agreement on the potential carcinogenic hazards of environmental factors, diet, and chemicals to humans. Technological developments of the last few decades have resulted in the introduction of thousands of new chemicals into the environment. Based on present experience, a number of these can be expected to be found carcinogenic. Indeed, the number of chemicals that are shown to have carcinogenic activity has continued to increase.

We are in an era of confusion and uncertainty as to the relative hazard of chemicals that humans have found to be of great benefit. Humans come into contact with thousands of chemicals in their daily life, and the relative role of each in contributing to the cancer problem is far from clear. The enormity of the task of identifying carcinogenic environmental chemicals, however, is clear when we realize that there are nearly 2 million known chemicals, of which more than 20,000 are produced and used in the United States. Another 500 to 700 new substances are introduced annually into commerce. They vary greatly in use, including industrial chemicals, consumer products, drugs, food additives, pesticides, and so forth. In 1972 alone the value of products of the chemical industry exceeded $1,200 billion. While a number of substances are known to cause cancer, the activity of the vast majority has not been adequately determined. From a review of literature data on the carcinogenicity testing of chemicals, about 1,000 of the approximately 6,000 tested have shown some sign of carcinogenicity (U.S. Department of Health, Education, and Welfare, 1941–1973). The number of important chemicals to which humans are exposed that are still untested remains large.

The linking in 1974 of vinyl chloride, a gas from which the second most widely used U.S. plastic is made, with liver cancer in humans (Creech and Makk, 1975) touched off new public concern and a series of regulatory actions unprecedented in history. Four years earlier Viola and co-workers (Viola, 1970; Viola et al., 1971) had reported that rats exposed to high levels of vinyl chloride developed skin, lung, and bone tumors. Viola's findings led other European researchers, Maltoni and Lefemine (1974), to conduct larger experiments that showed cancer induction at levels as low as 50 ppm. In the studies of Maltoni and Lefemine, liver cancers like that seen in humans were found. The U.S. Occupational Safety and Health Administration (OSHA) has now set a standard of 1 ppm for continuous occupational exposure. A new era of chemical awareness has been thrust forcefully on humanity by the vinyl chloride episode. This and other findings of cancer-causing chemicals in the environment (e.g., chlorinated compounds in water and arsenic) have stimulated a public demand for a more rigorous safety assessment of chemicals to which humans are exposed. Federal regulatory agencies are hard-pressed to come up with the best approaches to deal with human exposures to carcinogens. Indeed, the need for a unified and efficient approach to carcinogen testing and hazard assessment has never been more apparent. Decisions that must be made will have serious societal impact and should be arrived at only on the basis of the best data available to predict hazard.

Several federal agencies have legislated responsibilities to conduct research to detect and evaluate carcinogenic chemicals. The National Institute of Occupational Safety and Health (NIOSH) must determine hazards of chemicals to which humans are exposed in the workplace. Exposure levels are usually higher in occupational settings than in the general environment. Much, if not most, of the epidemiologic evidence for cancer (as well as other forms of toxicity) is based on the study of occupationally exposed populations. The Environmental Protection Agency (EPA) is concerned with chemicals present in the general environment—for example, the air and water. Assessing hazards of chemicals in the food supply or in pharmaceuticals is the purview of the Food and Drug Administration. The Consumer Protection and Safety Administration is concerned with consumer or household products, while the Energy Research and Development Administration must evaluate hazards resulting from energy-related activities, as from nuclear and fossil-fuel power plants, coal gasification processes, and so forth.

While other agencies must be concerned with all types of toxicity and the generation of data that can be utilized for hazard assessment, the National Cancer Institute has primarily been interested in detecting a chemical's capability for inducing cancer. The NCI has long had a program to identify environmental carcinogens; however, an increased emphasis resulted from passage of the National Cancer Act of 1971, which called for the further development of approaches to reduce the effectiveness of external agents in the causation of cancer (Rauscher, 1973). Two major goals of the NCI Carcinogenesis Bioassay Program are to identify and evaluate carcinogenic chemicals and to improve and validate methodology for testing.

In conceptual terms, toxicity testing usually takes the form of a multistep process. Initially tests are conducted to determine whether a toxic or carcinogenic effect exists. These may be followed by additional tests to confirm or evaluate the effects. Regulatory actions may result from the initial screening test or await the results of the follow-up studies. Possible tests and resultant actions are illustrated in Fig. 1. As conceived here, a presumptive test is typified by the usual animal bioassay screening test used by the NCI. Strong evidence from a screening test, such as carcinogenicity in both species or the induction of a tumor type rarely seen in the animals, may prompt immediate regulatory actions or in-depth evaluations. In situations where the evidence for carcinogenicity is less convincing, it may be best only to conduct tests to confirm the suspected effect.

In-depth evaluations will depend on the importance of the materials and the data needed for risk assessment. Studies could involve dose-response relations of carcinogenicity, metabolism and pharmacokinetics, or use of additional species more similar to humans, as well as epidemiology of persons exposed to the material. Two major factors must be considered in determining

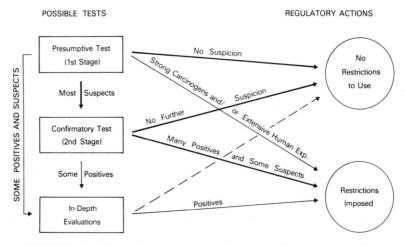

FIGURE 1 Possible carcinogenicity tests and corresponding regulatory actions.

the tests to conduct—time and money. Each chronic animal test is a long-term project 2-3 yr in duration. Whereas the initial presumptive test might cost $150,000, the in-depth test could cost two to five times that amount. To adequately test a single chemical could be a 5-6 yr process at a cost of close to $1 million. Indeed, the cost of research on such chemicals as vinyl chloride, arsenic, and asbestos has probably greatly exceeded that amount. Restricted by the available resources, the NCI program has stressed screening-type tests, anticipating that the industry or appropriate regulatory/research organizations will conduct the follow-up research. A point that cannot be overstressed is that the initial screening test may precipitate additional research or regulatory/societal activites of an enormous magnitude. It is, therefore, mandatory that they be conducted carefully and meaningfully. False results, whether positive or negative, can have a far-reaching impact on society.

In this chapter I will not attempt to compile and document the results of prior tests nor extensively discuss the various scientific issues involved. Neither can I present a discourse on activities related to the bioassay test, such as risk assessment. Rather, I will present the current concepts of a bioassay program as they pertain primarily to long-term *in vivo* animal tests with special emphasis on the screening assay for carcinogenicity. Some of the concepts have been implemented only in the last 1-2 yr by the NCI. It is essential for good science that procedures do not become overly rigid and irreplaceable, but remain capable of being continually modified as felt scientifically justified to improve the reliability and cost-effectiveness of bioassay tests. The procedures now used in conducting carcinogenicity tests will be briefly presented later in this chapter. Details are available in NCI Technical Report DHEW No. (NIH) 76-801 (NCI, 1976a). Extensive literature is available on various scientific and technical aspects of carcinogenicity testing, including excellent reviews by Magee (1970), Weisburger and Weisburger (1967), Clayson (1962), Shubik and Sice (1956), and Arcos et al. (1968). In addition, various governmental and private reports discuss philosophical considerations and methods of testing; among these are the International Union Against Cancer (UICC) Technical Report Series (Berenblum, 1969); Ad Hoc Committee on the Evaluation of Low Levels of Environmental Carcinogens (1971); Food and Drug Administration (1971); Canada, Ministry of Health and Welfare (1973), Golberg (1974), and National Academy of Sciences (1960).

History of the NCI Carcinogenesis Bioassay Program

Much of the early work at NCI was carried out in its intramural laboratories or independently under grant support. As with many other research organizations, progress was impeded by the same lack of coordination and unavailability of adequate resources, both scientific and fiscal. With the blossoming of the chemical industry, human exposure to increased types and concentrations of chemicals, and the dramatic increase in cancer, it became increasingly evident that a more coordinated effort was essential in carcinogenesis research and chemical testing. This need prompted the development of the Carcinogenesis Program.

The Carcinogenesis Program is responsible for planning, implementing, and managing the coordinated research program of the NCI on carcinogenesis by chemical and physical factors and on cancer prevention. This activity developed from the Carcinogenesis Studies Branch, established in March, 1961 as part of the Field Studies Area for intramural and collaborative investigations on carcinogenic factors, particularly as hazards in the human environment. In view of the limited intramural animal facilities and research staff, it was realized that contract support would be needed if major strides in identifying carcinogenic chemicals were to be made. Thus, beginning in 1962, much of the extensive bioassay testing and screening of potential environmental chemical carcinogens has been conducted by contracts with university, private, and commercial laboratories. Emphasis in the early years was placed on the following categories of compounds: (1) pesticides and agricultural chemicals; (2) pharmaceutical agents, including cancer chemotherapeutic agents; (3) industrial chemicals; (4) food contaminants, particularly mycotoxins, peroxides, and lactones; (5) fats and fatty acids; (6) metals and metallo-organic compounds; (7) air pollutants, including synthetic smog, asbestos, and metal oxides and salts; and (8) cigarette smoke. Additional contract support was awarded to study analytical methods for the identification of carcinogens and cocarcinogens, development of short-term bioassays, and mechanisms of carcinogenesis.

The foundation for many of the current program activities was largely developed in an extensive series of planning sessions undertaken in 1968–1969 (Cantarow et al., 1969). Those sessions served as the basis for outlining the research needs in the field of carcinogenesis, using the convergence technique to identify the major objectives and the linear array of subsequent phases leading to their implementation. Figure 2 illustrates the convergence plan. The initial objective was to identify population groups at risk from different types of cancer and to characterize individuals as to environmental factors and biological and functional parameters. To achieve this, three approaches were proposed: (1) the identification of carcinogenic chemicals by animal bioassays, (2) the identification of processes required for the carcinogenic action to develop corrective measures, and (3) the development of biological models for carcinogenesis bioassays and the characterization of carcinogenesis processes.

Initially it was necessary to select chemical agents to be tested or used for attempts at elucidating the mechanisms involved in carcinogenesis. It was realized that bioassay procedures should be standardized so that the chemical agents would be tested by defined and reproducible bioassay systems, each characterized for sensitivity to specific carcinogenic effects.

The plan calls for monitoring the various steps with the development of corrective measures to apply to the environment or to exposed humans. The

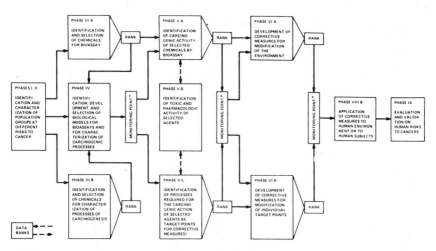

FIGURE 2 Summary of program plans—chemical carcinogenesis and prevention of cancer.

last phase deals with the evaluation and validation of the results of such corrective measures in humans and, it is hoped, decreased cancer risks.

The plan as outlined was aimed at a comprehensive approach to chemical carcinogenesis. It recognized the need for much more extensive bioassays than were then available, but also recognized that the animal results could not be directly extrapolated to predict with precision the hazards to humans. It was also realized that many carcinogens would be difficult to eliminate from the human environment for a long time to come, even after being identified. It was considered essential that efforts be made not only to identify and eliminate carcinogens where possible, but also to identify mechanisms of action, target tissues, and cellular/biochemical interactions, so that inhibitory or protective measures could be proposed. The identification of critical parameters of the carcinogenic processes of certain groups of chemicals, obtained in animal studies, represented the only direct link that could be applied to the study of the susceptibility of humans to comparable exposure conditions.

Animal models, capable of reproducing tumor types like those observed in humans, were necessary for the establishment of selectively sensitive bioassay systems that could be reproduced in several laboratories under standardized conditions. This was essential for an analysis of large amounts of data on carcinogenesis tests. A data retrieval and analysis system for carcinogenesis studies was considered essential to manage the large amounts of data envisioned. The program plan described represented a basis for the development of detailed operational plans that are now in use.

In 1962 the first NCI contract was awarded for carcinogen bioassay. During the following decade the program grew at a moderate rate, with less than 200 chemicals being tested in 1971. The major contract during that period, and the first large carcinogenesis screening contract, was established in 1963 for the bioassay of 130 pesticides and industrial chemicals in over 20,000 mice of two strains. Eleven of 120 compounds tested by feeding at high dose levels in mice were tumorigenic; most of these were pesticides. That study provided much of the knowledge and useful experience of logistics required in large-scale bioassay by a federal agency.

The rapid influx of financial support provided by the National Cancer Act of 1971 resulted in the award of several large testing contracts and a great expansion in chemicals entering bioassay tests in 1972–1973. It became apparent that such an intensified program presented managerial and logistical problems that required an expanded staff capability and the development of special program resources.

Drs. John and Elizabeth Weisburger were instrumental in developing the NCI's carcinogen testing program in the 1960s and 1971–1973. Most chemicals for which bioassays are now being completed were selected by the Weisburgers, as were the procedures used. The program peaked with approximately 550 compounds being tested in early 1974, about 350 by standard long-term tests with two species of rodents. The remainder were tested by various other protocols.

There has been a marked decline in the number of chemicals undergoing testing in the last 2 yr because of the following factors: stable budget, increased cost per bioassay test (due to inflation and more costly test procedures), inadequate pathology resources, and need for additional program staff to plan and monitor the studies. Currently about 325 materials are on standardized tests; however, as reports on many of these are nearing completion this number should fall precipitously in the next year.

Realization of the enormity of the task ahead, coupled with the untimely retirement of Dr. John Weisburger and the obvious need for expanded metabolism and toxicology studies, led to reorganization of the Carcinogenesis Program in March, 1973. Two new branches were created to manage the bioassay and metabolism programs: the Carcinogen Bioassay and Program Resources Branch (CBPR) and the Carcinogen Metabolism and Toxicology Branch. Dr. Elizabeth Weisburger was appointed chief of the latter branch and Dr. Norbert Page chief of the CBPR Branch.

This reorganization allowed for consolidation of management of carcinogenicity testing and resource development and also provided a much-needed impetus for the metabolism studies, which are of great importance in interpreting carcinogen hazards and understanding mechanisms of action. To cope with an inadequate allotment of staff positions to the program, it became necessary to recruit the services of a prime contractor to assist in managing the Bioassay Program. This concept, which had proved successful in Defense and NASA programs, was considered adaptable for the NCI. The NCI now has three prime contractors for the Carcinogenesis Bioassay, Cancer Therapy, and Tobacco and Health Programs.

Concurrent with the expansion of the Bioassay Program in the first half of this decade, two other aspects became apparent: (1) increased public awareness of and concern about environmental pollution and its potential role in the rise of cancer incidence, and (2) the need for improved liaison with other federal agencies. In response to the latter need, the Interagency Collaborative Group on Environmental Carcinogenesis was formed, and has been uniquely successful in coordinating activities among the various government agencies.

During 1974–1975 many of the current concepts for the Bioassay Program have evolved as the result of several activities as listed in Table 1. These activities will be discussed in the context of the various considerations necessary for conducting a large-scale bioassay testing program.

Current NCI Bioassay Program

The current NCI Carcinogenesis Bioassay Program is directed toward improving the technology for carcinogenesis bioassay tests as well as routine carcinogenicity testing of chemicals. At present the NCI program represents the most extensive federal screening program for environmental carcinogens, and is perhaps the largest in the world. Notwithstanding this, it plays only a minor role in the overall NCI program, with approximately 2% of the current NCI budget devoted to this effort. In the overall plan for reducing human exposure to cancer-inducing agents, the bioassay testing program provides leads to the epidemiologists to identify groups at potentially high risk due to exposure to known or suspected cancer-inducing agents.

While the discussion of the current NCI Carcinogenesis Bioassay Program will concentrate primarily on the standardized long-term animal bioassay tests, it should again be emphasized that the program provides for a necessary blend of both applied and basic carcinogenesis research. The mechanisms by which chemicals induce cancer must be understood if extrapolations of animal results

TABLE 1   Major Research and Developmental Activities of 1973–1975 (Carcinogenesis Bioassay Program)

Resource development
  Animal procurement/husbandry
  Chemical procurement/analysis/safety
  Information retrieval/dissemination
  Pathology support
    Standardized diagnosis/reporting
    Repository for tissues and slides
Review of past methods and development of standard procedures (guidelines)
Formalized chemical selection process
Carcinogenesis Bioassay Data System (CBDS)
Establishment of NCI Carcinogenesis (DHEW) Technical Report Series

---

to humans are to be reliably achieved. Thus the current program involves a broad attack on both aspects, with each benefiting from the results of the other. Only through such an integrated approach can the cancer problem be resolved. As in the development of any program one should strive to learn from the past—from both successes and failures.

As of January 1, 1976, about 540 materials were being tested, 325 by standardized protocols. These standard tests usually consist of exposing both sexes of two species of animals to a chemical alone for a major portion of their natural life-span. The route of exposure simulates (where practical) the normal route of human exposure. All animals are strictly monitored and given a detailed necropsy and microscopic examination. The final phase consists of a thorough tabulation, analysis, and presentation of the data, as well as the details of the experiment.

The remaining materials are being studied through less extensive special tests—for example, short-term tests such as the Strain A lung adenoma test in mice; cocarcinogenesis; initiation or promotion experiments; and nonspecific screening tests, such as intramuscular injection of materials. The extensive (and expensive) standardized carcinogenicity bioassays are considered the most indicative of the tests and the ones that might lead to important regulatory decisions or in-depth evaluation tests. The published NCI guidelines pertain to these standardized bioassay tests, as does the discussion that follows. Figure 3

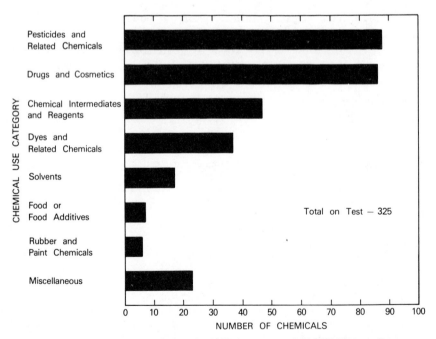

FIGURE 3 Chemicals on test by standard bioassay protocols in NCI Bioassay Program.

shows the various categories of chemicals and the relative number in each category being tested by standardized protocols. Of the 325 on standard tests, about 80% are mainly used as pesticides, drugs, chemical intermediates or dyes, and related chemicals. Many of these tests were initiated 2–3 yr ago and are now coming to completion, and a heavy burden is being realized in completing the pathology, analyzing data, and documenting results.

It should be recognized that each chemical test involves a large commitment in funds and time and constitutes a major research effort in itself. A typical test by current standards and protocols, from selection until results are reportable, requires at least 3 yr and costs in excess of $100,000. Mounting and controlling a coordinated and efficient program with hundreds of chemicals on test required the development of special resources to meet the program needs. Genetically defined specific-pathogen-free (SPF) animal colonies were established and provide a reliable animal supply for the program. Chemical resources were also developed to procure and analyze the chemicals to be tested. Pathology support contracts have been established to assist in completing the pathologic examinations, improving standards for diagnosis and reporting of lesions, and assuring high quality control.

To cope with the volume of data generated in a large-scale bioassay program, a computerized data system, known as the Carcinogenesis Bioassay Data System (CBDS) (Linhart et al., 1974), has been developed and is now in use. Data are routinely submitted through a series of data forms. The system is designed to tabulate, partially analyze, and provide data tables for each compounds.

The great majority of the actual testing and resource support is provided by contracts mainly with commercial organizations and universities, as illustrated in Fig. 4. In view of the logistical complexities of this operation, coupled with personnel/staffing problems, the NCI enlisted the services of a commercial organization as a prime contractor to help coordinate and monitor the program. Following extensive competition, Tracor Jitco, Inc. was selected as the prime contractor on March 1, 1974. Many of the ongoing NCI contracts, especially those with commercial laboratories, were assumed as subcontracts. Others have now been added as the result of competition in requests for proposals (RFPs). The concept of a prime contract, while relatively new for biological research, has been used successfully by the Department of Defense and NASA in electronics and physical research programs. Major scientific decisions are still the responsibility of the NCI. However, the prime contractor has both management and scientific staff to effectively coordinate the logistics of the bioassay operation and make most scientific decisions.

From experience gained in early studies at the NCI and other institutions, the bioassay protocol currently used in the NCI program evolved. Recent experience since the 1971–1972 expansion has provided the impetus for the revision of NCI methods and the publication of detailed guidelines.

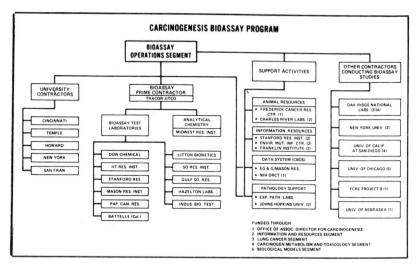

FIGURE 4 Organizations participating in Carcinogenesis Bioassay Program.

This has been a major undertaking in which many federal, university, and industrial scientists actively participated, either in workshops or by reviewing and commenting on the proposed guidelines. As the science progresses, test procedures will continue to be modified as felt necessary to comply with current state-of-the-art methods. Only by assuring high-quality science—animal care, chemistry, toxicology, and pathology—can we hope to promote the generation of the most reliable data possible, from which sound decisions can be made as to human health hazards.

PLANNING FOR CARCINOGENESIS BIOASSAY TESTS— ECONOMIC AND SCIENCE CONSIDERATIONS

In preparing for large-scale toxicity tests it is essential to plan for all required resources and activities well in advance. Perhaps the most important and difficult resource to obtain is experienced and qualified scientists and technicians. A successful bioassay operation requires a truly disciplinary approach with scientists in toxicology, chemistry, animal science, pathology, safety, statistics, data reporting, and administration working together in the design and conduct of the studies.

The phases and average time requirements to conduct a carcinogenesis study according to the current NCI guidelines are presented in Fig. 5. Contingency plans are necessary because events may occur to vary the actual time requirements. Whereas the 24-month treatment phase is usually fixed (except for toxicity or potent carcinogenic response), other phases are subject to variation because of shifting priorities for initiating or completing tests, unforeseen circumstances such as nonavailability of chemicals or animals,

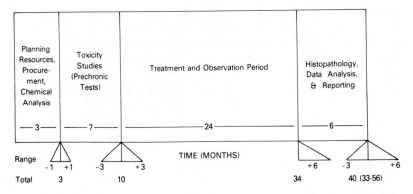

FIGURE 5 Phases and average time scale to conduct a standard carcinogenesis bioassay test.

uneven workloads in chemistry, pathology, and reporting, and so on. The costs by phase and time on study are graphed in Fig. 6. To utilize staff and laboratory space most effectively requires the programming of chemicals into and out of the test program so as to develop a steady-state condition in resource and personnel needs. In initiating carcinogenesis bioassay studies for the first time at a laboratory having the capability of starting and completing one chemical every 2 months, such as in Fig. 7, a steady-state condition in personnel requirements and space needs will not be reached for nearly 3 yr, as illustrated in Fig. 8. The initial workload involves primarily chemistry and toxicology. As animals are placed in chronic tests and as a steady state is reached, the effort in animal care and pathology becomes dominant. A

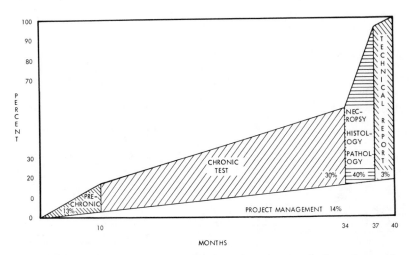

FIGURE 6 Cumulative cost by time and phase of a standard carcinogenesis bioassay using NCI guidelines.

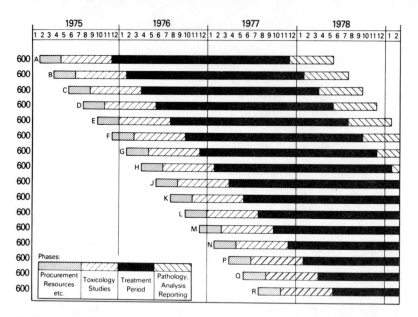

FIGURE 7 Buildup of effort required for various disciplines with continuous introduction of one new chemical into testing program every 2 months using standard protocol (NCI guidelines).

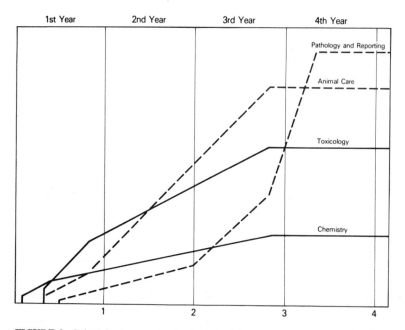

FIGURE 8 Schedule for conducting standard bioassays starting one chemical every 2 months.

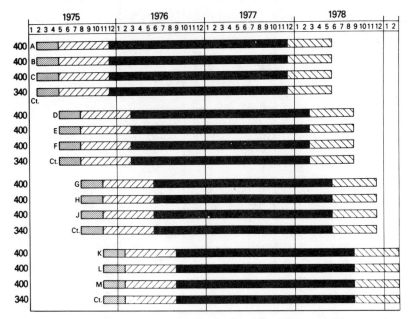

FIGURE 9 Schedule and number of animals utilized in conducting standard bioassays, starting three chemicals at a time at 2 month intervals and using a common control group.

non-steady-state condition can be disruptive to the test laboratory, resulting in periods of slack, periods of excessive requirements, delays in completion of pathology, reporting, etc., and general inefficiency.

A cost-saving alternative to starting one chemical at a time is to start two or more chemicals simultaneously with a common control, as illustrated in Fig. 9. In Fig. 9 three compounds are started simultaneously with the same control group. In multiple starts the square-root rule for control group size has been recommended (Dunnett, 1955). This calls for increasing the size of the control group by the square root of the number of chemicals; for example, for three test compounds with test groups of 50, the control group size should be $50 \times \sqrt{3}$, or 85 of each sex. The total number of controls is 340 for both species ($85 \times 2 \times 2$), as listed in Fig. 9. With separate testing, 600 controls would be required. Thus, a saving of roughly 260 animals $(1800 - 1540)$ or 14.4% is achieved by testing three compounds simultaneously. In doing this, it should be realized that proper randomization is required to assign animals to the treated and control groups and that the workload for necropsy will come in spurts, which may delay completing the pathology diagnoses. Management should decide whether personnel can be shifted to meet the sacrifice schedule and determine whether an actual cost savings will be realized. As demonstrated in Table 2, a great cost savings (10%) is realized by testing two chemicals with a common control. The gain in

TABLE 2 Savings by Using Common Control Groups (Based on Testing 12 Chemicals, Either Alone or in Six Groups of 2, Four Groups of 3, or Three Groups of 4)

No. of chemicals tested at a time	Sharing common control (same size)					Sharing common control (size $\times \sqrt{n}$)				
	No. of test animals[a]	No. of control animals[a]	Total animals[a]	Savings Per add'l. chemical	Total	No. of test animals[a]	No. of control animals[a]	Total animals[a]	Savings Per add'l. chemical	Total
1	1,200	600	1,800	–	–	1,200	600	1,800	–	–
2	1,200	300	1,500	16.7	16.7	1,200	420	1,620	10.0	10.0
3	1,200	200	1,400	5.5	22.2	1,200	340	1,540	4.4	14.4
4	1,200	150	1,350	2.8	25.0	1,200	300	1,500	2.3	16.7

[a]Numbers are for each sex and species, based on 50 animals per group and using two dose levels.

savings in going from two to three is considerably less (4.4%) and is probably not worth the attendant problems created in scheduling, animal supply, pathology completion, etc.

One can not overly stress the need for quality control. The results obtained from an experiment are only as good as the quality controls of the experiment itself. There are numerous aspects in a bioassay, any of which could drastically influence the relative value of the study. Quality control should be monitored closely in all of the following areas: (1) chemical procurement and analysis; (2) preparation—feed mixing, etc.; (3) animal science—disease prevention; (4) toxicology—determination of dose levels, onset of toxicity, clinical observations; (5) elimination of extraneous factors that can influence results, such as cross-contamination with other chemicals or biological agents; (6) conduct of necropsy; (7) histopathology evaluation; (8) data tabulation and verification; (9) statistical analysis; and (10) documentation of the study and results.

Regarding experimental design, program decisions should be made as to when to conduct a routine screening test for carcinogenicity as opposed to a more in-depth evaluation, which might involve dose-response relations, metabolism, species differences, etc. The main limiting factors are usually financial and staff, especially in pathology.

SELECTION OF CHEMICALS FOR TESTING

As mentioned earlier, a major goal of the Carcinogenesis Bioassay Program is to determine chemical and physical carcinogenic agents in the human environment. This is no small task in view of the vast number of chemicals to which humans are potentially exposed.

The number of possible chemical entities approaches infinity, with more than 3 million known chemical substances reported in the scientific literature to date; the rate of reporting new compounds continues to increase. Although most of these are laboratory or industrial curiosities and may never pose a serious threat to humans, the number of different chemicals in today's environment or being developed by industry still can be measured in the tens of thousands. Each year the number of new chemicals entering the environment increases the large array already present. This is obvious when one realizes the enormous growth in the chemical industry in the past few decades. By 1970 the total value of chemicals shipped in the United States was more than double that in 1958, reaching a level of approximately $50 billion per year (President's Science Advisory Committee, 1973). In 1971 a special committee appointed by the Surgeon General estimated that 20,000 chemicals, already in the environment with appreciable human exposure, should be tested for carcinogenicity (Ad Hoc Committee on the Evaluation of Low Levels of Environmental Chemical Carcinogens, 1971). It seems reasonable to conclude that current testing efforts have not kept pace with the rate of introduction of new chemicals and that a current estimate may well exceed 20,000. A recent survey by the Stanford Research Institute (McGee, 1975) estimated that 30,000 chemicals are produced in commercially significant quantities. Assuming that one-fourth have been adequately tested, which is probably high, that leaves well over 20,000 chemicals of unknown carcinogenicity.

Regardless of the actual number, it is apparent that government, private, and industrial resources are insufficient to test all chemicals. Therefore, a judicious selection process is required to utilize the available resources as best possible.

The process of selection must be founded on a systematic base, which takes into consideration a multitude of factors. Obviously, the most important criterion is that the individual chemicals selected should be those that pose significant threats to the people of the nation. As the NCI program is also directed to understanding mechanisms of action and establishing a basis for predicting carcinogenicity, some chemicals of less environmental importance may also be tested for purely scientific considerations; for example, chemical structure-activity relationships. Unfortunately, the current funding for the NCI Carcinogenesis Bioassay Program does not permit a great allocation of resources in this important area.

Following a program reorganization in 1973 a more formalized approach to chemical selection was initiated with the establishment of a Chemical Selection Working Group (CSWG). Those chemicals are selected for long-term animal bioassay that are believed to have immediate or potential human exposure of such magnitude that steps might be taken to restrict human exposure and risk of cancer in humans should the chemicals prove to be carcinogenic in the animal tests. Emphasis was placed on obtaining the most relevant and accurate information on which the decision to test could be scientifically based. A more structured and systematic search was instituted for information on prior chronic test results, other toxicology information, and estimates of current or projected human exposure. All sources of information were tapped, including literature publications, other government agencies, and the industries involved. The chemical selection process and sources of information are illustrated in Fig. 10. The CSWG has been composed of NCI staff or contract personnel with guest advisors on an ad hoc basis. As the CSWG set about its enormous task, certain procedures and the mass of information to be reviewed were found cumbersome. As this is an evolving process, innovations have been and will continue to be implemented wherever possible to streamline procedures and make the process more eficient.

Since the CSWG must make judgments of a scientific nature having extensive economic and political implications, it was found essential that a list of criteria be developed by which to move a chemical from the "nominated" status to "serious consideration." The set of criteria currently used are listed in Table 3. Not all criteria can be assessed due to lack of data for many

GENERAL OUTLINE OF OPERATIONS PROCEDURE FOR SELECTION OF CHEMICALS

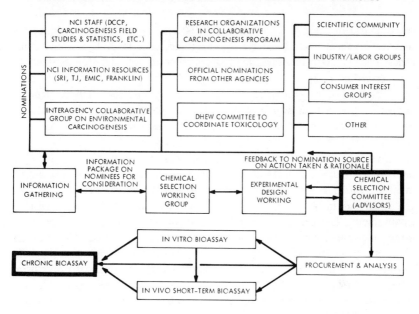

FIGURE 10 Procedures used and nomination sources in chemical selection.

TABLE 3 Criteria Used by the National Cancer Institute in Selecting
Chemicals for Carcinogenicity Tests

1. Production, occurrence, and use data
2. Human exposure data
   a. General population
   b. Occupational groups
   c. Pregnant women
   d. Infants, children, and other age-specific populations
   e. High-risk populations, e.g., genetically susceptible groups
   f. Other special populations
3. Anticipated human exposure based on projected new or increased uses of chemical
4. Existence of epidemiological clues that associate exposure with high cancer incidence rates
5. Evidence (or suspicion) of carcinogenicity from previous tests
6. Suspicion of carcinogenicity because of its structural relationship to known carcinogens
7. Member of a family or group of chemicals with high human exposure, but for which there has been little or no carcinogenicity testing
8. Physical-chemical properties that could alert to carcinogenicity
9. Mutagenicity properties, or biological effects found by other rapid screening tests
10. Suspected interactive effects such as promotional, cocarcinogenicity, etc.
11. Ability to take corrective actions if the substance is demonstrated to exert carcinogenic effects

compounds. In assigning a ranking for testing, some chemicals will be tested that fail to meet several criteria; for example, criteria 3, 4, 5, and 9. Indeed, others may be given low ranking or dropped from consideration as they fail to meet criterion 1, 2, or 3 while meeting another criterion, such as 6, 8, or 9, that might classify them as "suspect." It should be obvious from this discussion that a high degree of scientific thought and judgment goes into this decision-making process. Failure to test could lead to a false sense of security with potential detrimental consequences to humanity.

While numerous information resources are utilized by the CSWG, perhaps the major support activity is that provided by the Stanford Research Institute, under contract with the NCI. The SRI research effort is to acquire and analyze information on chemicals that impact humans and their environment. The procedures used by SRI are to divide human exposure into major and minor use classes and finally into product types. Chemicals have been assigned to four exposure categories: environmental, household, avocational, and occupational. The categories with examples of major uses are listed in Table 4. As of August, 1975, nine exposure modes have been investigated with 3,200 chemicals identified in 900 product types and representing 18,000 chemical-product combinations (McGee, 1975). A list of 27,000 chemicals has been prepared as a first approximation to the universe of chemicals that people come in contact with daily. The nine exposure modes are listed below:

Air pollutants	Over-the-counter drugs
Water pollutants	Cosmetics
Intentional food additives	Soaps and detergents
Pesticide residues in food	Trade sales paints
Prescription drugs	

TABLE 4   Categories and Major Use Classes

Category	Examples of major use classes
Environmental	Airborne pollutants
	Waterborne pollutants
	Food-chain contaminants
Household	Food and kindred products
	Soaps, detergents, and cleaning agents
	Household pesticides
Avocational	Graphic and fine arts
	Gardening and pet care
	Science and collecting
Occupational	Rubber and miscellaneous plastics manufacture
	Industrial inorganic and organic chemical manufacturing
	Medical and other health services

Three additional exposure categories are under development—agricultural chemicals, adhesives and sealants, and occupational exposure. SRI has used expert consultants from industry and academia, including carcinogenesis researchers, to improve its data base and quantify suspicion of carcinogenic activity. As the data are computerized and in a readily retrievable form, outputs can be in several forms, including lists of chemicals ranked by human exposure, activity value, group, and so forth; dossiers for individual chemicals; or product reports. Other types of output can be generated as the need arises. The data system developed primarily to assist the Carcinogenesis Bioassay Program has found several other applications: (1) in the NCI Cancer Control Program by identifying known carcinogens and assisting in the production of monographs that will recommend cancer control and prevention programs; (2) assisting the International Agency for Research on Cancer (IARC) in the selection of chemicals for study and providing production, use, occurrence, and exposure information on selected chemicals; and (3) providing information to the National Library of Medicine's Toxicology Information Program and the EPA Office of Pesticides Program.

Nominations for testing have come from various sources: NCI staff, other agencies, academic scientists, the SRI data base, concerned citizens, industry, congressional offices, and many others. One of the most reassuring and rewarding sources has been other government agencies, primarily through the Interagency Collaborative Group on Environmental Carcinogenesis (ICGEC). The ICGEC has also served to obtain additional data and information not readily available through other sources.

The names of chemicals that progress through the selection process and are tentatively selected for future testing are provided to other agencies and trade organizations. If no additional information is forthcoming, CSWG then submits the nomination to the Program Director for inclusion in the testing program. Actual testing will depend on the availability of financial and scientific and physical resources. As of January 1, 1976, over 1,500 specific chemicals were in the review process, with approximately 100 (6%) submitted to the segment for testing. Many others were in various stages of the selection cycle. In addition to consideration of individual nominations, the CSWG has selected chemicals based on an evaluation of classes or groups in terms of structural relationships or end uses. Outside working groups have assisted in these reviews. Classes of chemicals considered are:

Polycyclic hydrocarbons	Beryllium compounds
Plasticizers	Inorganic phosphates
Flame retardants	Soaps
Monomers	Esters
Azo dyes	Detergents and surfactants
Benzidine-based dyes	GRAS substances reviewed by
Hair dyes	FASEB Select Committee

Small halogenated hydrocarbons	Printing inks
Pesticides	Food additives
Vegetable gums	Alkyl chlorides
Polybrominated biphenyls	Alkyl nitrates
Polymers	Acylating agents
Liquid crystals	Alkylating agents

For pragmatic reasons, chemicals are assigned relatively lower priority if they are known to be constituents of the normal physiology or the normal human environment. Excluded from consideration would be such environmental chemicals as nitrogen, oxygen, rare gases, and carbon dioxide, to which human exposure could not be reduced in any event.

Form of Chemical to Test

Following selection, a decision as to the form of the chemical must be made. While opinions differ somewhat, it is generally agreed that the agents should be tested in the form and purity to which humans are exposed rather than a highly purified form. The obvious concern is that a product might be found to be carcinogenic as the result of the activity of a minor component or contaminant. It should also be recognized that a minor ingredient or contaminant may not itself be carcinogenic but may have serious toxicity that could influence the survival of the animals or the dose of the main compound that can be administered. On the other hand, it is conceivable that some commercial products that are mixtures may be carcinogenic due to synergism or cocarcinogenicity, whereas the highly purified product might be inactive.

Realizing all these possibilities, the prevailing opinion is that a chemical should be tested in a form as representative as possible of the "product of commerce," with analysis of the product to characterize its purity and ingredients. In some cases, the product of commerce is a relatively pure material; for example, in many pharmaceuticals or industrial chemicals. Often, however, the chemical is used in a wide array of mixtures or forms with purity varying from essentially 100% down to a few percent. This is especially true of many food chemicals and pesticide products. Sometimes a specific commercial product is predominant and might be tested as such; otherwise a "typical" mixture or perhaps purified material might be required. Such decisions obviously must be made only after review of the chemical's use and availability to the public. In the event that the test of a product of commerce shows it to be carcinogenic, it may be necessary to further test a highly purified form of the chemical and perhaps other product components in order to determine the actual chemical ingredient of concern.

Regardless of the form tested, it is essential that the material be well characterized and that a sample be retained for additional chemical analysis. A sufficient supply of the chemical should be obtained at the outset for the entire test wherever possible. In the event that the chemical is not sufficiently stable, it will be necessary to periodically replenish the supply, using the same composition as nearly as possible. Each batch should be well characterized. Storage methods should be such as to prevent deterioration or possible alteration.

METHODOLOGY OF LONG–TERM
CARCINOGENESIS BIOASSAY TESTS

Testing of environmental agents for carcinogenicity has reached a relatively sophisticated stage, based largely on the trials and errors of cancer researchers in the past decade. Even though much more is known now than a few years ago, many of the uncertainties of the past still exist. We are in full agreement with critics of past procedures. Carcinogenicity testing should keep pace with more sophisticated techniques, consistent with being as critical and comprehensive as possible. We should realize that the general acceptance of new procedures will be predicated on their applicability and predictive value. Assay procedures of the past have been used mainly to detect the carcinogenicity of a compound rather than for a study of dose-response relations and physiologic/metabolic alterations. This was based on the premise that a substance, when carcinogenic in animals by any test system, is likely to be carcinogenic in humans.

Artifacts in testing procedures can drastically alter the outcome of an experiment. Inasmuch as the results of a bioassay test can greatly influence public decisions on use or restriction of a compound, the test results should be unassailable. Anything less than a solid scientific experiment can not be accepted in today's climate.

The interpretation of results and their extrapolations may vary; however, tests for carcinogenicity are basically similar whether the compound is a food additive, drug, pesticide, or industrial chemical.

All carcinogenesis bioassay tests should strive for the following features: (1) sensitive and reliable animal test system; (2) optimal exposure conditions to reveal a carcinogenic response; (3) elimination of all extraneous factors that might influence the conduct of the test and the interpretation of the results; (4) in-depth pathology examination to detect the minute as well as the more obvious carcinogenic changes; and (5) complete documentation of all data to allow those responsible for interpretation of human relevance to make the best judgments possible.

There are many publications describing procedures for long-term animal tests for carcinogenicity. However, knowledge gained over the past few years, especially in the NCI Bioassay Program, has precipitated a very careful reevaluation of methods and their rationale. Based on such a review and following workshops and extensive critique by experts in carcinogenicity testing procedures, the NCI guidelines for carcinogen bioassay in small rodents (NCI, 1976a) were developed. A similar publication addressed more toward the carcinogenicity testing of drugs has also recently been published (Golberg, 1974). The NCI guidelines are intended to provide the investigator with specific operating procedures considered necessary for a good experiment rather than to review the scientific literature and methodology that prompted the recommended procedures. It should also be borne in mind that the NCI guidelines represent minimal requirements. Investigators obviously should vary or add procedures to meet the specific research needs.

The sections that follow describe some of the numerous considerations of a carcinogenesis bioassay study.

OBJECTIVES OF TEST

The methodology of long-term tests will depend on the objectives of the test and the use of the results. In some cases a simple indication of carcinogenic activity may suffice. In other cases the chemical may be of great benefit to society or impossible to eliminate from the environment, so that extensive studies elucidating the relative potency, cocarcinogen factors, pharmacokinetic relationships, species variations in response, and so on may be desirable. Such decisions on in-depth evaluation studies may be made at the first indication of carcinogenic activity from a more abbreviated or routine carcinogenesis bioassay test. In many cases the study might be conducted more in line with a complete toxicological assay of long-term or chronic effects. In no case, however, should other routine toxicological studies be included in an experiment which would detract from the usefulness of the study as a test for carcinogenicity.

It is often asserted that a substance will be carcinogenic if the animals are exposed long enough to it and at sufficiently high levels. Evidence does not substantiate this concept. The great majority of substances tested by the NCI have not been positive even when given for the majority of the animals' lifetime and in large doses. A good example supporting this fact is the large study conducted by Innes et al. (1969), in which only 11 of 120 chemicals—which had been selected for their possible carcinogenicity—were found definitely carcinogenic in the mouse.

NCI GUIDELINES

Since many chemicals in today's environment have great social and economic value, it is essential that the procedures used to determine their carcinogenicity be established on the best scientific bases that are practical. It is the purpose of the NCI guidelines to provide recommended procedures for carcinogenicity testing of environmental chemicals in small rodents. The guidelines were formulated on the basis of the experience of the NCI Carcinogenesis Bioassay Program, consultation with experts in the scientific disciplines applicable to long-term animal studies, and reviews of draft versions

TABLE 5   Major Recommendations in Current NCI Guidelines for
Carcinogen Bioassay in Small Rodents

Animals	At least two species, usually rat, mouse, or hamster; both sexes; weanlings started on treatment
Animal care	Improved facilities and care; filtered enclosed cages; sterilized bedding and feed
Chemistry	Analysis for purity, stability, and proper preparation; strict safety requirements
Route of administration	Same as usual human exposure, where possible
Doses and dose levels	At least two doses; highest = that tolerated
Treatment period	Major portion of natural life-span—24 months on study
Sample size	Fifty per dose/sex, including control groups
Pathology examination	Careful and complete gross and microscopic examination of all animals in study
Data reporting	All aspects including individual animal clinical effects, tumor and nontumor pathology results

by members of the scientific community at large. Included among the latter were investigators associated with universities, other federal agencies, and commercial and trade organizations. An attempt was made to incorporate as many of the reviewers' comments as were compatible with the intent of the review. As a result of this extensive review by scientists representing diverse interests in our society, it is felt that the guidelines will serve to standardize those aspects of a large-scale carcinogen bioassay which are essential to its scientific acceptability.

It should be recognized that differences in scientific approaches and end points, as well as economic considerations, exclude the use of any single set of procedures to meet the objectives of all carcinogen bioassay studies. Notwithstanding these differences, certain features are common to all well-designed and properly conducted long-term animal studies.

The NCI guidelines are used by the NCI Carcinogenesis Bioassay Program to screen environmental chemicals for carcinogenicity through their oral administration to small rodents. However, they may also be applicable, in part or in toto, to other long-term studies using different procedures or with other objectives or end points. The NCI guidelines do not address these variations, but recognize that deviations from the guidelines may sometimes be necessary for laboratories not specially equipped to conduct large-scale bioassay studies. Table 5 summarizes many of the key recommendations of the guidelines.

Briefly, the main aspects of the guidelines for screening are as follows:

1. Both sexes of two species, usually the rat and the mouse, are used. Animals should be started on test at an early age, usually as weanlings.
2. At least two dose levels should be used, the highest being the

maximum tolerated dose that does not cause life shortening or toxicity unrelated to tumor induction. The revised guidelines lengthened the preliminary toxicity test from 6 wk to 90 days in an attempt to better predict long-term tolerances.

3. Generally, each group consists of a minimum of 50 of each sex and at each dose level.
4. The period of exposure is 24 months with an additional observation period without treatment as optional. In the past, an 18 month exposure with an observation period of 3 months for mice and 6 months for rats was used.
5. The exposure route should, wherever possible, mimic that of human exposure. Most current studies, especially on environmental chemicals, are by the oral route, although a number of compounds recently selected are being administered by inhalation.
6. A detailed necropsy and histopathology examination of all animals is required with approximately 26 tissues routinely examined. This represents a great increase in the extent of pathology over that required in the earlier days in the program.

CHEMISTRY PROCEDURES

Prior to and during a carcinogenesis bioassay several chemical procedures should be used to assure that the results can be attributed to the chemical under assay and not to an impurity or degradation product.

Characterization of Test Material and Preparation

The purity, composition, and formulation of the test material and any solvent or vehicle should be determined prior to initiation of the test. While major impurities should always be known, identification of each minor impurity may not be practical unless the compound is found to be carcinogenic. To allow for that, a sample of the test material should be retained at least until the end of the experiment. For compounds exhibiting carcinogenicity the impurities should be well described in a report of the experiment.

Stability and Storage

The stability and storage requirements of each bulk test material should be determined prior to initiation of the long-term test. In addition, the bulk test material should be analyzed periodically during the course of the study to ensure that it has retained its original characteristics. Similar analysis of the test preparation should also be conducted under the same conditions in which it will be administered to the test animals—for example, in the feed or vehicle—and at a similar temperature and pH. Analysis of diet mixes should be conducted on stored as well as newly prepared treatment mixtures. In addition to initial concentration, such analysis will monitor the adequacy of methods used in preparation of the test material and instability or loss of test agent in the treatment preparation. The stability of the test preparation under defined conditions of storage and/or administration will determine the frequency at which fresh treatment mixtures must be prepared.

Determination of Proper Mixing

For diet preparations, complete homogeneity may sometimes be difficult to achieve, especially with low dietary concentrations. The concentration of the chemical in the diet should be determined from several locations. Periodic random sampling during the course of the study, as indicated earlier, should ensure that the proper mixing and formulation procedures are being used. While several types of diet mixers have been used successfully, the V-type shell blender has proved particularly effective in mixing while providing for optimal safety.

Treatment mixtures should be stored in inert, shatter-proof containers with air-tight covers. Each container should be clearly marked so that its contents can be easily and accurately identified, and storage containers should be located in a secure area free of congestion and with restricted access. An inventory of each treatment mixture should be maintained and records kept of its preparation and usage.

TEST ANIMALS AND ANIMAL SCIENCE

Selection of Animal Models

The ideal animal model for testing a chemical for carcinogenicity is one whose pharmacokinetics, metabolism, and biological (pathology) response are similar to those of humans. In addition, they must be available in large numbers, economical to maintain, hardy, and genetically stable. Since man is a heterogeneous species, having widely different metabolic profiles for various chemicals, animal differences are often discounted for more practical considerations. Economics thus usually becomes the deciding factor in selecting test animals. To guard against an atypical response, essentially all test guidelines and protocols require that at least two species be used in routine testing for carcinogenicity. Failure to detect carcinogenicity in either provides greater assurance that the compound is not carcinogenic to humans. Even this is far from failproof as several chemicals are considered carcinogenic to humans for which an animal model has yet to be demonstrated, a notable example being arsenic.

It is well established that many substances are themselves not carcinogenic but require metabolic conversion to a "proximate" carcinogenic chemical. From this viewpoint an animal that does not metabolize a chemical in the same way as humans could give "false negative" results. The extensive studies with the aromatic amine *N*-2-fluorenylacetamide (FAA) dramatically demonstrate this point. FAA in its parent form or when metabolized to the 7-hydroxy derivative (7-OH-FAA) is apparently not carcinogenic. It is another possible metabolite, *N*-hydroxy-2-acetylaminofluorene (*N*-OH-FAA), that is a proximate carcinogen. Of the species studied, the guinea pig and steppe-lemming do not show carcinogenicity when given 2-AAF and neither metabolize it to the *N*-OH-FAA metabolite. A strong correlation exists between *N*-hydroxylation and carcinogenicity with the rat, mouse, hamster, dog, and cat. Approximately 4–14% of 2-FAA administered to humans is biotransformed to the *N*-OH-FAA form, the remainder to 7-OH-FAA and glucuronides (Weisburger et al., 1964).

In the situation illustrated, the choice of the guinea pig as the sole test animal species could conceivably have produced a false negative response. Unfortunately, the relationship to metabolism and carcinogenicity is even more complex than previously realized. In a recent study Grantham et al. (1976) reported that a mouse strain (X/GF) that has an extremely low incidence of spontaneous tumors and is also resistant to many carcinogens is also resistant to 2-FAA although it *N*-hydroxylates FAA.

It is becoming apparent that the biochemical interactions involved in chemical carcinogenesis are complex and not well understood. Still, in selecting animal test species for a specific chemical a basic similarity in metabolism and pharmacokinetics would be of obvious importance.

The selection of species used in carcinogenesis studies has been largely determined by the necessity to continue the test for all or most of the life-span of the animal. While exceptionally powerful carcinogens may induce tumors in a short period, the usual carcinogenic response becomes evident only late in an animal's life. Indeed, most human cancers are not manifest for 10–20 yr after an exposure.

In practice, since test animals must be maintained for their life-span, only short-lived laboratory animals that can be economically housed in large numbers are routinely employed in carcinogenicity tests. The species most often used are rats, mice, and hamsters. Guinea pigs have not gained popularity because of their apparent resistance to carcinogenicity. While inclusion of a nonrodent such as the dog or monkey is ideal for species-to-species extrapolation, the requirement for large numbers maintained for 10–15 yr makes them impractical except for highly select situations.

In addition to the selection of species, the decision about strain is also highly controversial. Inbred strains offer greater uniformity of response, highly predictable spontaneous tumor incidence, and better repeatability in experiments. However, their homogeneity may also be a disadvantage in that they are more likely to be resistant to certain chemicals than are random-bred animals. The FDA Advisory Committee (1971) and the Canadian Ministry of Health and Welfare (1973) recommend random-bred strains, while Shimkin (1974) recommends the use of inbred strains.

The NCI guidelines do not specify either inbred or random-bred strains. Currently the major strain of mice used in the NCI Bioassay Program is an F1 hybrid cross between two inbred strains, the C57B1/6 female and the C3H male. This cross, commonly designated as the B6C3F1, was found highly successful in a large-scale pesticide testing program in the mid-1960s (Innes et al., 1969). It is a hardy animal with good survival, easy to breed, disease resistant, and has a relatively low spontaneous tumor incidence. Normally, at the 24 month sacrifice, at least 75% of the control mice are still alive. Table 6 lists the spontaneous tumor incidence found in over 2,300 animals necropsied as of this time. The spontaneous tumors of greatest incidence are of the lung and liver. The lung tumors were mainly adenomas, while 8.7% of the liver

TABLE 6 Percentage of Spontaneous Primary Tumors in B6C3F1 Mice[a,b]

Organ tissue	Males (1,132)[c]	Females (1,176)
Brain	< 1	–
Skin/subcutaneous	1.0	< 1
Mammary gland	–	< 1
Spleen	< 1	< 1
Lung/trachea	9.2	3.5
Heart	–	–
Liver	15.7[d]	2.5[e]
Pancreas	< 1	< 1
Stomach/intestines	1.3	< 1
Kidney	< 1	< 1
Urinary bladder	–	< 1
Testis[f]	< 1	NA
Ovary	NA	< 1
Uterus[f]	NA	1.9
Pituitary	< 1	3.5
Adrenal	< 1	< 1
Thyroid	1.1	< 1
Parathyroid	–	–
Pancreatic islets	< 1	< 1
Thymus	< 1	–
Body cavities	< 1	< 1
Leukemia/lymphomas	1.6	6.8

[a]Animals supplied by NCI with studies conducted at several laboratories.

[b]Studies terminated at 21–24 months. Data not adjusted for date of death.

[c]Number of animals necropsied.

[d]8.7% hepatocellular carcinoma.

[e]1.7% hepatocellular carcinoma.

[f]Includes accessory organs, such as seminal vesicles or fallopian tubes.

tumors were hepatocellular carcinomas, many of which were found metastasized to the lung. Most of the remaining hepatic tumors were adenomas, neoplastic nodules, or hemangiosarcomas.

The rats used at this time are primarily the Fisher 344 and Osborne-Mendel strains. Sprague-Dawley and Charles River CD rats have been used to a lesser extent. Tables 7 and 8 list the incidence of spontaneous tumors diagnosed as of this time in the current bioassay series. The most notable feature of the F/344 rat is the high incidence of testicular tumors in the male and pituitary tumors in the female. In both cases the tumors are benign and do not appear to detract from its usefulness as a general test animal. Advantages of the F/344 over the other strains are its smaller size, hardy vigor and good survival, disease resistance, and relatively low spontaneous tumor incidence in organs other than testis and pituitary.

TABLE 7   Percentage of Spontaneous Primary Tumors in
Fisher 344 and Osborne-Mendel Rats[a,b]

	Fisher 344		Osborne-Mendel	
Organ/tissue	Males (846)[c]	Females (840)	Males (112)	Females (149)
Brain	1.3	< 1	< 1	–
Skin/subcutaneous	5.7	2.5	4.5	3.4
Mammary gland	1.0	18.8	3.6	32.2
Spleen	< 1	< 1	3.6	–
Lung/trachea	2.4	< 1	–	–
Heart	< 1	< 1	–	1.3
Liver	1.2	1.3	–	1.3
Pancreas	< 1	< 1	–	1
Stomach/intestines	< 1	1.0	< 1	–
Kidney	< 1	< 1	6.3	3.4
Urinary bladder	< 1	< 1	–	–
Testis[d]	76.2	NA	–	NA
Ovary	NA	< 1	NA	2.0
Uterus[d]	NA	16.8	NA	4.0
Pituitary	10.2	29.5	8.0	15.4
Adrenal	8.7	4.0	11.6	2.0
Thyroid	5.1	5.6	3.6	12.7
Parathyroid	–	–	–	–
Pancreatic islets	3.2	1.3	2.7	1.3
Thymus	–	–	–	–
Body cavities	< 1	< 1	< 1	–
Leukemia/lymphomas	6.5	5.4	2.7	< 1

[a] Animals supplied by NCI with studies conducted at several laboratories.
[b] Studies terminated at 24 months. Data not adjusted for date of death.
[c] Number of animals necropsied.
[d] Includes accessory organs, such as seminal vesicles or fallopian tubes.

TABLE 8 Percentage of Spontaneous Primary Tumors in
Sprague-Dawley and Charles River CD Rats[a,b]

Organ/tissue	Sprague-Dawley		Charles River CD	
	Males (144)[c]	Females (145)	Males (183)	Females (184)
Brain	1.4	–	2.7	1.6
Skin/subcutaneous	2.8	1.4	6.6	3.8
Mammary gland	2.8	35.9	< 1	45.1
Spleen	–	–	< 1	–
Lung/trachea	–	–	1.6	3.8
Heart	–	–	–	–
Liver	–	–	1.1	2.2
Pancreas	< 1	–	–	–
Stomach/intestines	–	–	< 1	< 1
Kidney	–	< 1	1.6	–
Urinary bladder	< 1	< 1	< 1	–
Testis[d]	2.8	NA	4.4	NA
Ovary	NA	–	NA	1.1
Uterus[d]	NA	< 1	NA	3.3
Pituitary	11.1	32.4	33.3	57.6
Adrenal	1.4	2.8	7.7	4.3
Thyroid	–	2.8	3.8	–
Parathyroid	–	–	< 1	–
Pancreatic islets	< 1	–	2.7	–
Thymus	< 1	–	–	–
Body cavities	2.1	2.1	1.1	1.1
Leukemia/lymphomas	< 1	–	1.6	< 1

[a] Animals procured from commercial laboratories by NCI contractors.
[b] Studies terminated at 24 months. Data not adjusted for date of death.
[c] Number of animals necropsied.
[d] Includes accessory organs, such as seminal vesicles or fallopian tubes.

Within recent years the Syrian golden hamster has become adapted for long-term chronic studies. Its successful use as a carcinogenicity bioassay test animal has been demonstrated by Homburger (1972), Nettesheim (1972), and Shubik (1972).

In selecting animals for carcinogenicity testing one must be aware of the great differences in species and strains, not only in spontaneous tumors but in their response to carcinogenic chemicals. Weisburger and Weisburger (1967) presented data dramatically illustrating this problem. More recently Vesselinovitch et al. (1974), Matsuyama et al. (1972), and Martin et al. (1974) provided additional data on species differences in sensitivity.

Animal Science–Elimination of Extraneous Factors

Even the best designed chronic toxicity test can be lost or the reliability of the generated data severely compromised by the failure or breakdown of any single component. In addition to experimental design and reporting aspects, animal science factors that must be planned for are: animal quality, animal facilities and husbandry practices, clinical and pathology examinations, and data recording.

Animal quality. It serves no useful purpose either to purchase a low-quality microbially nondefined animal for a high-security barrier operation or to place germ-free animals into conventional (nonbarrier) facilities. The nature of the experiment and the risk that will be taken will dictate the quality of animal and environmental controls to be accepted. Purchased animals must be properly transported and quarantined on arrival to assure continued high quality.

Historically, poor animal care has been responsible for many toxicity studies being lost or severely compromised. For carcinogenicity testing competent animal husbandry is of the utmost importance.

Operational and extraneous factors can have dramatic effects on the successful completion of a carcinogenesis test as well as the interpretation and usefulness of the results. Among the most important are those listed in Table 9. While these factors have not been studied in sufficient detail, there is ample evidence that the diet itself as well as contaminants in the diet, bedding, water, or air can introduce variables or modifiers to the carcinogenic response. Other factors such as intercurrent infections, autolysis, and cannibalism can reduce the effective number of animals in the study and are largely preventable by the routine practice of strict hygiene and disease prevention measures and close clinical observation.

Several publications are available that provide detailed information and recommendations on animal facilities and their operations. Among these, the most current and comprehensive are (1) publications of the Institute of Laboratory Animal Resources of the National Academy of Sciences (1969,

TABLE 9 Husbandry Factors That Can
Influence Carcinogenesis Tests

1. Infectious diseases
   Microbiological
   Parasitic
2. Chemical pollutants in
   Feed
   Water
   Bedding
   Air
3. Operations management
   Cannibalism
   Autolysis
   Vermin infestation
   Diet
   Prevention of cross-contamination

1974, 1976); (2) the I. A. T. manual of laboratory animal practice and techniques (Short and Woodnott, 1971); (3) Canadian Council on Animal Care (1973); and (4) NCI guidelines for carcinogen bioassay in small rodents (NCI, 1976a). Recognizing that special conditions or situations pertain to chronic toxicity and carcinogenicity testing, the NCI supported the National Academy of Sciences in convening workshops and the development of the standards for long-term holding of laboratory animals (Institute of Laboratory Animal Resources, 1976).

Facilities. The physical design and maintenance of the animal facilities are of great importance in achieving the high standards of animal care and chemical and biological hazard control required for carcinogenesis bioassay studies. Even the best animals placed in poorly designed and maintained facilities will soon succumb to the level of their surroundings.

In constructing or modifying animal facilities to be used for long-term rodent studies, it is strongly urged that they be designed to allow for the most practical but effective barrier to the inadvertent introduction of infectious diseases or contaminants into the facility or between animal rooms. The minimum design recommmended at this time would be that allowing for a unidirectional flow of equipment, supplies, air, and personnel. Such a design is usually referred to as the "clean-dirty (return) corridor" concept. This concept has gained widespread acceptance. In such a design animal rooms have doors at opposite ends of each room. All materials are sterilized; personnel are fully enclosed in sterilized garments and enter only from the clean corridor and leave only by the dirty corridor. Once a person enters an animal room he is prevented from returning to the clean side or going to another animal room. He must leave the facility, take a shower, and dress in completely new clothing to reenter the clean area. Such a strict flow of materials and personnel through a corridor from which no access to other rooms is possible greatly reduces the potential for introduction of disease to the facility or rapid spread of a disease from one room to the other rooms or the entire facility.

Where such a corridor arrangement is not possible, the movement of clean and dirty equipment and materials should be scheduled to avoid backflow to cleaner areas. Animal rooms must be protected to reduce possible contamination between them. An example of an animal facility utilizing a clean-return system is that developed at the Frederick Cancer Research Center (Fig. 11). Other more elaborate designs, including germ-free (GF) isolator or specific-pathogen-free (SPF) barrier facilities, are also in use. However, the increased cost to operate and maintain such facilities is not considered practical for routine carcinogenesis tests. A committee of the National Academy of Sciences (1976) recently established a new classification for barrier systems based on methods and extent of contamination control. The classification consists of maximum, high, moderate, or minimal security and conventional systems. Minimal security or conventional systems are not considered acceptable for maintaining rodents for long periods.

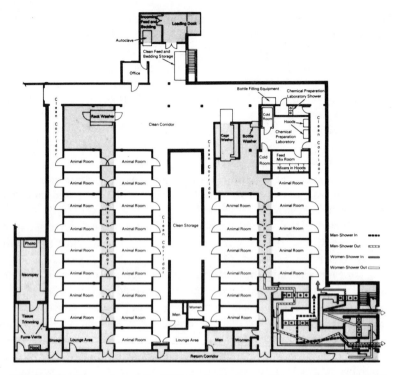

FIGURE 11 Floor plan of the NCI Frederick Cancer Research Center (FCRC)
Bioassay Test Facility (operated by Litton Bionetics, Inc.).

The animal facilities should be separated from the remainder of the
laboratories with access only to essential personnel. A special quarantine area,
effectively separated from the testing area, should be provided for holding
animals procured from outside the animal facility.

Ideally, for carcinogenicity testing, small rooms are recommended so
that a separate room can be used for each species and test agent. This allows
for better prevention and easier containment of a disease outbreak and
prevents inadvertent exposure of animals to low levels of other chemicals,
which could result if several chemicals were on test in the same room. This
also reduces the possibility of accidental mix-up in the test groups or
treatment administrations and the introduction of diseased animals into a
room in which studies are already under way. The increased cost incurred
from the use of small rooms is considered a warranted expense. In facilities
where large rooms must be used, a reasonable compromise is to use cages with
solid sides and bottoms and covered by filter tops.

All air entering and leaving the animal facilities should be adequately
filtered with 10–15 fresh-air changes per hour. The air pressure in the animal
rooms should be slightly positive to the dirty corridor and negative to the

clean one. Automatic control and recording of temperature and humidity in each room should be provided for, along with a monitoring system to alert the attendants to any deviations from the acceptable range.

Equipment/supplies. To complement an adequately designed facility it is essential that equipment and supplies be of suitable construction or composition and capable of effective sanitizing.

There have been numerous reports where ongoing studies have been lost because of unforeseen failures in the mechanical equipment (especially the air-conditioning system) or food supply problems (due to labor disputes, mill shortages, etc.). Rotated, reserve back-up supplies should be maintained to handle the latter situation. Air-conditioning failures can be due to such malfunctions as compressor failure or interruption of electricity. Access to an emergency power source with a generating capacity sufficient to power the animal facilities' air-conditioning and light systems should be available. Contingency plans for alternate air-conditioning ducts or compressors should be developed depending on the facility design.

Several rack/caging systems are commercially available that are capable of proper sanitization. Racks may be of either the shelf or the suspended-drawer type and sanitized either in place or moved to a wash area for cleaning. If a rack washer is not available, they can be scrubbed with a suitable detergent and hosed down under high pressure. Racks should be sanitized periodically, at least once every other week. Plastic or stainless steel cages with solid sides and bottoms covered with nonwoven polyester fiber filters constitute effective enclosures and provide for relatively efficient disease control and chemical containment measures. However, the gains from the additional environmental control may be partially offset by elevated cage humidity and ammonia levels, which might have detrimental effects in terms of respiratory disorders and hepatic enzyme induction. Bonnets or filter sheets should be replaced by sanitized ones at least once every 2 wk. Animals housed in cages with solid sides and bottoms should be changed to sanitized cages with fresh bedding as frequently as necessary, but not less than once weekly. Figures 12 and 13 illustrate the caging system in use by the Frederick Cancer Research Center. In this system filter sheets are used with the water spout protruding through the sheet into the cage. Wire mesh cages, which may be required for certain types of studies (e.g., inhalation), should be sanitized no less than once every 2 wk.

During the quarantine period and acute toxicity and repeated dose studies, animals may be caged together according to the weight-space specifications recommended by the National Academy of Sciences (Institute of Laboratory Animal Resources, 1974). However, for subchronic and chronic studies animals should be distributed from the outset as if they were in the upper weight range. This will obviate the need to later redistribute them to remain within the weight-space specifications. Even though the space-to-weight specification may be exceeded during the subchronic and chronic studies, no

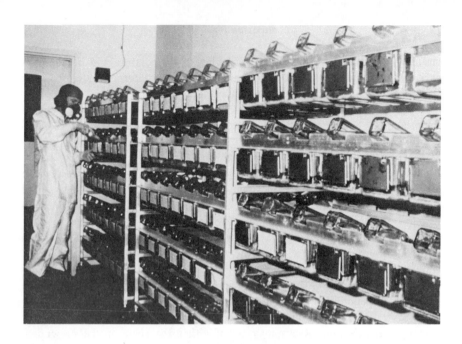

FIGURE 12 Mouse caging system and personnel safety measures used at the FCRC. Filter sheets are used to provide fully enclosed cages.

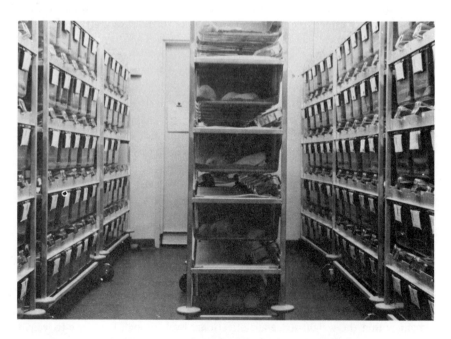

FIGURE 13 Rat caging system used at the FCRC.

cage should contain more than five animals. As animals die or are sacrificed, surviving animals should not be combined or redistributed among the cages.

Although mycotoxin-free ground corncob may be used for bedding, heat-treated hardwood chips are considered more desirable. Softwood chips or creosoted wood should not be used. The bedding should be sterilized. In studies in which open wire mesh cages are used, an absorbent material should be placed under them that effectively collects and holds waste matter.

Feeders that are adequately designed to prevent soiling, bridging, and scattering of the feed are acceptable when pellet-type rations are used. Although no feeder is completely satisfactory for meal feed, a hopper-type feeder that is firmly attached to the cage appears to cause the least problems. However, this type of feeder may still require daily "bumping" to dislodge bridged meal. The feeder developed by the National Center for Toxicological Research (Hunziker, 1975) would appear to be effective with minimal spillage. An open, unfixed feed cup should not be used, nor should the feed be placed directly on the cage floor. A sanitized feeder should be supplied at least once weekly.

A nutritionally balanced standard laboratory diet that supports normal growth and maintenance is essential (National Academy of Sciences, 1972). Other factors to consider in choosing a feed should include the constancy of its major ingredients and their sources, its moisture content, freshness, storage characteristics, and timely delivery. Nonnutritional intentional additives, such as antibiotics and estrogens, should be avoided. Periodic analyses of the feed for pesticides (chlorinated hydrocarbons, etc.), mycotoxin (aflatoxins, etc.), and industrial (polychlorinated biphenyls, etc.) contaminants are recommended. Whenever practical and consistent with the disease control program, the feed should also be sterilized, with care taken to assure that the nutrients are not degraded or the palatability of the feed altered. Feed should be provided as often as necessary, but not less than once weekly, to assure an adequate supply of fresh rations. When a test agent is given in the diet, its stability should also be considered as a factor in determining the frequency of feed changes. Semisynthetic diets may be preferred for some studies and have been recommended for use in all testing of drugs for carcinogenicity (Newberne, 1974). As of this time the increased cost has prevented general implementation of this recommendation.

Water systems should be capable of providing an adequate, continuous supply of fresh, pathogen-free water. Each cage should be supplied at least twice weekly with a filled sanitized water bottle, stopper, and sipper tube. The bottles should be filled and the stoppers and sipper tubes inserted into them only outside the animal rooms. Empty or partially full water bottles should be replaced rather than refilled. When an automatic watering system is used, the valve end should be located in such a manner as to prevent accidental flooding of the cage.

Operations. The key to a successful animal care operation is a well-trained and motivated caretaker staff interested in and concerned for the health of the individual animals and their role in quality research. As in design considerations, operations should strive to prevent entrance of extraneous factors at all levels of containment, from facility to animal room to individual cage.

Lack of or improper quarantine with inadvertent introduction of disease to a facility can jeopardize chronic studies that may have been under way for many months. Strict procedures in this regard are essential. Newly arrived animals should be taken, in their unopened shipping containers, directly to the quarantine area. Animals that are unsuitable by reason of size, health, or another criterion should be immediately discarded. Animals should be quarantined a minimum of 7 days, after which they should be reexamined and those unsuitable discarded. A small, randomly selected number of animals from each shipment should be sacrificed and examined for parasites and enteric pathogens. When an epizootic disease is found among the animals, the entire shipment from which they came should be discarded. The quarantine area should be disinfected prior to the receipt of additional animals. Professional judgment must be exercised to determine when minor losses may be attributed to the stress of shipment or normal attrition of young animals.

Access to the animal facilities should be restricted to individuals essential to the operation. Both professional and technical personnel should receive adequate animal care and personal hygiene training. Those with disease conditions that may affect the animals' health should be excluded from the animal rooms.

Attention should also be given to personnel and supplies entering the facility or animal rooms to prevent introduction of disease. Actual measures should conform to the disease prevention plan—barrier or conventional operation, etc. Sterilization of food and bedding as well as personnel showering, while warranted in barrier and clean-dirty corridor facilities, may not be practical for many conventional operations.

Clinical examinations. Astute clinical observations can alert the investigator to the early onset of an infectious disease or degeneration of health due to the test compound. As each animal in a chronic study represents a great investment in time and money, all losses, whether due to disease, unwanted toxicity, autolysis, or cannibalism, must be avoided. The cost of careful and frequent clinical examinations is a warranted expenditure, not only to reduce animal losses but to provide data of use in evaluating the test and results obtained. A viability check of every animal should be made once in the morning and once in the late afternoon on a 7-day-a-week basis by competent laboratory animal technicians. Animals in poor health or with life-threatening conditions should be isolated. Those whose condition makes it unlikely that they will survive another 24 hr should be sacrificed and immediately necropsied.

Every animal should be palpated and carefully examined at least once a week. In addition to an examination for abnormalities of hair coat, eyes, mouth, teeth, nose, and ears, the animals should be palpated for body masses and observed for neurological conditions. Animal weights should be measured at day 1 of the study and thereafter at 2–4 wk intervals. The frequency should be increased when large numbers of tumors are evident or when an apparent deterioration in the animals' health is detected. Ideally, weights should be recorded for individual animals. The use of balances coupled with an automatic recording system, as illustrated in Fig. 14, facilitates weighing and clinical examinations.

Food consumption, while of limited value in monitoring a study, nevertheless provides useful information in determining dose administered in feed and food consumption effects. An alternative to continuous measurement is used by the NCI. Food consumption is measured on a representative sampling of each test group 1 wk per month.

The same examination and weighing schedule as well as procedures should be used for all test animals, including controls. Whenever individual animal data are to be routinely recorded, each animal should be marked at the outset of the study by using a standard method of identification such as ear notching, toe clipping, or tagging.

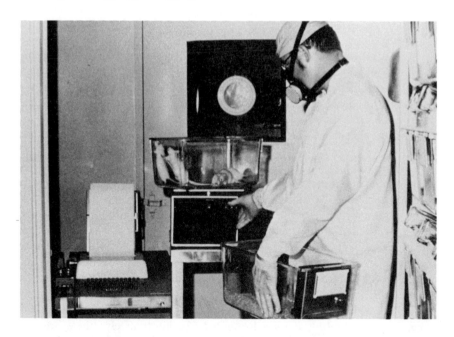

FIGURE 14 Technician weighing rats with automatic recording balance system at the FCRC. Clinical signs are also recorded in code form.

EXPERIMENTAL DESIGN ASPECTS

The objective of a carcinogen bioassay screening experiment is to detect the carcinogenic potential of a compound. It is intended that results obtained with small groups of laboratory rodents aid in predicting the potential hazard of a compound to which millions of people might be exposed. An environmental agent causing 1-2% cancer in the general public could result in over 2-5 million cases, considered an unacceptable risk to most. Unfortunately, the usual bioassay with small numbers of animals cannot detect a low incidence of that magnitude. To overcome this, the usual procedure employed is to maximize the likelihood of finding moderate to weak carcinogens by the use of higher dose levels for a long period of time. One should keep in mind that certain experimental design aspects, such as high doses or unusual routes, may in some cases create a modifying effect or unusual metabolic pathway that conceivably could result in an effect not qualitatively found under normal circumstances. A practical .approach to the problem is viewed as one where the experimental design simulates as closely as possible the human exposure situation but maximizes the probability of detecting a low-incidence response. The design to maximize detection of carcinogenicity might be to expose animals beginning *in utero* and continuing for life at the highest tolerated dose levels.

Route of Exposure

As a general rule, the test agent should be administered by a route that duplicates or closely simulates the one by which human exposure occurs. Entirely unrealistic and artificial situations should be avoided in order that the results be amenable to evaluation in terms of the potential human health hazard. Many factors should be considered in selecting the route of exposure, such as the pharmacokinetic characteristics of absorption, metabolism, and excretion.

There may be many compounds to which humans are exposed by several different routes or mode of entry to the body. For example, a pesticide that may be inhaled or absorbed through the skin during occupational exposure may also gain access to the body through food and the water supply. Will animal tests conducted by one route serve as an adequate test for carcinogenicity regardless of the route for humans? Will liver cancer occur to the same extent after inhalation of a compound as it does after oral administration with absorption into the portal circulation and direct exposure to the liver, the first organ encountered? Does a compound administered by the oral route and inducing gastrointestinal cancer (perhaps a direct contact effect) pose a health hazard when inhaled? Unfortunately, these are real questions for which limited data are available for prediction. In deciding on the route of exposure to use, one must consider not only the human use or exposure but also specific properties of the chemical, such as solubility, absorption, physiological effects, organs affected, metabolism, dose and length of treatment, and potential safety hazard to technicians.

Except for certain drugs, nearly all chemicals gain entry to the body by the oral route, inhalation, or absorption through the skin. Other routes may have certain special advantages directed toward merely screening for carcinogenic activity with no intent to facilitate quantitating the hazard to humans.

Weisburger and Weisburger (1967) described in detail the various considerations involved in each route of exposure. Several of their recommendations will be mentioned in the following discussions of the various routes of exposure.

Oral route. The oral route is used extensively in bioassay tests as it simulates the main human exposure route for many compounds and is technically an easy method of administering a compound in animal bioassays. Substances can be administered orally by several methods, such as in the diet mix, water, pills, or capsules or by intubation or gavage. Each method has certain advantages and disadvantages, and a decision as to the method used depends largely on the compound to be tested.

While the NCI generally prefers to mix the compound in the feed (diet) whenever possible, as it usually simulates more closely the human exposure pattern, gastric intubation is also utilized to a great extent. Capsules or water mixtures are not commonly used. The introduction of the test agent by gastric intubation offers greater hazard control, better quantitation, the need for less test agent, fresher preparations, easier storage, and increased animal handling. Its disadvantages are that generally there is less than maximum intake of the test agent, a solvent is usually required, mortality may be increased, and animals need to be closely matched by weight. Diet mix offers a greater total intake of the test agent and may more closely simulate the mode of human exposure. Its disadvantages are that contamination may be difficult to control, the homogeneity of the mix is not assured, decomposition of the test agent may occur during storage or while in the feeder, the palatability of the feed may be affected, and the quantity ingested by each animal may vary. The advantages and disadvantages of giving the test agent in water are similar to those encountered when the diet mix is used as the mode of administration.

Diet mixture can be used in virtually all species so long as the mixture is not unpalatable and it is recognized that absorption kinetics may vary with different species.

It is important that the chemical be mixed into the feed so that the diet is homogenous throughout. The method used to achieve a homogenous mixture may vary with the form of the chemical and the dosage level. While in many cases it may be possible to blend the chemical directly into the feed, in other cases it will be necessary to first premix the compound into a small aliquot or concentrate of feed or other substance to assure proper final mixing. For powdered or crystalline chemicals a dry granular ingredient of the feed such as starch or sugar can be used, with mixing best achieved in a mortar. Sometimes the compound can be dissolved in a volatile organic solvent such as acetone, which then can be distributed over the granular portion of the diet. Following evaporation of the solvent, concentrate can then be mixed into the final diet mix. With oil-soluble compounds it may be best to first dissolve the compound in the lipid constituent of the diet, such as corn oil. The premix can then be homogenized into the bulk diet mix by means of a V-blender or commercially available food mixer such as used in large food operations.

Some compounds may react with the feed ingredients or undergo decomposition, which could lead to erroneous results. It is therefore important that diet mixtures be prepared frequently enough to prevent such deterioration or loss of the chemical as well as spoilage of food. For stable compounds mixing at 2–4 wk intervals may suffice, with prepared diets stored in vermin-proof coolers and chemical analysis conducted to assure proper mixing of diet and its stability during storage.

Feeders, designed to minimize spillage, should be filled with fresh diet mix frequently, a minimum of once per week and more often in the case of unstable materials. Addition of water or milk to the feed is considered undesirable as it may lead to spoilage and bridging of feeders.

Intubation or gavage may be used in cases in which the chemical may be too volatile, unstable, or reactive to mix in the feed. It has advantages in that the dosage can be accurately controlled, and chemical hazard or exposure of other animals can be reduced. This method requires more technicians and may result in some loss of animals (especially very young ones) through trauma at the time of intubation (Magee, 1970). This latter problem is not of great concern as technicians can readily learn the technique of intubation so as to minimize the animal losses. In fact, the intubation method has been used even for newborn and infant mice and rats (Klein, 1959; Miller and Dymsza, 1963), and its use with neonatal animals has now become routine. Animals adapt to accept the procedure provided the proper technique is used. With adequately trained personnel, perforation of the esophagus or stomach and intratracheal insertion does not present a major problem (Moreland, 1965). Illustrations of gastric intubation of rats and mice are presented in Fig. 15.

There are several advantages of this method over dietary mixes. If necessary, the solution can be prepared immediately prior to use. The increased need for technicians to individually treat animals is partially offset by not needing to mix and store dietary preparations.

The vehicle used can vary with the chemical to be administered. Water-soluble compounds can be administered in aqueous solutions. Caution must be exercised as some water-soluble compounds are reactive in water; for example, beta-propriolactone to proprionic acid. If necessary, alcohol can be added to the water for increased solubility. For compounds not soluble in

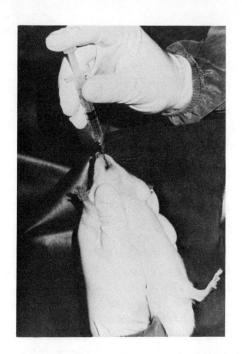

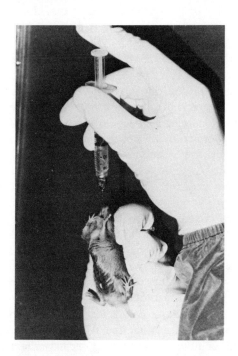

FIGURE 15 Gastric intubation of chemicals
in rat (top) and mouse (bottom) (FCRC).

129

water other vehicles have been used, including food oils and suspensions containing gum tragacanth, arachis, gelatin, or methylcellulose. A vehicle used by the NCI known as steroid suspending vehicle (SSV) is useful for many water-insoluble compounds (Weisburger and Weisburger, 1967).

It should be borne in mind that administering excessive amounts of oils may contribute significantly to the dietary intake of lipids as well as cause diarrhea. Regardless of the vehicle used, it must be free of contaminants that themselves might be carcinogenic or have an unwanted physiologic effect and lead to erroneous conclusions. A discussion of vehicles can be found in Clayson (1962), Hueper and Conway (1964), Magee (1970), and Weisburger and Weisburger (1967).

With the intubation method higher instantaneous levels will be achieved as compared with intake via diet. While this simulates immediate ingestion of chemicals such as many drugs, it obviously varies from the human exposure to a chemical in the food or water supply. While quantitative differences in absorption, blood, and tissues levels can occur, their influence on a carcinogenesis bioassay is not considered of major importance. Perhaps of more concern is the possibility of acute toxicity, which can reduce the total dosage that can be administered. For practical purposes the compound may be administered on a 3 or 5 time per week basis rather than a 7-day per week schedule. While this may enhance toxicity and decrease long-term survival, the total chemical administered is less and may reduce the sensitivity of the test for some carcinogens.

Administration as a water mixture is restricted to nonvolatile water-soluble, water-stable, and nonreactive chemicals. The addition of alcohol to the water may increase the solubility for some compounds (Magee, 1970). As with diet mixtures, unpalatability can be a problem for treated water. From the technical viewpoint considerably less effort is required in preparing and supplying the animals with treated water than with diet mixtures.

Capsules and pills are sometimes used, but because of obvious difficulties in administration they are feasible only for larger species such as dogs. The compound can be measured directly into a capsule or compressed into a pellet or pill. When necessary, inert compounds can be used as filler material.

Skin application. Cutaneous application was the first technique to be used successfully in inducing cancer in experimental animals (Yamagiwa and Ichikawa, 1915). Since that time it has gained widespread popularity as a test system to assay chemicals for carcinogenicity. It has obvious relevance to assay chemicals for which exposure to humans is by the dermal route, such as certain drugs and cosmetics. It has also gained acceptance for screening other chemicals as well as determining cocarcinogenic, promoting, and initiating activity. It should be recognized that the skin in most species is not very permeable to aqueous solutions and also may not have the necessary enzymes to activate some carcinogens. Such cutaneous application is used mainly for organic lipophilic materials, with the size of the molecules and the related absorption a limiting factor (Weisburger and Weisburger, 1967). Carcinogenic chemicals of large, insoluble molecules may not be reactive in the cutaneous system and may present false negative results.

The species of choice has generally been the mouse, as its skin epithelium has been generally more responsive to tumor formation than that of the rat (National Academy of Sciences, 1960). Some scientists feel that the rat and guinea pig are of limited value for this purpose (Golberg, 1974). Magee (1970), however, feels that there is no inherent difference in the capacity of mouse, rat, and hamster skin to undergo malignant change. This is based on the work of Fare (1966), who demonstrated that azo dyes were potent skin carcinogens in the rat but inactive in the mouse, while Graffi et al. (1967) found the rat, mouse, and hamster highly susceptible to skin carcinogenesis by skin application of N-nitrosomethylurea.

The advantages of the skin application method are mainly in the ability to observe and establish with greater precision the time of development of local cancer or of precancerous lesions and the ability to alter treatments so as to test for promotion or initiating activity. It should be recognized that some compounds may be absorbed and induce systemic effects. Among the disadvantages are the labor involved in clipping and repeated treatments, the lack of quantitation of exposure, and possible chemical hazard/contamination concerns. Because of species difference in absorption and the small amounts of the test compound that can be applied to the skin of rodents, it may be desirable to test some compounds by the oral route although the usual human exposure is by dermal application (Friedman, 1974).

Many liquids can be applied directly to the skin. More often, however, vehicles or solvents are necessary. Among various solvents that have been used acetone is the most common, followed by toluene, benzene, and heavy mineral oils (Weisburger and Weisburger, 1967; Magee, 1970). Proper control and test groups are necessary to determine whether the solvents themselves might possess initiating or promoting activity. The technique of applying chemicals to the skin is relatively easy to learn. Application in early studies was mainly by brush, although a pipette or dropper is now used frequently as it allows for more precise quantitation of the exposure. Usually the hair must be removed prior to the start of treatment and during the course of the experiment. Clippers not lubricated with mineral oils are highly recommended over chemical depilatory agents. Both promotion and initiating activity can be determined by use of skin tests. Boutwell (1964) provided a good review of this assay method for promotion activity. To determine promotion activity, the test material is applied subsequent to a small initiating dose of a known skin carcinogen. An enhancement effect is considered evidence of promotion activity. 7,12-Dimethylbenz[a]anthracene is often used as the carcinogen with one to three doses applied in a 1 wk period. After 1-2 wk, repeated applications of the test material are given. To determine initiating activity the reverse order is used, with the test material given first or on an alternating basis. Perhaps the most widely used promoting agents have been croton oil and its active constituents (Van Duuren et al., 1963; Hecker et al., 1964; Arrayo and Holcomb, 1965). Dodecane and mixtures of sulfur compounds (Horton et al., 1965), Tween 60 (Setala, 1969), anthra-1,8,9-triol (Bock and Burns, 1963), and some essential oils (Roe, 1965) have also been utilized as promoters.

Respiratory exposure. The lung is the most prominent site for cancer in humans and many chemicals gain entrance into the body by inhalation. However, until recently, the respiratory route for carcinogen bioassay was not routinely used for two main reasons: (1) animal models have not been established that simulate closely human respiratory exposure, and (2) the cost for facilities and maintenance of inhalation equipment is considerably greater than that for other types of carcinogenesis tests. Inhalation facilities for long-term tests generally have not been available. There has been increasing evidence that various inhaled materials are of importance in the causation of cancer; for example, arsenic, bis(chloromethyl) ether, vinyl chloride, asbestos, and tobacco smoke. Recently several other chemicals to which humans are exposed by inhalation—namely, chloroform, trichloroethylene, and ethylene dibromide—have been implicated as causing cancer in animals when tested by the oral route, and might also be tested by inhalation. As the result of increased interest in assay of materials that are inhaled, inhalation facilities have been severely taxed. Only minor expansion of such testing laboratories has occurred until recently because of the expense required to conduct such tests and the limited number of inhalation toxicologists available.

There are considerable differences in the inhalation of particulate material into the deep lung of small rodents and humans. Humans are more likely to inhale through the mouth than rodents, thereby bypassing filtration by the nasal passages. Nasal inhalation, along with smaller nasal passages, results in particulates above 1 μm in size being essentially excluded from rodent lungs, whereas that is not the case for humans. The problem is not as crucial with chemical vapors, although some settling out on dust particles is still likely to occur. A series of excellent conferences on experimental respiratory carcinogenesis has been held by the Atomic Energy Commission with the partial support of the NCI (Atomic Energy Commission, 1970a, 1970b, 1973; see also Karbe and Park, 1974). These conferences followed the first major conference on respiratory carcinogenesis, which was held in Perugia, Italy, in 1965 (Severi, 1966).

Laskin and Sellakumar (1974) concluded that the present state of our knowledge indicates that the common laboratory rat most closely meets the requirements of the ideal animal model for inhalation studies. This conclusion was based on the induction of a squamous cell carcinoma of bronchogenic origin (similar to that in humans and rarely occurring spontaneously in rats). Recently, however, the hamster has been gaining support for the same reason.

Various types and configurations of chambers or exposure rooms have been used for inhalation toxicology, depending primarily on the species to be employed. For rodents, the usual chamber design has been such that groups of animals are placed into an entire chamber with a volume of several cubic feet. Thus, the animal is completely immersed in an atmosphere containing the chemical. For larger animals, such as the dog, rabbit, and primates, larger chambers have been used, or face masks or other devices employed so that the animals face, mouth, and/or nostrils only are exposed to the test agent. Similar devices have also been developed for rodents (Karbe and Park, 1974). To comply with safety requirements, a common practice now is to commit chambers to a chronic test with animals kept in the chambers continuously although exposure to the chemical may be for only a 6–8 hr period per day. Regardless of the system, it is essential that the concentration of chemical be analyzed frequently to assure proper exposure. Provisions must also be made for feed and water as well as removal of excreta.

In view of the technical difficulties in satisfactorily exposing the rodent's lung to chemicals by inhalation, several artificial methods, including intranasal, intratracheal, and intrapulmonary injection, or implants have been used successfully to assure penetration of the test materials into the deep lung. Of these, the intratracheal injection experiments by Saffiotti et al. (1968) have perhaps been the most successful. In those studies Syrian golden hamsters, which had received 15 weekly intratracheal instillations of hematite particles impregnated with benzo[a]pyrene, developed a high incidence of respiratory tract cancers, many of bronchogenic origin similar to those of humans. Other advantages of this technique are that no special solvents or colloids are required other than the hematite dust particles, with relatively little injury or inflammation of the lung. By this method, a suspension of the test compound can be deposited directly into the trachea with movement into the deep lung. In addition to iron oxide (hematite) particles, other carrier materials such as colloidal gelatin, casein, saline, and charcoal have been used to enhance deposition, retention, and intimate contact of the test chemicals with the pulmonary tissues.

Intraperitoneal injection. While this route has been widely used in general pharmacology and toxicology, it has not gained as wide use in carcinogenicity testing. Perhaps the major reason is that it is not the usual route of human exposure for most chemicals, except perhaps some pharmaceuticals. Unstable or sensitive compounds can be administered by the intraperitoneal route that can not be administered by other means. Nevertheless, it has certain advantages that should be considered, such as rapid absorption and quick exposure of the liver. Most chemicals are absorbed relatively rapidly from the peritoneal cavity, even many that are insoluble in water. This route thus provides rather quick systemic exposure. In some cases, however, relatively insoluble materials or oil solutions may be absorbed slowly, providing for rather constant exposure.

In using this method, several disadvantages should be recognized: it is likely that some of the material will not be accurately injected into the peritoneal cavity even by the most experienced of technicians; some compounds may be more toxic with less total exposure to the chemical by this route than by other parenteral routes due to rapid absorption; complications such as adhesions and infections are difficult to avoid in long-term administrations; there is difficulty in detecting locally induced peritoneal tumors; and there is considerable species variation in sensitivity. A wide variety of vehicles or solvents can be used for peritoneal injection, including various food oils, propylene glycol, trioctanoin, methyl cellulose, water, saline, gelatin, and alcohol solutions. Care should be taken to assure freedom of the solvents from carcinogenic chemicals. The frequency of injections will often depend on the duration of the total exposure period.

Subcutaneous injection. This route has been widely used, mainly because of the ease of administration, slower absorption, and lower toxicity than in the intraperitoneal or intravenous routes. It appears to be one of the most sensitive routes for assay of some chemicals, with which only a few injections are necessary for the induction of cancer; for example, some carcinogenic hydrocarbons and other relatively insoluble compounds. Various solvents or vehicles have been used, including food oils such as arachis, corn, peanut, olive, or mineral oils, trioctanoin, saline, water, and dimethyl sulfoxide. In view of the sensitivity of this test system, it is essential that the solvents be as free from carcinogenic impurities as possible. This may require purification if a highly pure commercial product is not obtainable. The amount of diluent will usually depend on the size of the animals. The frequency of treatment is dependent on the rate of absorption. As a practice, injections should not be made at the same site more often than twice a week (Mori, 1965). For some chemicals the test material can be compressed into small pellets for subcutaneous implantation. Diluents such as cholesterol and paraffin have been used. These pellets have the advantage of slow, continuous release of the chemical as it elutes from the pellet.

The use of the subcutaneous test for carcinogenicity has been highly controversial, based primarily on the induction of local sarcomas by substances normally found in the body and in a normal diet, such as sucrose, glucose, sodium chloride, and distilled water. In addition, some chemicals positive by the subcutaneous route have not been carcinogenic by other routes. An explanation usually offered for these results is that sarcomas are induced by a physical rather than chemical mechanism. Regardless of possible false positives, the subcutaneous route has considerable merit. In using it, however, the investigator must be aware of the difficulties in interpreting the results, especially if local sarcomas are induced. In all tests adequate controls and several dose levels are essential for evaluation of a true effect.

Both rats and mice can be used; however, the subcutaneous tissue of the rat is generally considered the more sensitive. Newborn or infant animals appear to be more sensitive than adults.

Other routes. In addition to the routes previously discussed, others, such as intravenous, intramuscular, intranasal, intrapulmonary, and various types of implantation, are used for special situations. As in the case of subcutaneous sarcomas, extrapolation of the results obtained with atypical routes to predict human hazard is very difficult.

Doses and Dose Levels

As currently conceived, much of the NCI Carcinogenesis Bioassay Program is related to the testing of chemicals for carcinogenic activity and the investigation of methodology for carcinogenicity testing rather than toxicological assessment of hazard. However, the finding of carcinogenic activity from the screening test may be of sufficient concern that regulatory actions are initiated. With this in mind, in selecting the doses and dose levels one should consider not only the main objectives of the test, but also the ultimate utilization of the test results. A test to assay for carcinogenic activity conceivably might require only a single, well-selected dose, whereas for risk estimation, several dose levels with dose-response analysis, metabolism studies, etc., may be required.

In the concept of an initial assay for carcinogenic activity, one should strive to maximize the sensitivity as well as selectivity of the carcinogenesis test. In other words, we must be efficient in detecting carcinogenicity if it exists (few false negatives), while at the same time avoiding the introduction of effects not representative of realistic situations (few false positives). False positive results could cause considerable economic harm to a producer and might result in the substitution of an even more hazardous alternative. False negatives could permit a harmful chemical to remain at large, with the consequences to be discovered later only after great human suffering.

It is a generally acceptable procedure in toxicology to determine an "effect" level, regardless of the parameter to be evaluated. If an effect is found, additional tests at lower levels are employed to facilitate establishing a "no effect" or "acceptable risk" level.

It is argued that induced neoplastic lesions are irreversible and conform to a linear, no threshold, dose-response relationship similar to that graphed for chemicals A and B in Fig. 16. While this may be true for many (perhaps most) chemicals, this argument neglects to account for biological considerations that could result in a nonlinear dose-response relationship.

On a theoretical basis, there are at least three possible mechanisms by which a curve similar to that of chemical D conceivably could result: (1) as the latent period for many carcinogens is inversely related to dose, animals at the lower levels simply may not live long enough for the cancer to be manifested; (2) high lose levels might exceed the body's capacity to efficiently detoxify or eliminate a carcinogenic chemical (sometimes referred to as metabolic overloading); and (3) high doses might result in increased conversion of an inactive chemical to a carcinogenic metabolite.

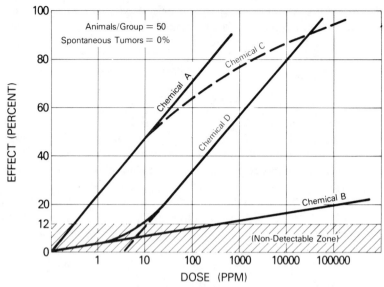

FIGURE 16 Differences in the ability to detect carcinogenicity depend on the relative strength of the carcinogen, as illustrated by differences in slope of dose-response curves.

Indeed, Hefner et al. (1975) provided evidence that this may occur with vinyl chloride. According to Kraybill (1974), other chemicals including methyl parathion, melangesterol acetate, and selenium may demonstrate metabolic differences related to dose. On the other hand, the efficiency of increasing exposure might decrease on a per dose basis for some chemicals. This could occur if the body's ability to absorb or retain a chemical becomes saturated. As an example, strontium-90, when ingested, follows basically the same kinetics of absorption from the intestinal tract as calcium. After reaching a certain level in the gut, further ingested strontium will not be absorbed but will pass on through the gut. There are examples of other materials that may be absorbed, but after the protein-binding capacity of the blood becomes saturated may be quickly eliminated through the kidneys or intestinal tract, so that a lower percentage can be metabolized to harmful metabolites. In these situations, the dose-response curve could appear like that of chemical C.

From Fig. 16 if one assumes linearity it can be seen that a single dose yielding 90% response might be greatly misleading as regards potential hazard. In the case of chemical C it would greatly underestimate hazard at lower doses, while with chemical D it would overestimate the low-dose response.

The conservative approach to bioassay is to maximize sensitivity by using the highest dose possible. In so doing, we should be cognizant that this might create results that may be difficult to extrapolate to low-level effects.

As was illustrated in Fig. 1, the results of the initial or presumptive test could lead to confirmatory or in-depth studies that might "evaluate" the possible modifying effects previously mentioned. From lack of a better method, the use of the highest dose possible to test for carcinogenicity is still considered necessary. Such doses have been referred to as "maximum tolerated" or "maximum test" doses (MTD).

As it is essential that the animals survive sufficiently long to allow induced cancers to become observable, the limiting factor in establishing the upper test level (MTD) is usually the animal's ability to tolerate the chemical for long-term exposure without death or substantial life-shortening. It should also be borne in mind that excessive levels might impose nonlife-shortening but also unacceptable physiologic stresses that might affect a tumorigenic response; for example, excessive weight loss, nutritional or endocrine imbalance, and immunologic depression. The dosage levels should be selected with this in mind.

It is generally conceded that the maximum dose can produce slight toxic effects, such as depression of weight gain, so long as it is compatible with prolonged survival and permits valid interpretation of the experimental results. Weisburger and Weisburger (1967) were willing to accept 10–20% deaths due to toxicity. In practice, however, choosing dose levels that might allow that degree of mortality often resulted in an even greater mortality, with an unacceptable death loss due to toxicity or a necessity to change the dose level.

For routine carcinogenicity testing, a minimum of two dose levels is recommended by the NCI. The second dose level has been viewed as insurance in the event of unanticipated animal mortality from toxicity at the higher dose. It also has some value in estimating a dose-response relationship. In practice, the second dose has usually been one-half or one-fourth of the MTD.

For highly important compounds it may be desirable to have several dose levels to obtain a graded dose-response relationship, which may be helpful in assessing carcinogenicity. For testing of drugs, the routine use of three dose levels has been recommended (Golberg, 1974; World Health Organization, 1969).

To predict the maximum tolerated dose level, preliminary toxicity studies are usually necessary. Three types of tests, depending on prior knowledge of toxicity in the test species, may be desirable in order to arrive at the estimated MTD. These are outlined in Table 10. Initially a simple single-dose, acute toxicity study is used to locate the lethal range. As this rarely will predict tolerance to continuous dosing, it is often followed by another study in which treatment is for a 14 day period to further define the dose range for longer-term exposure. The final prechronic toxicity test (known as the subchronic test) entails a 90 day treatment period. From the results of this subchronic test, tolerance to life-span or 24 month treatment is predicted.

The NCI initially used 6 wk treatment for the subchronic test. This proved inadequate to reliably predict long-term survival or latent toxicity and resulted in several studies being aborted or the dose levels reduced. Burchfield

TABLE 10 Preliminary Toxicity Tests Used to Arrive at Maximum Tolerated Doses for Chronic Test[a,b]

Toxicity test	No. of animals per group	No. of dose levels	Treatment period	Additional observation period	Clinical examinations
Acute study	5	3	Single-dose or 1 day	14 days	Mortality Relevant clinical signs Weight at start and end
Repeated-dose study	5	5	14 days	1 day	Mortality Clinical signs Weekly weights Selected toxicity tests
Subchronic study	10	5	90 days	1 day	Mortality Clinical signs Weekly weights Selected toxicity tests

[a]Route of administration: same as that to be used in chronic study.
[b]Pathology examination: Necropsy of all animals. Microscopic examination of all controls and highest dose level without mortality. (In subchronic study, microscopic examination of next highest dose level also.)

et al. (1974) reviewed the dose levels used in testing a series of pesticides and concluded that a maximum tolerated dose for the chronic test could have been achieved by using one-fourth of the 6 wk tolerated dose level.

The Frederick Cancer Research Center (FCRC) is conducting a series of experiments to assess the length of the subchronic test needed to accurately predict long-term tolerance and the maximum tolerated dose. From the data obtained to date, a 6-8 wk test will fail to predict the MTD with the majority of chemicals, while the results of 90 day (13 wk) subchronic tests are considerably more predictive of chronic toxicity. As considerable variability exists for various chemicals due to differences in pharmacokinetics, irreversible organ damage, and numerous other biological factors, each with variable temporal manifestations, a set length for a subchronic test will not be satisfactory for all chemicals. Indeed, the FCRC studies indicate that for some chemicals a subchronic test of 20-30 wk (or perhaps even longer) would be required to provide a close estimation of 2 yr tolerance.

In some cases, the chronic toxicity level will plateau or decrease with continued exposure, as illustrated in Fig. 17; however, animals may develop an apparent tolerance to some chemicals so that they might be exposed to even higher levels as time progresses.

Current NCI guidelines recommend a much greater emphasis on toxicity testing, including longer treatment and more extensive clinical/pathology examination than were employed in the past. A minimum exposure of 90

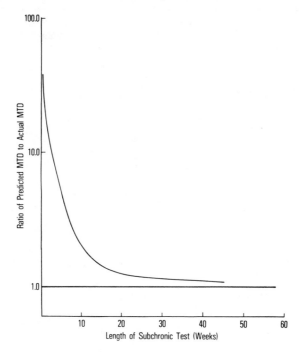

FIGURE 17 Relationship of maximum tolerated dose for chronic exposure to length of subchronic treatment test.

days is now used, with the test chemical administered by the same route and treatment schedule to be used in the long-term study. In addition, a careful analysis is made of clinical signs of toxicity, weight depression, and pathology lesions in order to estimate the highest dose level that can be used in the long-term carcinogenicity study. Pharmacokinetic data of body retention would obviously be of benefit in better predicting latent toxicity.

Once chronic dose levels are established, they are changed only when absolutely necessary to ensure the integrity of the study. The changes in toxicity tests and method of determining MTD have been in effect since the guidelines were adopted in January, 1974. Experience to date indicates that the new method of dose selection has resulted in considerable improvement in estimating the MTDs, especially with rats. Difficulty is still being encountered in estimating tolerance in mice, even with a 90 day subchronic test.

Considerably variability exists in long-term toxicity to chemicals, as one might expect. Table 11 lists the maximum dose levels used by the NCI for bioassay of a series of pesticides. The range of MTDs varied from 50,000 (5% of diet) to less than 1 ppm. The data available at this time do not correlate the dose level used with the probability of finding a carcinogenic effect.

Class/chemical	Dose levels[b] (ppm)			
	Mouse		Rat	
	Male	Female	Male	Female
Organochlorine insecticides				
Chlorobenzilate	3,200	2,350	8,500	6,000
Methoxychlor	3,500	2,000	850	1,500
DDD (TDE)	3,300	1,700	825	825
Dicofol	525	225	950	750
DDE	290	290	900	500
Toxaphene	200	200	1,100	1,000
Lindane	160	160	470	270
DDT	45	175	600	400
Chlordane	55	65	400	250
Chlordecone (Kepone)	23	40	24	26
Heptachlor	15	20	80	50
Aldrin	10	5	55	60
Endosulfan	7	4	1,100	1,000
Dieldrin	5	5	50	50
Endrin	3	5	5	5
Photodieldrin	0.6	0.6	10	5
Organophosphate insecticides				
Tetrachlorvinphos (Gardona)	16,000	16,000	8,500	8,500
Malathion	16,000	16,000	8,500	8,100
Dichlorvos (DDVP)	635	635	325	325
Dimethoate	375	500	310	380
Phosphamidon	125	160	160	160
Parathion	125	160	60	45
Azinphosmethyl (Gusathion)	60	125	150	125
Methyl parathion	80	125	40	40
Other insecticides/related materials				
Perthane	5,000	6,000	7,000	7,000
Piperonyl butoxide	3,000	3,000	10,000	10,000
Piperonyl sulfoxide	3,000	6,000	700	700
Dioxathione	550	900	180	90
4-Dimethylamino-3,5-xylyl N-methyl-carbamate (Zectran)	650	130	420	675
Azobenzene	400	500	400	400
Fungicides				
Phthalamide	50,000	13,000	30,000	15,000
Captan	16,000	16,000	6,000	6,000
2,4,6-Trichlorophenol (Omal)	10,000	14,500	10,000	10,000

TABLE 11 Maximum Tolerated Doses Used in Carcinogenicity Bioassays
of Pesticides (Diet Mixtures)[a] (*continued*)

| | Dose levels[b] (ppm) | | | |
| | Mouse | | Rat | |
Class/chemical	Male	Female	Male	Female
Fungicides (*continued*)				
Daconil	5,400	6,000	10,140	10,140
Pentachloronitrobenzene (quintozene)	5,000	8,000	11,000	15,500
Sodium dimethyldithiocarbamate	4,000	4,000	2,500	2,500
Ethyl tellurac (tetrakis)	3,000	5,000	600	300
Ethyl tuads	2,000	500	600	600
Lead dimethylthiocarbamate (Ledate)	50	50	50	50
Herbicides/plant regulators/miscellaneous				
Chlorambin (Amiben)	20,000	20,000	20,000	20,000
Pichloram	5,100	5,100	14,850	14,850
Trifluralin	4,000	5,400	8,200	8,200
Nitrofen	4,700	4,700	3,600	2,600
Chlormequat (CCC)	2,000	2,000	3,000	3,000
Monuron	2,000	2,000	1,500	1,500
Calcium cyanamide	2,000	2,000	400	200
CDEC (Vegadex)	2,000	1,900	500	500
Molluscicide				
Niclosamide (Bayluscide)	550	550	28,000	28,000

[a]Material mixed in diet and fed *ad libitum* continuously for 18–24 months.

[b]Approximate weighted average of highest dose level (MTD). Lower dose level usually ½ MTD. In some cases the dose(s) were adjusted during the experiments to achieve maximum tolerance. Initial dose levels were selected on the basis of short-term toxicity (6–8 wk) tests.

Duration and Frequency of Treatment

For the greatest confidence in a "negative" result, a test agent should be administered continuously for the majority of an animal's life-span. The NCI considers that 2 yr is a practical treatment period in rats and mice, although the animals currently used in the program may survive on the average another 6–12 months. Treatment periods of 15–18 months are considered adequate for the shorter-lived hamsters. Recent reviews by Golberg (1974) and Page (1976) point out that there is general agreement by federal agencies and scientific groups that exposure of rodents should be for the life-span or a minimum of 2 yr.

The National Academy of Sciences (1960) also recommends a 2 yr treatment for dogs. In my opinion and that of the FDA Advisory Committee (1971), this is totally inadequate for carcinogenicity testing in such a long-lived species. An acceptable exposure/observation period for dogs is considered to be 7-10 yr, an age equivalent to about 45-60 yr in humans. For diet/water treatments continuous exposure is considered desirable and practical. With other routes practical considerations may dictate interrupted treatments. For example, inhalation treatment for 6-8 hr per day on a 5 day/wk schedule is usual. Regimens requiring special handling of animals, such as parenteral injections, are usually on a 5 day/wk basis. With some compounds intermittent exposures may be required because of toxicity. Various types of recovery can occur during exposure-free periods, which may either enhance or decrease chances of carcinogenicity. In view of the objective of assessing for carcinogenicity as the initial step, intermittent exposures on a 3-5 day/wk basis is considered practical for most compounds.

Observation Period

Following cessation of treatment, continued observation may be warranted before termination of the experiment. This period is considered desirable because (1) induced lesions may progress to more readily observable lesions, and (2) morphologically similar but noncarcinogenic proliferative lesions that are stress-related may regress. Neoplastic or "neoplastic-like" lesions that persist long after removal of the stimulus are considered of serious consequence, from the hazard viewpoint. Many expert morphologists, however, feel able to diagnose and determine the biological nature of tumorous lesions existing at the time of treatment without the added benefit of a treatment-free period.

In determining the length of an observation period, several factors must be considered: period of exposure, survival pattern of both treated and control animals, nature of lesions found in animals that have already died, tissue storage and retention of the chemical, and results of other studies that would suggest induction of late-occurring tumors. The usual length of a treatment-free observation period is at least 3 months in mice and hamsters and 6 months in rats. An alternative would be to terminate the experiment or individual groups on the basis of survival experience.

Pathology

It is essential to include in carcinogenicity tests adequate consideration of pathology. To plan and conduct an animal bioassay with meticulous care and then permit an inadequate pathology evaluation is ludicrous. The same is true when the pathologist is presented with autolyzed tissues or useless animals because of improperly designed or monitored experiments. Pathology must be planned for before initiation of the experiment with the pathologist participating in the selection of the animal models and design and monitoring of the studies. Like the toxicologist, the pathologist can function as a generalist in assessing changes occurring early in an experiment and alert the test director to effects that might jeopardize the successful completion of the study. The two essential ingredients to success in the pathology phase are good tissues and qualified personnel. A lack of either will predispose the experiment to failure.

The complete pathology examination consists of several separate steps: macroscopic examinations, histologic preparation of tissues, microscopic diagnosis, recording and tabulation of lesions, and evaluation of the experiment. As currently conducted by the NCI, this is a very major aspect of a carcinogenesis bioassay, representing approximately 40% of the overall cost for the study (Fig. 6).

Quality control at all steps in this process is of the utmost importance. A careful microscopic evaluation cannot make up for inadequate gross necropsy or histologic preparation. In simple terms, the pathologist reviewing the tissue slides can only report on the lesions placed before him. Important lesions may not be observed or may be lost at one of several steps: necropsy, trimming and fixation, paraffin blocking, or slide preparation.

As many important chemically induced lesions may appear to be similar to lesions that can occur spontaneously in aged animals, it is of the utmost importance that the pathologist receive professionally prepared tissue slides. Not only is it necessary that the trimming and fixation be properly conducted, but tissue sections must be sliced and stained with precision. Artifacts such as tearing or cooking of the tissues can easily be introduced by technicians. The histologic procedures as described by Sanders (1972) are recommended.

Assigning a well-trained and concerned animal pathologist responsibility for the complete pathology process as well as a major role in designing and conducting the experiment obviates many of these problems.

While there seems to be little controversy regarding the need for a careful and thorough gross necropsy, considerable disagreement exists as to the extent of microscopic examination needed for routine bioassay tests. In January, 1974, the NCI pathologists introduced an expanded protocol that not only instituted more thorough necropsy procedures but also required the microscopic examination of approximately 30 tissue sections plus blood smear, tissue masses, and gross lesions from each animal in the study. The enormity of this task can be better visualized when one realizes that for a routine test using 600 animals per study, at least 18,000 tissues will require examination. A pathologist not only conducts microscopic evaluations but also supervises gross necropsy, prepares reports on the results, and engages in other

TABLE 12   List of Tissues to Be Microscopically Examined
According to NCI Bioassay Protocol

Gross lesions	Stomach
Tissue masses/suspect tumors	Small intestine (one section)
and regional lymph nodes	Colon
Blood smear (if desired by	Liver
pathologist)	Gall bladder
Mandibular lymph node	Pancreas
Mammary gland	Spleen
Salivary gland	Kidneys
Sternebrae, femur, or vertebrae	Adrenals
including marrow	Bladder
Thymus	Prostate
Trachea	Testes
Bronchi	Ovaries
Lungs	Uterus
Heart	Brain (three sections)
Thyroid	Pituitary
Parathyroid	Eyes
Esophagus	Spinal cord (if neurological signs are present)

aspects of the study. A usual allotment for microscopic study is 50% of his time. At that rate a pathologist can diagnose the tissues for no more than three to four tests per year. Currently this single aspect has delayed completion of studies initiated in 1972–1973 and represents one of the limiting factors preventing expansion of the Bioassay Program. The tissues required in the NCI guidelines are listed in Table 12.

At the time tests were initiated on several hundred chemicals in 1971–1973, the protocols required the examination of far fewer tissues from only a portion of the test animals. Even with those protocols the pathologists would have been hard-pressed to keep up with the workload as the studies were terminating. The introduction of the greatly expanded examination of all animals resulted in a backlog of considerable magnitude. At a rate of four chemicals per pathologist per year, a cadre of 25 pathologists would be required to complete the examinations for 100 chemicals per year. Following the large influx of new chemicals into the testing program in the period 1971–1973, a great reduction in initiation of new tests was necessary to allow the pathologists to reduce the backlog. As this has essentially been accomplished, the program has now plateaued at the steady-state condition as recommended at the beginning of this chapter.

Differences of opinion exist as to the number of animals in an experiment as well as tissues of each animal that should be routinely examined in a carcinogenesis or chronic toxicity test. Many guidelines use such terms as "complete" or "adequate" examination, leaving the selection of tissues up to the responsible pathologist's judgment (FDA, 1971; Magee, 1970; WHO, 1961). Abrams et al. (1965) felt that 18 different tissues should be routinely examined. Realizing the impracticality of a microscopic examination of all organs, the WHO (1961) recommended an initial examination of only five organs (lungs, liver, spleen, kidneys, and urinary bladder), plus organs showing gross lesions, for evaluating drugs for carcinogenicity. Most recently a joint subcommittee of the Food and Drug Administration and the Pharmaceutical Manufacturers Association (1973) recommended microscopic examination of all major tissues for only the high-dose and control groups supplemented by gross lesions from other dose groups. Benitz (1970) supports this procedure. Zbinden (1976), recognizing that a compromise was needed between an all-encompassing evaluation of all possible tissues and a superficial examination, assigned the tissues into priority classes according to the frequency with which morphological changes are likely to occur. First priority consisted of organs in which gross changes were observed plus 9–11 organs or tissues (depending on sex) that would be routinely examined. This comprised the liver, kidney, lung, adrenal glands, heart, spleen, thymus, testis (or ovary), epididymis, bone marrow, and mesenteric lymph node. Another and larger group of tissues would be routinely examined in high-dose animals and some of the controls (second priority). Lower doses would be examined only when dictated by results from the high-dose group. The third-priority group would receive examination only as indicated for clinical or scientific reasons.

It is likely that the NCI requirements are among the most stringent of all at this time. There can be little doubt that a very thorough examination may be required to detect early small lesions, those in small organs, and those that have metastasized and are in a minute form. Kyriazis et al. (1974) illustrated the futility of a cursory examination to detect small metastatic foci of liver tumors in the lung. A simple examination of randomly selected lung lobes revealed only 4 and 0% metastatic foci of diethylnitrosamine-induced hepatocellular carcinomas in male and female B6C3F1 mice, respectively. Sections of the whole lung at two different levels detected foci in over 20% of animals with liver cancer. Additional sections might have detected an even higher metastatic rate.

On the other hand, the argument can be made that the extensive microscopic examination required by the NCI reduces the number of chemicals that can be evaluated, thereby jeopardizing the detection of important carcinogens because of the inability to test more chemicals. Perhaps the returns gained by the complete (30 tissue) examination are diminishing returns. Data to support one method over another simply are not available at this time. It is hoped that as the NCI data base grows to include a wide variety of chemicals, the cost-effectiveness of very detailed pathology examinations can be better evaluated.

Another technical issue debated frequently is whether it is desirable for the pathologist to diagnose tissues that have been coded so that he has no prior knowledge of the treatment. Fears and Schneiderman (1974) argue that coding or "blind reading" can reduce the potential for investigator bias, protect those reading slides from charges of bias, and increase the validity of the results to critiques and reviewers. They feel that the blind technique can be easily implemented and would avoid errors associated with the influence of subjective factors.

Weinberger (1973) admits that bias can unconsciously creep into the observations of the pathologist. However he feels that the need for blind evaluation is less important than requirements that the pathologist be technically skilled, objective, imaginative, and creative. In his opinion the blind technique might become overly rigid, keep the pathologist in ignorance of other aspects of the study, and deprive the pathologist of knowledge of diseases occurring in the untreated control group that he could use as a baseline to measure changes in the treated animals.

Zbinden (1976) is even more adamant in opposing the blind technique, claiming that it would be wasteful and impractical, forcing the pathologist to look at large numbers of tissues with extraordinary care. He prefers that the pathologist save time by concentrating on lesions not present in the controls. Of concern also is the possibility that lack of interest or enthusiasm might result, with the investigator becoming indifferent, which might be worse than potential bias. In the opinion of Zbinden, fear of making a false decision might subconsciously suppress the noting of slight changes.

While the FDA Panel on Carcinogenesis (1971) recommends conducting both gross and microscopic examinations "blind" or without knowledge of treatment, the NCI Bioassay Program has not chosen to implement this requirement as yet.

Among the most perplexing problems in predicting hazard to humans based on animal pathology results is that of the biological significance of liver tumors in the mouse. Several chemicals, especially organochlorines, have apparently induced hepatocellular carcinomas and hepatic nodules in the mouse without a similar response in the rat. Among the chemicals eliciting this type of response have been important pesticides, such as DDT, dieldrin, chlordane, and heptachlor, and economically important solvents, such as trichloroethylene, chloroform, and perchloroethylene. Grasso and Crampton (1972) and Roe and Tucker (1974) are perhaps the most adamant in challenging the validity of liver cancer in the mouse as a predictor of carcinogenic activity in humans. The reasons presented included the presence of viruses and the high background incidence of liver tumors in untreated controls. Considerable disagreement also exists as to the biological nature and classification of liver nodules or tumors (Butler, 1971; Grasso and Crampton, 1972; Tomatis et al., 1973).

Grasso (1974) proposes that tissue injury and repair may be important in the development of hepatic nodular lesions. As examples he illustrates the effects of carbon tetrachloride and chloroform in producing extensive necrosis as well as an apparent increase in liver tumors. Other factors have also been suggested, such as sex hormones and diet.

The World Health Organization (1974b) considers that it would be unwise to classify a substance as a carcinogen solely on the basis of increased liver tumors. It is their recommendation that long-term feeding studies in at least one other species be conducted in an effort to resolve this issue.

In an attempt to evaluate this problem, Tomatis et al. (1973b) surveyed the available literature to correlate the induction of liver tumors in mice with the capability of the chemical to induce tumors in the rat and hamster. From the survey of 58 chemicals a strong positive correlation existed when the chemical induced tumors of the liver and other sites in both sexes. Tomatis et al. concluded that the induction of liver tumors in the mouse should be considered as valid as the evidence obtained in the rat and/or the hamster at any site. This review also illustrated that target organs may differ in the rat and/or hamster from those in the mouse.

As there is no universally accepted nomenclature with simple terminology, it is important that morphological changes be described in detail, especially those considered to be treatment-related. Wherever possible the pathologist should attempt to determine the biological nature of the lesions. Such aspects as morphogenesis, primary lesions, and reversibility might be considered in assessing the biological significance of the lesions. Needless to say, accurate records and data presentations are essential aspects of a pathology review.

Age at Inception of Test

For routine screening tests for chemicals of unknown carcinogenicity the NCI guidelines recommend starting animals on treatment as young as possible, preferably no older than weanlings. As commercially obtained animals are shipped by the breeder within a few days after weaning (3–4 wk for most rodents) and quarantined for 1–2 wk, they are thus 5–6 wk of age before they can be placed on treatment.

It is likely that some chemicals may be carcinogenic to fetal tissues while inactive in newborns or adults. In other cases the fetus or infant may not have the metabolic competence to transform a chemical to an active metabolite and the adult may be more sensitive. Until recently, only chemicals known to produce tumors in adults or newborn animals have been employed in transplacental or *in utero* exposures, and thus an assessment of the extent of specific fetal sensitivity has not been possible (Tomatis, 1974; Tomatis et al., 1973a).

In general, however, it has been conceded that prenatal, neonatal, and infant rodents have a higher susceptibility than adults. This is predicated on the active organogenesis that occurs in the fetus or newborn for most organs. At that time its cells are immature, have a high rate of macromolecular synthesis, are actively proliferating, and are sensitive to transformation and thus more prone to carcinogenesis. Tumors of the nervous system, while quite difficult to induce in adults, are readily inducible by prenatal exposure. This is probably related to the active prenatal development of the nervous system (Zulch and Mennel, 1973; Druckrey, 1973; Ivankovic, 1973; Kommineni et al., 1970).

The differing age sensitivity for liver tumors is of particular interest. From the very fine studies of Vesselinovitch and his colleagues, it appears that the fetal and neonatal livers of both the rat and the mouse are considerably more sensitive to hepatocarcinogenesis than those of weanlings or adults. Their studies were with aflatoxin, urethan, ethylnitrosourea, and benzo[a]pyrene (Vesselinovitch et al., 1972, 1975; Kommineni et al., 1970; Vesselinovitch, 1973).

The mouse, previously found tolerant to hepatocarcinogenic effects of aflatoxin (Wogan, 1969), developed liver cancer when aflatoxin was administered to infant mice (Vesselinovitch et al., 1971). Kyriazis and Vesselinovitch (1973), in a study of the biological behavior of neonatal and adult mouse liver tumors induced by ethylnitrosourea, found that the liver tumors from neonatal exposed mice not only were easily transplanted (75% compared to 30%) but were biologically more active than those of the adults. They grew rapidly, were highly metastatic, and resulted in quick death to the host. Mohr et al. (1973) determined that the days 12–15 of gestation are the decisive period for the Syrian hamster, during which the fetus is most susceptible to induction of respiratory tract tumors by diethylnitrosamine.

The data indicate that prenatal, neonatal, and infant animals are more sensitive, in some cases, than adults to carcinogenesis even from minute exposures. It would also appear that the induction time is generally shorter, with greater malignancy. Even with mounting evidence for these differences, the working group on inception and duration of tests at the Conference on Carcinogenesis Testing in the Development of New Drugs (Tomatis, 1974) did not recommend *in utero* or neonatal exposures as a general procedure.

Diethylstilbestrol (DES) administered to pregnant women has resulted in an increased risk of vaginal adenocarcinoma in daughters 7–29 yr later (Herbst et al., 1975). This effect had not been predicted as no animal studies of DES *in utero* had been conducted. Recently, Rustia and Shubik (1976) have confirmed the effect in hamsters treated *in utero* with DES. Data are now becoming available from a series of experiments in Japan that provide further evidence for increased sensitivity for carcinogen detection by *in utero* or newborn treatment. The results also illustrate the increased sensitivity for adults in some cases. In the Japanese studies a series of chemicals of various classes, previously tested by routine adult carcinogenesis tests, are being further evaluated by a battery of short-term *in vitro* and *in vivo* tests, including the newborn and transplacental methods. Results on 33 chemicals have now been reported (Odashima, 1976). In comparing the results of adult, newborn, and transplacental methods, complete agreement was not obtained in 13 cases (39%). Of the 16 "adult negatives," seven were active by either newborn or transplacental methods: four of these by newborn only, one by transplacental only, and two by both methods. Of the 17 "adult positives," three were not detected by either newborn or transplacental techniques, one other was missed by the newborn method, and two more were not detected by the transplacental method. In assessing these false negatives one must realize that the exposure to the chemical was much less than in the adult studies. *In utero* treatments were for 3 days whereas newborns were treated for 4 days only. As with previous results, these data do not permit one to clearly recommend one method over another.

It is obvious, however, that to obtain maximum sensitivity and not miss an important age-related effect, exposure should be during all phases of the animal's life. This would require treatment of the pregnant mother and continuing exposure of offspring during infancy and adult life. Such a "true lifetime" exposure is recommended by the FDA (1971) for the carcinogenesis testing of food additives and pesticides. The *in utero* treatment has the added feature that such an exposure might also detect teratogenic properties.

Statistical Considerations

The statistician, like the toxicologist and the pathologist, has a most important role in the design and interpretation of the test. In designing bioassay studies careful attention to proper biometrical aspects are necessary to assure the maximum reliability of the test and integrity of the results available for analysis. Design aspects of particular importance are: determination of experimental groups, number of animals per group, and randomization procedures to use in assigning animals to test groups.

In testing a chemical it is necessary to limit the experiment to the study of a single variable, exposure to the test agent. In order to analyze for an effect, spontaneous disease, tumors, and survival of the treated groups may need to be statistically compared with those normally encountered in the test animals. Even with inbred strains the incidence of spontaneous diseases and tumors and their latency period can vary and may be influenced by such factors as diet, temperature, caging conditions, and vehicle (if used). It is therefore mandatory that appropriate comparison or matched control groups accompany the treated groups in the experiment. Except for the specific treatment, all experimental groups should be identical in every respect, including source and conditions of maintenance. Matched controls should receive a vehicle if one is used in treatment groups.

In addition to the appropriate matched controls located in the same room as the test groups, it is also desirable to have a group of untreated animals in a room free of any chemical testing where an inadvertent exposure to a test agent is assured. These untreated controls may suggest effects in the matched controls caused by the vehicle or any low-level contamination in the animal room. Positive controls may also be desirable to assess sensitivity of the test animals to a carcinogenic stimulus. This issue is considered further in the next section.

All animals for a bioassay test should be from the same animal shipment, assigned to the experimental groups by established randomization procedures, and maintained identically except for exposure of treated groups to the test chemical. A table of random numbers is used by some investigators, while others have used weight distribution as the main criterion. The NCI guidelines describe a method of assigning animals to the appropriate groups by use of a random number scheme in which weight distribution is also considered. Regardless of the design of an experiment, randomization of animals is necessary to ensure that unintentional biases are not introduced into the experiment.

The number of animals to be used in the experimental and control groups should be that necessary to yield statistically reliable results. In arriving at the sample size, one should have an estimate of the expected incidence of spontaneous tumors in the control group and a decision as to the desired sensitivity of the test. Another important factor is the percentage of animals that are expected to survive to tumor-bearing age (sometimes referred to as "effective number of animals").

As illustrated by Table 13, both the experimental group size and the spontaneous tumor incidence in the controls greatly influence the number of

TABLE 13   Incidence of Tumors in Treated Groups Required for
Significance ($p = 0.05$) Depending on Experimental
Group Size and Spontaneous Tumors in Controls[a]

Incidence of tumors in controls (%)	No. of animals per group[b]				
	10	25	50	75	100
0	50%	20%	12%	8%	6%
10	70	40	28	24	21
20	80	52	40	36	34
30	90	64	52	47	45
40	100	72	62	58	55

[a]Calculations based on tabulations of Mainland and Murray (1952).
[b]Controls and treated groups of same size.

tumors required in the treated groups for a significant result of $p = 0.05$. In practice, one usually cannot predict in advance whether tumors that may be induced will be a generalized elevation of total tumors or will be of a cell type practically nonexistent in the controls. Therefore, for practical purposes most carcinogenicity testing protocols, including the NCI's, recommend 50 animals per group. With a group size of 50, 28% of the experimental group must have tumors for statistical significance ($p = 0.05$) when 10% of the controls also possess the same tumor(s). In situations where a very rare tumor is induced (0% in controls), only 12% incidence is needed for significance at the $p = 0.05$ level.

A factor that affects the ability of a bioassay to detect carcinogenicity is the relative strength of the carcinogenic activity. As simplistically illustrated in Fig. 16, chemicals can vary greatly in carcinogenic potency. Using 50 animals, an exposure to a few parts per million of chemical A could detect activity, whereas with chemical B the exposure required must be several thousand parts per million. Increasing the group size to 100 might allow detection of chemical B at 100 ppm. A weak carcinogenic agent such as chemical B could be responsible for a 1-2% incidence of cancer in humans and escape detection by the current bioassay test. As pointed out by Friedman (1969), an effect that occurs in only 1% of the test animals will be entirely missed 37% of the time even if 100 animals are used in each test and with a 0% incidence in the controls. Any spontaneous incidence in controls further diminishes the capability of detection.

POSITIVE CONTROLS

Positive controls or "carcinogen controls" are animals treated with a chemical of known or established carcinogenic activity. They are included in a carcinogenesis testing program and administered under standard test conditions—species, strain, sex, age, and husbandry—used for testing chemicals of unknown activity.

The inclusion of positive or carcinogen controls is recommended because it (1) establishes that the test animals are capable of responding in a predictable manner to a known carcinogenic stimulus, which provides a degree of confidence that tests with unknown agents can be acceptable as valid experiments; (2) provides for a check of the instability of the animal model (i.e., genetic drift); (3) reveals inadvertent inclusion of extraneous factors that might influence the outcome of carcinogenicity tests, such as chemical and biological contaminants that might affect the enzyme systems or metabolism of the test animal; (4) monitors technical procedures in use, such as diet mixture, treatment administration, animal care and monitoring, pathology, data handling, and chemical safety; and (5) allows comparability of research results within as well as between laboratories and between *in vivo* and *in vitro* test procedures. Conclusions as to the relative sensitivity of different bioassay systems to a specific class of chemicals might be evaluated by testing with equal dose levels.

Inclusion of positive controls cannot be recommended for each unknown chemical to be tested. Rather, their application seems more appropriately related to the testing of a series of compounds. They could be spaced in such a manner that a new positive control would be included in the testing program periodically—for example, every 12–24 months or when drastic modifications are made in the test procedures, such as a change in test animal or diet.

In testing of drugs for carcinogenicity, the World Health Organization (1969) recommends inclusion of a positive control group when testing a drug similar in structure or biological effect to a known carcinogen; however it considers a positive control superfluous when the carcinogen susceptibility of the test animals is known. The Panel on Positive Controls in the Conference on the Carcinogenicity Testing of New Drugs (Weisburger, 1974) felt that periodic in-house tests with select standard carcinogens should be conducted.

The failure of a positive control to give an expected response should cast suspicion on the validity of other simultaneous tests of unknown chemicals where no carcinogenicity was evident. The selection of the positive control ideally should be on the basis of chemical similarity to the agents of unknown carcinogenic properties under test. However, in a large testing program where chemicals having diverse structures and biological activities are being tested, proper consideration of structure may not be possible. For large-scale testing programs of orally administered agents, the most common carcinogens used appear to be N-2-fluorenylacetamide (2-AAF), diethylnitrosamine (DEN), safrole, and 3-aminotriazole. The target organs for 3-aminotriazole are primarily the thyroid and liver, whereas the other three are primarily liver carcinogens. DEN and 2-AAF are potent carcinogens, whereas safrole and 3-aminotriazole are less potent. Among other compounds used are uracil mustard, nitrogen mustard, urethane, 7,12-dimethylbenz[a]anthracene, N-dimethylstilbenamine, and N-methyl-4-diethylaminoazobenzene and N-methyl-N'-nitro-n-nitrosoquanidine.

It should be recognized that there are species/strain differences in the response to some of the positive controls. Thus, the sensitivity of the animals in use should be considered in selecting the positive control.

While the NCI guidelines recommend only a single dose level, it may be desirable to use several dose levels in order to equate the response to procedural design aspects, such as concentration, method of administration, and length of exposure. While a low dose might mimic the weak response of unknown materials, the higher dose could serve to quickly verify the consistency and sensitivity of response of the test systems or test animals. The use of multiple dose levels of a positive control might also allow for the semiquantitative interpretation of results with the unknown compounds.

The number of animals required for positive controls, especially at high dose levels, may be less (20-25) than in regular test groups for some strong carcinogens such as 2-AAF and DEN.

Regardless of the positive control used, precautions should be taken to minimize exposure of personnel or other animals in the laboratory. The use and handling of the positive control chemical should be carefully monitored and conform to proper safety precautions.

CHEMICAL HAZARDS AND IMPLICATIONS TO CARCINOGEN TESTING PROGRAM

The Carcinogenesis Bioassay Program tests chemicals to determine their potential for oncogenic activity. Hence for the majority of the time when they are being prepared and administered to animals their carcinogenic hazard is not known. Once the results of a test are realized it is too late to undo any exposure of laboratory personnel or environmental contamination that may have occurred. It is true that the great majority of tests are negative; however, one must use routine safety measures in order to protect against the "surprises" that can occur.

Laboratory operations must comply with the intent of the Occupational Safety and Health Act, which mandates that employers have a general duty to provide a safe and healthful workplace for employees. Threshold limit values (TLVs) or OSHA standards for permissible exposure levels do not exist for most chemicals on bioassay tests.

High levels of exposure are given to animals as a feature of the experiment's design. Thus, a bioassay test facility must be viewed as a potentially hazardous work area. Legal and moral reasons dictate that personnel exposures be minimized as much as possible. The key to chemical safety is "containment."

Total containment, while difficult, can be achieved, albeit at astronomical cost. Containment safety cabinets similar to those developed for highly infectious agents could be used for treatment of animals with chemicals. The cost for such an operation with chemicals would be much greater as contamination procedures are usually more difficult than with biological agents.

As the great majority of chemicals are not a significant hazard, such stringent measures are considered infeasible and an unwarranted expense for routine tests. A reasonable compromise is to impose safety measures in the form of "effective containment" and good chemical safety work practices. Essential aspects of safety are: (1) adequately designed and operated facilities; (2) effective protective clothing and equipment; (3) proper education and attitude in chemical safety measures; and (4) frequent and effective safety monitoring.

Facilities should be designed to contain the chemical at all points in the laboratory operation, thus minimizing the possibility of exposure. Movement of air, personnel, and equipment should be such that a chemical will not be spread from one room to another or to the rest of the facility or the outside environment should a spill occur.

In the bioassay laboratory the area of greatest potential hazard is in the chemical preparation or diet mixing room. Improper ventilation or spill at that point could result in a high concentration in the room and correspondingly high exposure to personnel. Strict controls are essential, including the use of ventilated safety cabinets for weighing and mixing processes. For large bioassay operations and in the handling of highly toxic materials, fully contained and ventilated safety suits are recommended. Figures 18 and 19 illustrate safety equipment in use in a maximum security chemical preparation laboratory.

Prepared diet mixtures should be stored in a safe and well-ventilated area. It is preferable but not always practical to add the diet mix to the

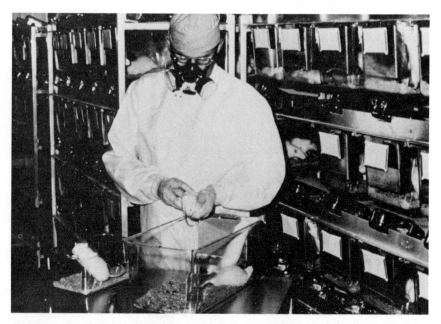

FIGURE 18 Technician conducting routine clinical examination of rats. Activated charcoal respirators and protective clothing are used in animal rooms as safety measures (FCRC).

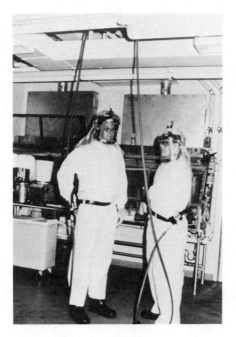

FIGURE 19 Fully contained safety suits are used in the mixing area for preparation of diet/chemical mixtures (FCRC).

animal cages or to dose animals with volatile chemicals under an exhaust hood to prevent exposure of technicians to aerosols or vapors.

Fully contained (filtered) caging systems help to confine the chemical and prevent contamination of the animal room. Even with these precautions workers should be protected with appropriate laboratory clothing, gloves, and masks to prevent inhalation of dusts or vapors that are likely to be present even with use of totally enclosed cages (Fig. 20). No eating or smoking should be permitted, and all personnel should thoroughly shower when leaving the facility. In the interest of technician safety, animals are taken off compound 1 wk prior to sacrifice. Adequate measures should be enforced for the disposal of refuse, animal carcasses, unused feed, soiled bedding, etc. in order to minimize exposure to other workers and the environment. Wherever possible, bagging and incineration of combustible chemical refuse is recommended.

Concern is often expressed regarding positive control or known carcinogens as their use might involve an unnecessary exposure of laboratory personnel. As indicated earlier, positive controls may be a desirable experimental design feature. Their inclusion should be limited to only that essential to meet the experimental needs. Laboratory personnel are subject to exposure

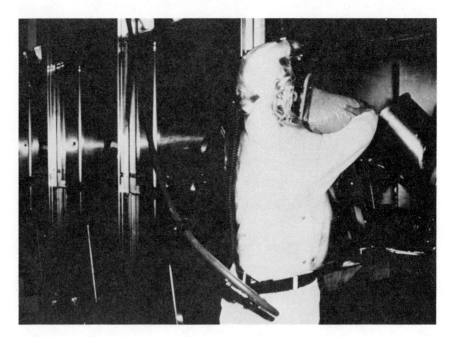

FIGURE 20   In addition to having technicians wear fully contained safety suits, feed
blenders are enclosed in ventilated hoods (FCRC).

to a known carcinogen, and unless an employer shows that he is using all reasonable measures to protect his employees, special legal issues could arise. Certain chemicals are regulated by the OSHA, and while laboratories may be exempt from the standards at this time, it would seem prudent and proper to adhere to the requirements as best possible.

REPORTING AND INTERPRETATION OF TEST RESULTS

One of the most perplexing problems confronting scientists in evaluating carcinogenicity testing results is inadequate documentation of the tests. The usual methods of publication in scientific journals or conference proceedings do not permit presenting the details of experimental conditions or observations made on each animal included in the test. It is often difficult to evaluate the significance of the findings and the limitations and completeness of the test. As a result, regulatory scientists often must rely solely on the investigators' conclusions. In many cases, current editorial practice precludes the presentation of negative results. Yet these are important results that should be known not only to provide a data base to estimate safety of the compound but also to prevent unnecessary duplication of testing.

Considering the cost to conduct bioassay tests and the potential for important public decisions regarding the use of the chemical tested, complete and accurate reporting is an essential element of carcinogenicity testing. In the course of conducting a bioassay test, the investigator collects a large mass of data that are never published and for all practical purposes are lost to the scientific community.

It is important in the initial planning for a carcinogenicity test that one determine in advance the data elements to be collected, their ultimate use in evaluating the experiment, and the details to be published. Because of the importance and scope of the effort, a plan for the collection of information should be devised before the start of the carcinogenesis test. As a minimum, the information recommended by the International Union Against Cancer (Berenblum, 1969) should be collected and available for review and presentation at the end of the study. This includes detailed information on the chemicals, preparations, animals, experimental methods, clinical and pathologic findings, and observations.

Methods of Data Collection

With the advent of computer technology, a gradual transition from manual methods of data recording to automatic data processing (ADP) systems has taken place. The need for and extent of ADP systems is predicated primarily on the size of the carcinogenicity testing program. For small operations manually maintained logbooks may represent the most practical approach. The key to a successful logbook system is ease, accuracy, and completeness in recording and retrieving data.

When dealing with many studies and large numbers of animals, manually maintained logbooks can become bulky and difficult to manage. To prepare reports necessitates the extraction, review, consolidation, and tabulation of large amounts of data from the logbooks. The enormity and time-consuming nature of such hand operations have been overcome to a great extent by the use of ADP techniques.

Several major biological research centers have ADP systems in use. Two of the most recent and perhaps most extensive systems for collecting and retrieving toxicology and carcinogenicity data have been developed by the NCI and the National Center for Toxicological Research (NCTR). The systems vary considerably in approach due to the differences in their testing programs. Whereas the NCI Carcinogenesis Bioassay Program involves testing of many chemicals in a network of laboratories throughout the United States, with variations in the size and sophistication of the operations, the NCTR program is currently an in-house operation with data generated on fewer chemicals under essentially comparable conditions. While both systems can be used for management and reporting, emphasis in the NCI system is directed more toward sophisticated data collection, analysis, and reporting, while the NCTR system has superior capability in "real-time" management of the ongoing experiments. Thus, the data systems requirements have been tailored in somewhat different directions.

The NCI ADP system, known as the Carcinogenesis Bioassay Data System (Linhart et al., 1974), is used primarily by the NCI Carcinogenesis Bioassay Program to collect, retrieve, tabulate, analyze, and report bioassay test data. It also serves to manage and monitor the status and progress of individual bioassay studies as well as the total effort of the Bioassay Program. Data are usually input through a series of forms prepared by the bioassay contractors and submitted to the NCI, where they are processed for entry into a computer. In some cases, data input is by data terminals in the laboratory providing direct entry to the CBDS or automatically punched tapes or cards. Because of their cost the direct entry methods cannot be employed universally in the program at this time. The pathology results for each animal are submitted on data sheets and coded by using the systematized nomenclature of pathology (SNOP) (Committee on Nomenclature and Classification of Disease, 1965). Essentially all of the information recommended by the UICC (Berenblum, 1969) are collected. Data output is provided by monthly monitoring or status reports, or data tables and the analysis of results which can be incorporated into a technical report series now being used by the NCI's Carcinogenesis Program.

In contrast to the NCI's data system the NCTR system minimizes the use of data entry forms by having data input terminals in each animal room. An outstanding feature of the NCTR system is the real-time daily monitoring capability for reviewing clinical data such as changes in body weight fluctuations, disease outbreaks, mortality, etc. The method of recording pathology involves the use of a precoded form with data entered by darkening the appropriate blocks. The form is then optically scanned by machine and data are directly entered into the computer. While this simplifies the pathologist's role in recording his observations, it does not permit the recording of descriptive information regarding the lesions observed.

As can be seen from this discussion, both systems described have their own unique features, advantages, and disadvantages. Any system devised should be developed to address the needs of the laboratory or program, computer equipment available, and fiscal/personnel resources that can be committed. In any event, it should be borne in mind that the usefulness and integrity of the data output is only as good as the accuracy of the data input. It is necessary to monitor data prior to their entry into the system. Computer assistance by error checks and data compatibility features can help to prevent an unacceptable error rate.

Reporting of Bioassay Results

Earlier reporting of carcinogenesis test results primarily through publications in scientific journals or conference proceedings suffered mainly from two serious problems: (1) available space limited or precluded complete documentation of experimental conditions, observations, and individual animal data; and (2) negative results were often not considered of sufficient interest to warrant publication. As a solution to these problems the UICC (Berenblum, 1969) recommended two possible approaches: (1) preparation of detailed reports by the investigators to be kept by them and made available on request, with the ultimate establishment of a central repository system where all such reports could be permanently deposited; or (2) establishment of a periodic publication or "Bulletin of carcinogenesis tests" which could present the complete data in tabular form or summary tables of the data with reference to the availability of the complete data.

After due consideration of the reporting needs, journal policies, U.S. government regulations pertaining to publications, and data available from the Carcinogenesis Bioassay Data System, a carcinogenesis staff study concluded that the most promising solution would be the preparation of technical reports presenting the complete documentation of the testing of each chemical, including the individual animal data, statistical analysis, discussion, and conclusions. These technical reports will be printed and available to the public through the U.S. Government Printing Office. Routine distribution will be to all libraries, government agencies, and cancer research centers with announcements as to the availability made in cancer research journals. The first technical report on a chemical test pertained to the carcinogenesis bioassay of trichloroethylene (NCI, 1976b).

The usual publication in scientific journals is still encouraged. However, even journal articles should provide sufficient details of the experimental design to allow readers to make their own assessment of the thoroughness of the study and validity of conclusions drawn by the author. The technical report series could logically be tied to a regular "Bulletin of carcinogenesis tests" as recommended by the UICC. Due to current government policy such a recurring periodical might best be undertaken by a nongovernment organization.

The results and information on the program should be available to the public, regulatory agencies, industry, and other interested groups as soon as they become available. The release of information is a particularly difficult situation. There is an important ethical issue as to the appropriate time when government officials and the public should be notified of early suspicious results. As illustrated in Fig. 21, a tumorogenic response may be evident as early as 12 months (chemical A). At other times, such as with chemical D, the outcome will not be evident until late or perhaps not until terminal sacrifice of the animals. To delay public notification of highly suspicious preliminary findings until a final detailed report is compiled, reviewed, and published may result in the continued exposure of the public to potentially hazardous compounds.

Caution must be exercised regarding early release of information. An

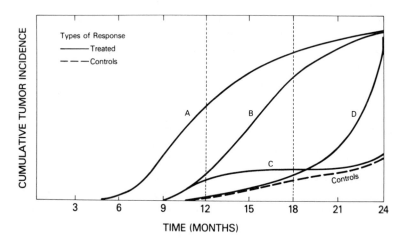

FIGURE 21 Time patterns of tumor response; cumulative tumor incidence is shown on an arbitrary scale (courtesy of U. Saffiotti and N. Page).

early indication of carcinogenicity may not be confirmed when all the results are finally tabulated and analyzed. Such a premature and erroneous release could cause great economic and technological harm to the industry and public. Thus, care must be exercised as to when preliminary reports should be released. In the case of chemicals B and C it would appear that a tumorogenic response is evident for both at 12 months. However, in the case of chemical C this response was not sustained and the end result was not a positive response. The NCI has a procedure to release "Preliminary carcinogenesis reports" simultaneously to the public at large by announcing their availability by press release and in the *Federal Register*. A review of the ethical considerations in preliminary reporting has been presented by Saffiotti and Page (1975).

In addition to reports on individual testing results, activities are under way to review and abstract carcinogenesis test data from literature reports. The single most extensive review is that of the "Survey of compounds which have been tested for carcinogenic activity" (PHS No. 149 Series) published by the National Cancer Institute (U.S. Department of Health, Education, and Welfare, 1941-1973). Surveys covering the literature up to 1971 have been published, while that for 1972-1973 is now in preparation. As of this time, approximately 6,000 chemicals have been tested. Approximately 1,000 of these have shown carcinogenic activity. This survey is useful as a guide to the literature and does not attempt to evaluate the results.

Following up on the PHS No. 149 Series are monographs published by the International Agency for Research on Cancer (WHO) on the evaluation of the carcinogenic risk of chemicals to man (IARC, 1972-1976). With the fiscal and literature support of the NCI, the IARC convenes expert scientific panels to review and evaluate published data on selected chemicals. As the result of their deliberations, monographs are prepared covering the chemical properties, production, use, occurrence, animal research results, observations in humans, conclusions as to carcinogenicity, and an extensive reference list. As of July, 1976, ten monographs covering 272 agents have been published.

Evaluation and Interpretation of Results

The objective of an initial carcinogenicity bioassay screening test is to determine an agent's potential for carcinogenic activity in an animal system. It is not intended to provide data on which to predict, with any degree of certainty, the relative hazard to humans.

Considerations in the extrapolation of animal test results to predict effects in humans are indeed extensive and beyond the scope of this chapter. Of obvious concern, however, are the required extrapolations from high to low doses within the animal models and from animal species to humans. Before considering possible implications for human health, it is necessary that we first carefully evaluate the results to determine the nature of the evidence in the animal tests.

Initially, it is necessary to review the experimental design to determine whether the studies were properly designed and executed. Such an initial assessment will indicate deficiencies that may exist in the data base and that must be considered. Among the initial considerations must be the selection and source of animals, adequacy of randomization procedures, assignment of controls, chemical analysis, and animal husbandry methods.

Following an initial review of experimental design, a very careful examination of clinical records, weight, food consumption, and survival data is necessary to assess the "goodness" of the experiment. The presence of intercurrent infections or environmental factors must be assessed for any possible contributory influence on the experiment.

Having evaluated the adequacy of the design and conduct of the experiment, attention can now be directed to assessing the data to determine whether a carcinogenic response is evident. Interpretation is based on a comparison of the treated and control groups. Among the factors to be considered are: total numbers of tumors, specific tumor type, time of appearance (latency), multiplicity and malignancy of the tumors, and dose-response trends.

In order to assess for these effects, it is obviously necessary that the pathology lesions have been properly recorded with tumors adequately tabulated and categorized. Evaluation is a team effort, with the pathologist, toxicologist, and statistician all reviewing the data.

In many cases, the differences between treated and control animals is so great that the statistician need only conduct simple group comparisons to substantiate an effect. In other cases, especially with weak carcinogens, it may be necessary to analyze for competing risks, time to tumor development,

N. P. Page

system effects, etc. in order to adequately assess for a carcinogenic response. It is essential that the pathologist and toxicologist provide the statistician with guidance as to lesions to consolidate and analyze.

It is necessary to determine whether the observed lesions are treatment-related. Essentially all induced tumors can also occur as spontaneous neoplasms since they originate from the same somatic cells. While the astute pathologist may be certain that there are subtle biological features that, to him, constitute a difference from what is seen in controls, often the analysis must end up with the statistician demonstrating that the differences are real and not the result of normal variability of the controls.

Ultimately it will be necessary to reach one of the following decisions: the test clearly indicates a carcinogenic response, the results are suspicious, there is no evidence of carcinogenicity, or the test is inconclusive in either direction.

Finding a statistically significant increase in all groups of both species makes the decision quite simple. As the number of significant groups decreases, so does the confidence in the final statement. With each test there is a probability of a false decision, either negative or positive.

The sensitivity of the routine test is limited so that a negative experiment cannot be regarded as having shown that no carcinogenic effect exists. As indicated in Table 13, at least 28% of the treated animals in each group of 50 are required for significance ($p = 0.05$) if 10% of the controls possess the tumor(s) of interest. Only when an elevated incidence of 18% is observed will the effect be statistically significant. At the 90% confidence intervals, 2.3 cancers per 1,000 test animals could not be detected, an unacceptable health risk (FDA, 1971). A 1% incidence of cancer in a group of 100 test animals (and 0% spontaneous incidence in controls) would be entirely missed 37% of the time (Friedman, 1969).

While the inability of the bioassay test to detect weak carcinogens is often discussed, very little is said about the possibility of false positives. Consider the spontaneous incidences of tumors for the B6C3F1 mouse and F344 rat as presented in Tables 6 and 7. Assuming barely borderline significance ($p = 0.05$) in a single group of the eight treated groups in a routine bioassay, the probability of a false positive or spurious effect could be 0.06–0.09 for mice and 0.17–0.23 for rats (Fears et al., 1976). The probability of a false positive if both doses of one sex and species are barely significant and the other six groups are negative drops to less than 0.025. Obviously, the probability of a false positive becomes even more remote as more groups show an effect. These probabilities of false positives further disappear if the statistical significance becomes very high, as where there are very great differences in tumor incidence between the treated and control groups.

From the biological viewpoint, a barely significant increase of a common tumor type in a single group could hardly justify making a positive statement. In practice, the usual response is to see effects in several groups of one species or in both species. Thus, the issue of statistical false positives is one limited to unusual situations.

While there is a possibility of statistical false negatives or positives, there are certain biological aspects that might even be of more concern and influence the interpretation of the data. If dose levels are excessive, the toxic effects of the chemical might result in early lethality that could mask a carcinogenic response and result in a false negative. On the other hand, some unrealistic positive conclusions might result from unusual metabolic changes occurring at high doses, which are not typical of those seen at the lower levels.

In assessing the overall meaning of the experiment all aspects of the study, including design, conduct, and data evaluation, must be assessed in reaching a conclusion as to carcinogenicity.

CONCLUSIONS—RESEARCH NEEDS

Among the major needs in a carcinogenicity bioassay of environmental chemicals are: reliable short-term screening tests, improved and definitive *in vivo* animal tests, comprehensive and accurate reporting, and better methods for extrapolating animal test results to humans.

Considerable effort is under way throughout the world to develop short-term, inexpensive, reliable screening tests that can be used as predictors of carcinogenicity. Indeed, tests having a variety of different end points have been exploited, including: accelerated tumor formation, chromosomal aberrations, mutagenesis, DNA repair synthesis, teratogenesis, *in vitro* cell transformation, reaction with nucleic acids, and cytological alterations. Stoltz et. al. (1974) have reviewed the numerous short-term tests and feel that the most promising are those involving mutagenesis, DNA repair synthesis, and *in vitro* cell transformation. The results of a recent international workshop on screening tests (IARC, 1976) would seem to support their conclusions.

Among the *in vitro* tests, perhaps those developed by Ames and McCann (Ames et al., 1973a, 1973b; McCann et al., 1975, 1976) have gained the widest popularity. The Ames test consists of subjecting mutant tester strains of *Salmonella thyphimurium* to minute quantities of a test compound. Strains were selected for their sensitivity and specificity in being reverted back to prototrophy by mutants. A positive result is indicated by growth of revertent bacteria around the site of the chemical. The addition of microsomal enzymes of rat (or human) liver extends the sensitivity of the system to detect a wide variety of carcinogens that require enzymatic activation. Among these are aflatoxin, benzo[a]pyrene, and 2-acetylaminofluorene. The quantity of chemical necessary for detection is so small that mutagenic metabolites have been detected in urine samples (Durston and Ames, 1974). Obvious advantages of this system are low cost, quick testing, and sensitivity to minute quantities of the chemical.

In order for *in vitro* mutagenicity tests to be accepted as screening tests for carcinogens, they must be reliable with a low percentage of false positives and false negatives. While great strides have been made in developing and evaluating these short-term tests, they have yet to be proved sufficiently reliable to replace long-term animal tests. However, they show promise of being developed to the point of screening for candidates for the long-term tests. In addition, activity in the short-term tests (especially mutagenicity) can be used to further substantiate the significance of carcinogenic activity in the animal test.

It is likely that standard long-term bioassays will continue to represent the definitive test for carcinogenicity in the foreseeable future. As such we must recognize their limitations, seek to improve their reliability and useful-ness, and devise cost-savings methods where possible. Much has been done in the past couple of years to improve the standard bioassays. However, improvements are still needed to provide for: a defined, contaminant-free diet; reducing the pathology workload without affecting the ability to detect small, important lesions; use of lower dose level(s) to allow for an assessment of dose reponse and altered physiology; and comparative/correlative metabolism studies.

Carcinogenesis test results have a major impact on societal decisions concerning the use of important chemicals. Thus it is essential that the tests and their results be reported completely and accurately. Several government and industrial laboratories are now issuing comprehensive reports similar to the NCI technical reports. These follow in general the recommendations of the UICC (Berenblum, 1969). Such detailed reporting of important carcinogenicity tests should be encouraged on an international basis. In the interest of public health the announcement of test results should be made at the earliest possible time. The mechanism of issuing alerts or preliminary reports has considerable merit and should be encouraged so long as the results are clearly definitive and made available to all affected parties at the same time.

Animal bioassays are conducted in order to predict possible hazard to humans. As yet there is no simple method to extrapolate from high doses to low ones and from animal species to humans. Understanding the basic mechanisms of the carcinogenic response and species differences in the pharmacokinetics and metabolism of the chemical tested would be of obvious benefit in assessing human risk. Only through well-designed and well-conducted tests, coupled with astute scientific evaluation and interpretation, can carcinogenicity bioassays be exploited to their full potential in protecting the public's health.

REFERENCES

Abrams, W. B., Zbinden, G. and Bagdon, R. 1965. Investigative methods in clinical toxicology. *J. New Drugs* 5:199–207.

Ad Hoc Committee on the Evaluation of Low Levels of Environmental Chemical Carcinogens. 1971. *Evaluation of environmental carcinogens.* Report to the Surgeon General (NIH-77762). Washington, D.C.: Department of Health, Education, and Welfare.

Ames, B. N., Lee, F. D. and Durston, W. E. 1973a. An improved bacterial test system for the detection and classification of mutagens and carcinogens. *Proc. Natl. Acad. Sci. U.S.A.* 70:782–786.

Ames, B. N., Durston, W. E., Yamasaki, E. and Lee, F. D. 1973b. Carcinogens are mutagens: A simple test system combining liver homogenates for activation and bacteria for detection. *Proc. Natl. Acad. Sci. U.S.A.* 70:2281–2285.

Arcos, J. C., Argus, M. F. and Wolf, G. 1968. In *Chemical induction of cancer,* vol. 1, pp. 303–463. New York: Academic Press.

Arrayo, E. R. and Holcomb, J. 1965. Structural studies of an active principle from Croton tiglium L. *J. Med. Chem.* 8:672–675.

Atomic Energy Commission. 1970a. *Inhalation carcinogenesis,* eds. M. G. Hanna, P. Nettesheim, and J. R. Gilbert. AEC Symp. Ser. No. 18.

Atomic Energy Commission. 1970b. *Morphology of experimental respiratory carcinogenesis,* eds. P. Nettesheim, M. G. Hanna, and J. W. Deatherage. AEC Symp. Ser. No. 21.

Atomic Energy Commission. 1973. *Radionuclide carcinogenesis,* eds. C. Sanders, R. Busch, J. Ballou, and D. Mahlum. AEC Symp. Ser. No. 29.

Benitz, K. F. 1970. Measurements on chronic toxicity. In *Methods in toxicology,* ed. G. E. Paget, pp. 82–131. Oxford: Blackwell.

Berenblum, I. 1969. *Carcinogenicity testing.* UICC Tech. Rep. Ser., vol. 2. Geneva, Switzerland.

Bock, F. G. and Burns, R. 1963. Tumor-promoting properties of anthralin (1,8,9-anthratriol). *J. Natl. Cancer Inst.* 30:393–400.

Boutwell, R. K. 1964. Some biological aspects of skin carcinogenesis. *Progr. Exp. Tumor Res.* 4:207–250.

Boyland, F. 1969. The correlation of experimental carcinogenesis and cancer in man. *Progr. Exp. Tumor Res.* 11:222–234.

Burchfield, H. P., Storrs, E. E. and Kraybill, H. F. 1974. In *Pesticides, environmental quality and safety,* suppl. vol. 3, eds. F. Coulston and F. Korte. Stuttgart: George Thieme.

Butler, W. H. 1971. Pathology of liver cancer in experimental animals. In *Liver cancer.* IARC Sci. Publ. No. 1, pp. 30–41.

Canada, Ministry of Health and Welfare. 1973. *The testing of chemicals for carcinogenicity, mutagenicity, and teratogenicity.*

Canadian Council on Animal Care. 1973. *Care of experimental animals, a guide for Canada.*

Cantarow, A., Klein, M. and Greenfield, R. 1969. Survey of need for support of research in chemical carcinogenesis. Report to the National Advisory Cancer Council from the Discussion Group on Chemical Carcinogenesis.

Clayson, D. B. 1962. *Chemical carcinogenesis,* pp. 55–100. London: Little, Brown.

Committee on Nomenclature and Classification of Disease. 1965. *Systematized nomenclature of pathology.* Chicago: College of American Pathologists.

Creech, J. L., Jr. and Makk, L. 1975. Liver disease among polyvinyl chloride production workers. *Ann. N.Y. Acad. Sci.* 246:88–99.

Druckrey, H. 1973. Chemical structure and action in transplacental carcinogenesis and teratogenesis. In *Transplacental carcinogenesis,* eds. L. Tomatis, U. Mohr, and W. Davis. IARC Sci. Publ. No. 4, pp. 44–58.

Dunnett, C. W. 1955. A multiple comparison procedure for comparing several treatments with a control. *J. Am. Stat. Assoc.* 50:1096–1121.

Durston, W. E. and Ames, B. N. 1974. A simple method for the detection of mutagens in urine: Studies with the carcinogen 2-acetylaminofluorene. *Proc. Natl. Acad. Sci. U.S.A.* 71:737–741.

Fare, G. 1966. Rat skin carcinogenesis by topical applications of some azo dyes. *Cancer Res.* 26:2406–2408.

Fears, T. R. and Schneiderman, M. A. 1974. Pathologic evaluation and the blind technique. *Science* 183:1144–1145.

Fears, T. R., Tarone, R. E. and Chu, K. C. 1976. Error rates for carcinogenicity screens. *Cancer Res.* Submitted.

Food and Drug Administration Advisory Committee on Protocols for Safety Evaluation. 1971. Panel on Carcinogenesis report on cancer testing in the safety of food additives and pesticides. *Toxicol. Appl. Pharmacol.* 20:419–438.

Food and Drug Administration/Pharmaceutical Manufacturers Association. 1973. *Preclinical testing of drugs for carcinogenic potential.* Joint FDA/PMA Subcommittee Report.

Friedman, L. 1969. Symposium on the evaluation of the safety of food additives and chemical residues: III. The role of the laboratory animal study of intermediate duration for evaluation of safety. *Toxicol. Appl. Pharmacol.* 16:498–506.

Friedman, L. 1974. Dose selection and administration. In *Carcinogenesis testing of chemicals,* ed. L. Golberg, pp. 21–22. Cleveland, Ohio: CRC Press.

Golberg, L., ed. 1974. *Carcinogenesis testing of chemicals.* Cleveland, Ohio: CRC Press.

Graffi, A., Hoffman, F. and Schutt, M. 1967. N-methyl-N-nitrosourea as a strong topical carcinogen when painted on skin of rodents. *Nature (Lond.)* 214:611.

Grantham, P. H., Mohan, L. C. and Weisburger, E. K. 1976. Metabolism of N-2-fluorenylacetamide in X/GF mice: Lack of correlation between biochemical interaction and carcinogenicity. *J. Natl. Cancer Inst.* 56:649–651.

Grasso, P. 1974. *Neoplastic and nodular hyperplasia in mouse liver. Strain differences in natural incidence and response to carcinogens,* pp. 210–240. Surrey, England: British Industrial Biological Research Association.

Grasso, P. and Crampton, R. F. 1972. The value of the mouse in carcinogenicity testing. *Food Cosmet. Toxicol.* 10:418.

Hecker, E., Bresch, H. and V. Szczepanski, C. 1964. *Angew. Chem.* 76:225.

Hefner, R. E., Jr., Watanabe, P. G. and Gehring, P. J. 1975. Studies of the fate of inhaled vinyl chloride monomers (VCM) in rats. *Ann. N.Y. Acad. Sci.* 246:135–148.

Herbst, A. L., Poskanzer, D. C., Robboy, S. J., et al. 1975. Prenatal exposure to stilbestrol. A prospective comparison of exposed female offspring with unexposed controls. *N. Engl. J. Med.* 292:334–339.

Higginson, J. and Muir, C. S. 1973. In *Cancer medicine,* eds. J. F. Holland and E. Frei III, pp. 241–306. Philadelphia: Lea & Febiger.

Homburger, F. 1972. The use of the Syrian golden hamster in chronic toxicity testing. *Progr. Exp. Tumor Res.* 16:152–175.

Horton, A. W., Bingham, E. L., Burton, M. J. G. and Tye, R. 1965.

Carcinogenesis of the skin. III. The contribution of elemental sulfur and of organic sulfur compounds. *Cancer Res.* 25:1759.

Hueper, W. C. and Conway, W. D. 1964. In *Chemical carcinogenesis and cancers,* pp. 403–604. Springfield, Ill.: Thomas.

Hunziker, J. 1975. A new feeder system for quantitating actual toxicant consumption by mice during feeding studies. *J. Lab. Anim. Sci.* 25(1):85–87.

Innes, J. R. M., Ulland, B. M., Valerio, M. G., Petrucelli, L., Fishbein, L., Hart, E. R., Pallotta, A. J., Bates, R. R., Falk, H. L., Gart, J. J., Klein, M., Mitchell, I. and Peters, J. 1969. Bioassay of pesticides and industrial chemicals for tumorigenicity in mice: A preliminary note. *J. Natl. Cancer Inst.* 42:1101–1114.

Institute of Laboratory Animal Resources. 1969. *Rodents: Standards and guidelines for the breeding, care, and management of laboratory animals.* Washington, D.C.: National Academy of Sciences.

Institute of Laboratory Animal Resources. 1974. *Guide for the care and use of laboratory animals.* DHEW Publ. No. (NIH) 74-23.

Institute of Laboratory Animal Resources. 1976. Long-term holding of laboratory rodents. *ILAR News* 19(4).

International Agency for Research on Cancer. 1972–1976. *IARC monographs on the evaluation of carcinogenic risk of chemicals to man.* Vol. 1 (1972); vol. 2 (1973), *Some inorganic and organometallic compounds;* vol. 3 (1973), *Some polycyclic aromatic hydrocarbons and heterocyclic compounds;* vol. 4 (1974), *Some aromatic amines, hydrazine and related substances, N-nitroso compounds and miscellaneous alkylating agents;* vol. 5 (1974), *Some organochlorine pesticides;* vol. 6 (1974), *Sex hormones;* vol. 7 (1974), *Some anti-thyroid and related substances, nitrofurans and industrial chemicals;* vol. 8 (1975), *Some aromatic azo dyes;* vol. 9 (1975), *Some aziridines, N-, S-, and O-mustards and selenium;* vol. 10 (1976), *Naturally occurring substances;* vol. 11 (in press), *Epoxides and miscellaneous industrial chemicals.* Lyons, France: World Health Organization.

International Agency for Research on Cancer. 1976. *Screening tests in chemical carcinogenesis,* eds. R. Montesano, H. Bartsch, and L. Tomatis. IARC Sci. Publ. No. 12.

Ivankovic, S. 1973. Experimental prenatal carcinogenesis. In *Transplacental carcinogenesis,* eds. L. Tomatis, U. Mohr, and W. Davis. IARC Sci. Publ. No. 4, pp. 92–99.

Karbe, E. and Park, J. F., eds. 1974. *Experimental lung cancer: Carcinogenesis and bioassays.* New York: Springer-Verlag.

Kennaway, E. L. 1955. The identification of a carcinogenic compound in coal-tar. *Br. Med. J.* 2:749–752.

Klein, M. 1959. Influence of low dose of 2-acetylaminofluorine on liver tumorigenesis in mice. *Proc. Soc. Exp. Biol. Med.* 101:637–638.

Kommineni, V. R. C., Greenblatt, M., Mihailovich, N. and Vesselinovitch, S. D. 1970. The significance of perinatal age periods and doses of urethan on the tumor profile in the MRC rat. *Cancer Res.* 30:2552–2555.

Kraybill, H. F. 1974. Unintentional additives in food. In *Environmental quality and food supply,* eds. P. L. White and D. Robbins, pp. 173–184. New York: Futura.

Kyriazis, A. P. and Vesselinovitch, S. D. 1973. Transplantability and biological behavior of mouse liver tumors induced by ethylnitrosourea. *Cancer Res.* 33:332–338.

Kyriazis, A. P., Koka, M. and Vesselinovitch, S. D. 1974. Metastatic rate of liver tumors induced by diethylnitrosamine in mice. *Cancer Res.* 34:2881–2886.

Laskin, S. and Sellakumar, A. 1974. Models in chemical respiratory carcinogenesis. In *Experimental lung cancer: Carcinogenesis and bioassays,* eds. E. Karbe and J. F. Park. New York: Springer-Verlag.

Linhart, M. S., Cooper, J., Martin, R. L., Page, N. P. and Peters, J. A. 1974. Carcinogenesis bioassay data system. *Comput. Biomed. Res.* 7:230–248.

Magee, P. N. 1970. Tests for carcinogenic potential. In *Methods in toxicology,* ed. G. E. Paget, pp. 158–196. Philadelphia: Davis.

Mainland, D. and Murray, I. M. 1952. Tables for use in fourfold contingency tests. *Science* 116:591–594.

Maltoni, C. and Lefemine, G. 1974. Carcinogenicity to bioassays of vinyl chloride. I. Research plan and early results. *Environ. Res.* 7:387–405.

Martin, M. S., Martin, F., Justrabo, E., Michiels, R., Bastien, H. and Knobel, S. 1974. Susceptibility of inbred rats to gastric and duodenal carcinomas induced by N-methyl-N′-nitro-N-nitrosoguanidine. *J. Natl. Cancer Inst.* 53:837–839.

Matsuyama, M., Suzuki, H., Ito, M., Yamada, S. and Nagayo, T. 1972. Strain differences in carcinogenesis by urethan administration to suckling rats. *Gann* 63:209–215.

McCann, J. and Ames, B. N. 1976. A simple method for detecting environmental carcinogens as mutagens. *Ann. N.Y. Acad. Sci.* 271:5–13.

McCann, J., Spingarn, N. E., Kobori, J. and Ames, B. N. 1975. Detection of carcinogens as mutagens: Bacterial tester strains with R factor plasmids. *Proc. Natl. Acad. Sci. U.S.A.* 72:979–983.

McGee, A. A. 1975. A research program to acquire and analyze information on chemicals that impact on man and his environment. In *Papers on a seminar on early warning systems for toxic substances.* EPA 560/1-75-003, pp. 151–153. Washington, D.C.: Environmental Protection Agency.

Miller, S. A. and Dymsza, H. A. 1963. Artificial feeding of neonatal rats. *Science* 141:517.

Mohr, U. 1973. Effects of diethylnitrosamines on fetal and suckling Syrian golden hamsters. In *Transplacental carcinogenesis,* eds. L. Tomatis and U. Mohr. IARC Scientific Publ. No. 4. Lyon, France: International Agency for Research on Cancer.

Moreland, A. F. 1965. In *Methods of animal experimentation,* ed. W. I. Gay, vol. 1, p. 1. New York: Academic Press.

Mori, K. 1965. Induction of pulmonary and uterine cancers and leukemia in mice by injection of 4-nitroguanoline 1-oxide. *Gann* 56:513.

National Academy of Sciences. 1960. Problems in the evaluation of carcinogenic hazard from use of food additives. Publ. No. 749. *Cancer Res.* 21:429–456, 1961.

National Academy of Sciences. 1972. Committee on Animal Nutrition. *Nutrient requirements of laboratory animals.* Washington, D.C.

National Academy of Sciences. 1975. *Principles for evaluating chemicals in the environment.* Publ. No. ISBN-0-309-02248-7. Washington, D.C.: National Academy of Sciences.

National Cancer Institute Carcinogenesis Technical Report Series No. 1. 1976a. *Guidelines for carcinogen bioassay in small rodents,* J. A. Sontag, N. P. Page, and U. Saffiotti. DHEW Publ. No. (NIH) 76-801.

National Cancer Institute Carcinogenesis Technical Report Series No. 2. 1976b. *Carcinogenesis bioassay of trichloroethylene.* DHEW Publ. No. (NIH) 76-802.

National Cancer Institute Meeting Report. 1975. Report of a workshop on classification of specific hepatocellular lesions in rats. *Cancer Res.* 35:3214-3223.

Nettesheim, P. 1972. Respiratory carcinogenesis studies with the Syrian golden hamster. A Review. *Progr. Exp. Tumor Res.* 16:185-200.

Newberne, P. M. 1974. Report of Discussion Group No. 2, Diets. In *Carcinogenesis Testing of Chemicals,* ed. L. Golberg, pp. 17-20. Cleveland, Ohio: CRC Press.

Odashima, S. 1976. The cooperative development in Japan of methods for screening chemicals for carcinogenicity. In *Screening tests in chemical carcinogenesis,* eds. R. Montesano, H. Bartsch, and L. Tomatis. IARC Sci. Publ. No. 12, pp. 61-79.

Page, N., Chairman. 1976. Report of the Subtask Group on Carcinogen Testing to the Interagency Collaborative Group on Environmental Carcinogenesis.

Passey, R. D. 1922. Experimental soot cancer. *Br. Med. J.* 2:1112-1113.

Pott, P. 1775. Chirurgical works 5, p. 63, London. In *Potter, M., Natl. Cancer Inst. Monogr.* 10:1-13, 1963.

President's Science Advisory Committee. 1973. *Chemicals and health.* Publ. No. (NSF 73-500). Washington, D.C.: Government Printing Office.

Rauscher, F. J. 1973. *New frontiers in cancer: Development of the National Cancer Program Plan (NCPP),* pp. 711-720. Seventh National Cancer Conference Proceedings. Philadelphia: Lippincott.

Rehn, L. 1895. Blasengeschwulste bei Fuchsin-Arbeiten. *Arch. Klin. Chir.* 50:588.

Roe, F. J. C. 1965. Spontaneous tumors in rats and mice. *Food Cosmet. Toxicol.* 3:707.

Roe, F. J. C. and Tucker, M. J. 1974. Recent developments in the design of carcinogenicity tests on laboratory animals. In *Experimental model systems in toxicology and their significance to man, Proc. Eur. Soc. Study Drug Toxic.* 15:171-177.

Rustia, M. and Shubik, P. 1976. Transplacental effects of diethylstilbesterol on the genital tract of hamster offspring. *Cancer Lett.* 1:139-146.

Saffiotti, U. and Page, N. P. 1975. Releasing carcinogenesis test results: Timing and extent of reporting. *Proc. AACR ASCO* 17:208.

Saffiotti, U., Cefis, F. and Karp, L. B. 1968. A method for the experimental induction of bronchogenic carcinoma. *Cancer Res.* 28:104-124.

Sanders, B. J. 1972. *Animal histology procedures.* DHEW Publ. No. (NIH) 72-275.

Setala, K. 1960. Progress in carcinogenesis, tumor-enhancing factors, bio-assay of skin tumor formation. *Progr. Exp. Tumor Res.* 1:225-278.

Severi, L., ed. 1962. *The morphological precursors of cancer.* Perugia, Italy: Division of Cancer Research.

Severi, L., ed. 1966. *Lung tumors in animals, Proceedings of the Third Quadrennial Conference on Cancer, University of Perugia, June, 1965.* Perugia, Italy: Division of Cancer Research.

Shimkin, M. B. 1974. In *Carcinogenesis testing of chemicals,* ed. L. Golberg, p. 15. Cleveland, Ohio: CRC Press.

Shimkin, M. B. 1975. In *Cancer epidemiology and prevention,* ed. D. Shottenfeld, p. 60. Springfield, Ill.: Thomas.

Short, D. J. and Woodnott, D. P., eds. 1969. *The I.A.T. manual of laboratory animal practice and techniques.* Springfield, Ill.: Thomas.

Shubik, P. 1972. The use of the Syrian golden hamster in chronic toxicity testing. *Progr. Exp. Tumor Res.* 16:176–184.

Shubik, P. and Sice, J. 1956. Chemical carcinogenesis as a chronic toxicity test: A review. *Cancer Res.* 16:728–742.

Stoltz, D. R., Poirier, L. A., Irving, C. C., Stich, H. F., Weisburger, J. H. and Grice, H. C. 1974. Evaluation of short-term tests for carcinogenicity. *Toxicol. Appl. Pharmacol.* 29:157–180.

Tomatis, L. 1974. Report of Discussion Group No. 4: Inception and duration of tests. In *Carcinogenesis testing of chemicals,* ed. L. Golberg, pp. 23–27. Cleveland, Ohio: CRC Press.

Tomatis, L., Mohr, U. and Davis, W., eds. 1973a. *Transplacental carcinogenesis.* IARC Sci. Publ. No. 4.

Tomatis, L., Partensky, C. and Montesano, R. 1973b. The predictive value of mouse liver tumour induction in carcinogenicity testing—A literature survey. *Int. J. Cancer* 12:1–20.

U.S. Department of Health, Education, and Welfare. 1941–1973. *Survey of compounds which have been tested for carcinogenic activity.* PHS Publ. No. 149, 1st ed. (1941); 2nd ed. (1951, 1963); suppl. 1 (1957); suppl. 2 (1969); 1961–1967 vol. (1973); 1968–1969 vol. (1971); 1970–1971 vol. (1974); 1971–1973 vol. (in press). Washington, D.C.: Government Printing Office.

Van Duuren, B. L., Arroyo, E. and Orris, L. 1963. The tumor-enhancing and irritant principals from Croton tiglium L. *J. Med. Chem.* 6:616–617.

Vesselinovitch, S. D. 1973. Comparative studies on perinatal carcinogenesis. In *Transplacental carcinogenesis,* eds. L. Tomatis, U. Mohr, and W. Davis. IARC Sci. Publ. No. 4, pp. 14–22.

Vesselinovitch, S. D., Mihailovich, N., Rao, K. V. N. and Itze, L. 1971. Perinatal carcinogenesis by urethan. *Cancer Res.* 31:2143–2147.

Vesselinovitch, S. D., Mihailovich, N., Wogan, G. N., Lombard, L. S. and Rao, K. V. N. 1972. Aflatoxin B1, a hepatocarcinogen in the infant mouse. *Cancer Res.* 32:2289–2291.

Vesselinovitch, S. D., Rao, K. V. N., Mihailovich, N., Rice, J. M. and Lombard, L. S. 1974. Development of broad spectrum of tumors by ethylnitrosourea in mice and the modifying role of age, sex and strain. *Cancer Res.* 34:2530–2538.

Vesselinovitch, S. D., Kyriazis, A. P., Mihailovich, N. and Rao, K. V. N. 1975. Conditions modifying development of tumors in mice at various sites by benzo(a)pyrene. *Cancer Res.* 35:2948–2953.

Viola, P. L. 1970. *Proc. 10th Int. Cancer Congr., Houston.* Abstract 29.

Viola, P. L., Bigotti, A. and Caputo, A. 1971. Oncogenic response of rat skin, lungs and bones to vinyl chloride. *Cancer Res.* 31:516–522.

Weinberger, M. A. 1973. The blind technique. *Science* 181:219–220.

Weisburger, J. H. 1974. Inclusion of positive control compounds. In *Carcinogenesis testing of chemicals,* ed. L. Golberg, pp. 29–34. Cleveland, Ohio: CRC Press.

Weisburger, J. H. and Weisburger, E. K. 1967. Tests for chemical carcinogenesis. In *Methods in cancer research,* ed. H. Busch, vol. 1, pp. 307–398. New York: Academic Press.

Weisburger, J. H., Grantham, P. H., Vanhor, E., Streigbigel, N. H., Rall, D. P. and

Weisburger, E. K. 1964. Activation anu detoxification of N-2-fluorenylacetamide in man. *Cancer Res.* 24:475–479.

Wogan, G. 1969. Metabolism and biochemical effects of aflatoxins. In *Aflatoxin–Scientific background, control, and implications,* ed. L. Boldblatt, pp. 151–186. New York: Academic Press.

World Health Organization. 1961. Evaluation of the carcinogenic hazards of food additives. *WHO Tech. Rep. Ser. 220.*

World Health Organization. 1964. *Prev. Cancer Tech. Rep. Ser.,* p. 276.

World Health Organization. 1969. Principles for the testing and evaluation of drugs for carcinogenicity. *WHO Tech. Rep. Ser. 426.*

World Health Organization. 1974a. Pesticide residues in food. *WHO Tech. Rep. Ser. 545.*

World Health Organization. 1974b. Assessment of the carcinogenicity and mutagenicity of chemicals. *WHO Tech. Rep. Ser. 546.*

Yamagiwa and Ichikawa. 1915. *Mitt. Med. Fak. Tokio* 15:295.

Zbinden, G. 1976. *Progress in toxicology, special topics,* vol. 2, pp. 7–11. New York: Springer-Verlag.

Zulch, K. J. and Mennel, H. D. 1973. Recent results in new models of transplacental carcinogenesis in rats. In *Transplacental carcinogenesis,* eds. L. Tomatis, U. Mohr, and W. Davis. IARC Sci. Publ. No. 4, pp. 29–44.

Chapter 5

ROLE OF ANALYTICAL CHEMISTRY IN CARCINOGENESIS STUDIES

H. P. Burchfield, Eleanor E. Storrs, and E. E. Green
Gulf South Research Institute
New Iberia, Louisiana

INTRODUCTION

Analytical chemistry together with pathology and toxicology plays a key role in carcinogenesis studies. Without it we would still believe that the chimney sweeps of London developed cancer of the scrotum from a nonspecific irritant in soot. We would be unaware that residues of DDT, dieldrin, and other hard pesticides had built up in the environment and were stored in the tissues of most of the world's population. We would not know that some carcinogens are deactivated by metabolic processes while others become activated. It would not have been discovered that some compounds when released into the environment are converted by sunlight, microorganisms, and plants into substances with different physical and toxicological properties.

In conducting carcinogenesis bioassay studies, we would be unable to properly characterize the compounds under test and determine whether carcinogenicity is caused by the principal active ingredient or an impurity. We would have no way of determining whether the desired amount of chemical had been added to experimental diets and whether the chemical in the diet was stable on storage. We would not be able to determine the body burden of chemicals in test animals or demonstrate the presence of metabolites. We could not analyze urine and feces to determine if the animals were being overdosed. Finally, we could not monitor the test environment for the presence of potentially carcinogenic contaminants.

Without analytical chemistry, our knowledge of chemical carcinogenesis would be confined to knowing only that people working in certain industries, eating certain diets, and living in certain areas have an abnormally high incidence of cancer.

Analytical chemistry does not describe cancer at the tissue level, as does pathology. However, it is gradually helping to disclose the events that occur at the molecular level to induce cancer. Without analytical chemistry, the science of chemical epidemiology would not exist.

IDENTIFICATION OF CARCINOGENS IN THE ENVIRONMENT

Analytical chemistry can play several roles in the identification and measurement of carcinogens in the environment. It can be used to identify carcinogens in situations where epidemiology studies have demonstrated a high incidence of cancer. It can be used for the measurement of persistent compounds in the environment and human tissues, which then can be evaluated for carcinogenicity. Finally, when carcinogens have been identified or persistent compounds have been demonstrated to be carcinogenic, analytical methods can be used for monitoring the environment for their presence to determine if hazards exist.

Relating the Incidence of Cancer to Unknown Carcinogens

The chemical epidemiology of cancer began in London in 1775 when Percivall Pott described the occurrence of cancer of the scrotum in English chimney sweeps. Coal was mined in the Midlands and had been introduced in the previous century for heating dwellings. Chimney pots poked into the smoky London skyline much as they do today, and many sweeps were needed to keep the chimneys free of soot. Baths and changes of clothing were infrequent among the working classes of early Imperial Britain, so presumably the "soot wart" described by Pott was caused by continuous long-term exposure to products of the combustion of coal. In Denmark and other countries where chimney sweeps were required to bathe frequently and wear protective clothing, scrotal skin cancer was relatively rare (Butlin, 1892). The first induction of cancer in mice and rabbits by coal tar was achieved by Yamagiwa and Ichikawa (1915, 1918) in Japan; but many workers still believed that it was caused by nonspecific irritation. However, in 1930, Kennaway and Hieger were able to induce cancer with a pure compound, dibenz[a,h]anthracene, and in 1933 Cook et al. isolated the carcinogen benzo[a]pyrene (BaP) from coal tar.

Cook et al. were aided greatly in this effort by the fact that BaP has a characteristic fluorescent spectrum with bands at 400, 418, and 440 nm (Fig. 1). These same bands were common to the tars and mineral oils that produced cancer in industrial workers and experimental animals. The authors made the assumption that these bands were characteristic of the carcinogen, or a substance closely associated with it that was contained in the coal tar. In this they were correct. Therefore, an important technique of analytical chemistry, fluorescence spectroscopy, provided the clue that made it possible to isolate a key compound that was the cause of scrotal cancer in chimney sweeps a century and a half earlier.

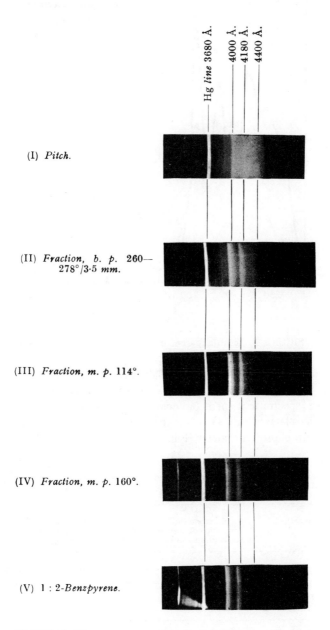

(I) *Pitch.*

(II) *Fraction, b. p. 260—278°/3·5 mm.*

(III) *Fraction, m. p. 114°.*

(IV) *Fraction, m. p. 160°.*

(V) 1 : 2-*Benzpyrene.*

FIGURE 1 Fluorescence spectra of pitch fractions (Cook et al., 1933).

absorption spectrum
excitation spectrum
Detector response
250
300
350
400
(nm)

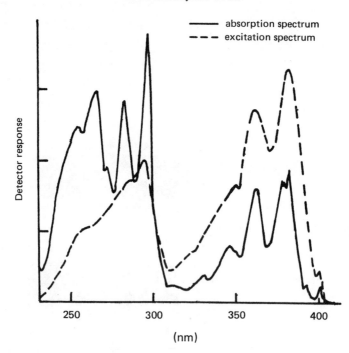

FIGURE 2 Benzo[*a*]pyrene in pentane (Sawicki et al., 1960).

Although the first isolation of BaP was accomplished only 42 yr ago, analytical techniques have advanced remarkably since then. Compare the fluorescence spectra obtained on coal tar fractions and BaP recorded on photographic plates (Fig. 1) with the spectrum of BaP obtained with a modern spectrophotofluorometer (Fig. 2).

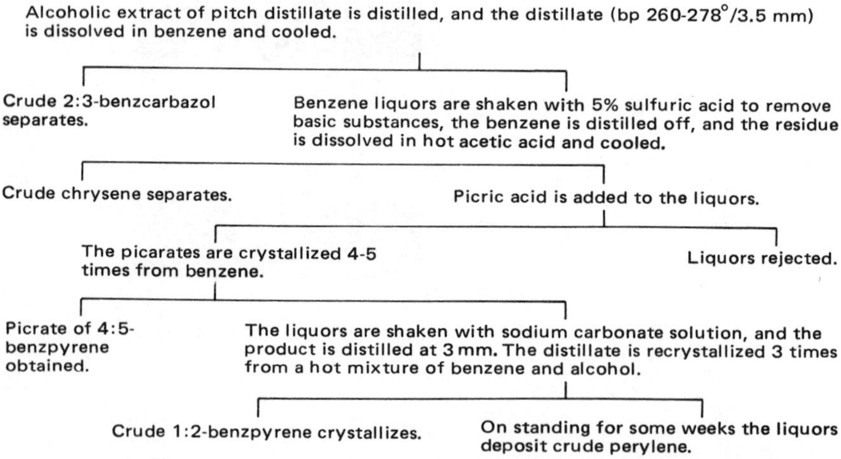

Alcoholic extract of pitch distillate is distilled, and the distillate (bp 260-278°/3.5 mm) is dissolved in benzene and cooled.
Crude 2:3-benzcarbazol separates.
Benzene liquors are shaken with 5% sulfuric acid to remove basic substances, the benzene is distilled off, and the residue is dissolved in hot acetic acid and cooled.
Crude chrysene separates.
Picric acid is added to the liquors.
The picarates are crystallized 4-5 times from benzene.
Liquors rejected.
Picrate of 4:5-benzpyrene obtained.
The liquors are shaken with sodium carbonate solution, and the product is distilled at 3 mm. The distillate is recrystallized 3 times from a hot mixture of benzene and alcohol.
Crude 1:2-benzpyrene crystallizes.
On standing for some weeks the liquors deposit crude perylene.

FIGURE 3 Procedure for isolating BaP from Pitch (Cook et al., 1933).

The amounts of materials used and methods for isolating carcinogens have changed remarkably over the past four decades. Cook et al. (1933) initiated their work with 2 tons of medium soft pitch that would have required carbonization of 25-100 tons of coal. The fractionation procedure they used is outlined in Fig. 3. Extraction and crystallization of picrates of polynuclear arenes (PNA) were the primary techniques employed. Advances in separation techniques have made it possible to isolate these compounds by liquid-solid chromatography, gas-liquid chromatography (glc), and high-pressure liquid chromatography (hplc) using a few grams of tar at most.

Recently, techniques have been developed for the simultaneous analysis of BaP and other PNAs in air particulates by gas chromatography and hplc using a spectrophotofluorometer for a detector (Burchfield et al., 1971, 1974). Particulate matter is stripped from the air by passing it through a fiber glass filter, and only 100 mg of the shredded filter is required for analysis. The PNAs are stripped from the filter with a stream of heated nitrogen and collected on a precolumn (Fig. 4). The PNAs are then separated by glc and measured fluorometrically. Alternately, these compounds can be extracted from the fiber glass filter with solvent using an ultrasonorator to facilitate removal of PNAs and the extract then separated into its components by hplc. BaP can be separated from BeP (benzo[*e*]pyrene) by this latter method, although this pair is very difficult to resolve by gas chromatography (Fig. 5).

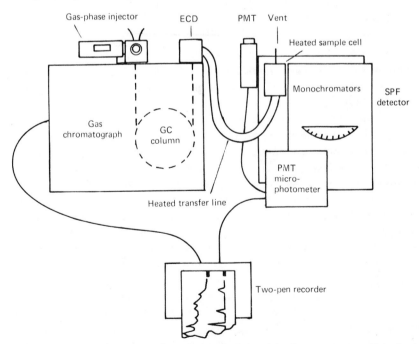

FIGURE 4 Gas-phase injector/gas chromatograph with electron capture detector (ECD) and spectrophotofluorometric (SPF) detector combination (Burchfield et al., 1974).

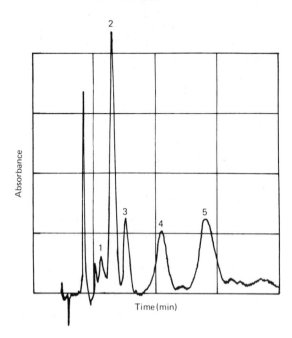

FIGURE 5 High-pressure liquid chromatography of polynuclear aromatic hydrocarbons. (1) Pyrene; (2) triphenylene; (3) benz[a]anthracene; (4) benzo[e]pyrene; (5) benzo[a]pyrene.

However, other pairs of compounds that can be separated by glc are difficult to separate by hplc. Therefore, use of glc and hplc for achieving separations combined with gas-phase and liquid-phase spectrofluorometry for detection can be used to determine nanogram quantities of most mixtures of these compounds isolated from the environment.

Great strides have also been made in methods for the identification of environmental carcinogens. In 1933 the classic method used by Cook et al. for identification was to synthesize the unknown compound by an unequivocal procedure. The synthetic product was mixed with a portion of pure natural product and the melting point of the mixture was determined. If the two compounds were identical, no depression of the melting point was observed. This is still a valid method for confirming identity, but it is tedious since many steps are often required during synthesis and losses are encountered at each step.

Identifications are now made far more rapidly using much smaller amounts of materials through use of commercially available analytical instrumentation. The combined results obtained by infrared spectroscopy, mass spectrometry, and nuclear magnetic resonance spectrometry will usually suffice for structure determination of most organic compounds. Of course, the identities of many PNAs had already been established before advanced analytical instruments became commercially available.

Nevertheless, the newer methods are very useful for monitoring carcinogens in industrial smoke, automobile exhaust, and other environmental samples. Identification techniques are still required since different compounds may sometimes have the same retention volumes when analyzed by gas chromatography, for example. Sometimes they can be resolved by using different column packings and tentatively identified by measuring relative retentions on several columns. However, this is not unequivocal proof of identity. The best confirming evidence now available is use of a mass spectrometer (ms) as a chromatographic detector. As each peak elutes from the column, its mass spectrum can be determined and compared with that of an authentic specimen of carcinogen.

Computer-controlled gas chromatograph mass spectrometers are considerably more efficient for obtaining data and using it for identification of unknown compounds than manually operated ones. Each peak can usually be scanned several times during separation of the components of a mixture by glc. Even if some compounds are not resolved on the chromatographic column, they can be detected selectively in the same peak by mass spectrometry. Thus the mass spectrometer serves as a selective glc detector. If the compound(s) giving rise to the peak is unknown, electron impact is used for fragmentation since production of a large number of ions is useful for structure determination. If the identities of the compounds are known with reasonable certainty and the peak represents a mixture of compounds, chemical ionization is preferred for fragmentation since the $(M + 1)^+$ ion is the principal one produced and assignment of fragments to specific compounds is simplified. All of this data is stored in a computer during chromatography. It can be displayed oscillographically anytime afterward for structural analysis or for comparison with mass spectra of known compounds. Handling of the data by computer is much more rapid and accurate than operator-controlled analysis. The amount of data that can be generated by the ms-glc or more generally ms-gc system is in fact so large that interpretation of results by the individual operator becomes impractical except when a small section of the chromatogram is of interest.

Relating Environmental Contaminants to Cancer

In the case of the PNAs, carcinogenicity was observed first, and identification of the active agents and development of rapid methods for monitoring them in the environment required 200 yr of research. In the case of DDT and other chlorinated hydrocarbon insecticides, events took place in the reverse order within a greatly compressed time span. DDT was first introduced into the United States in the early 1940s and a colorimetric method was developed for its measurement in 1945 (Schechter et al.). It soon became apparent that DDT was a hard pesticide that accumulated in the environment, in the tissues of occupationally exposed workers, and in the tissues of the general population (Edmundson, 1972).

The downfall of DDT and related compounds began when it was found that chlorinated hydrocarbon insecticides could be measured rapidly, selectively, and with very high sensitivity by using a gas chromatograph equipped with a microcoulometer (Coulson et al., 1960) or an electron capture detector (Lovelock and Lipsky, 1960). The former detector could be used to measure these materials at the nanogram level (10^{-9} g) with high selectivity, and the latter at the picogram level (10^{-12} g) but with lower selectivity (Fig. 6). These methods made it possible to selectively measure DDT and its metabolites DDE and DDD in soils, water, and air, and in the tissues of plants, animals, and humans at very low levels. Using the same procedures, a variety of other compounds, including isomers of hexachlorocyclohexane, heptachlor epoxide,

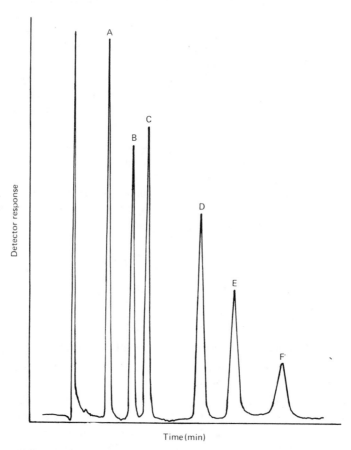

FIGURE 6 Electron capture gas chromatogram of pesticide standards. (A) Lindane; (B) heptachlor; (C) aldrin; (D) DDE; (E) DDD; (F) *p,p*-DDT.

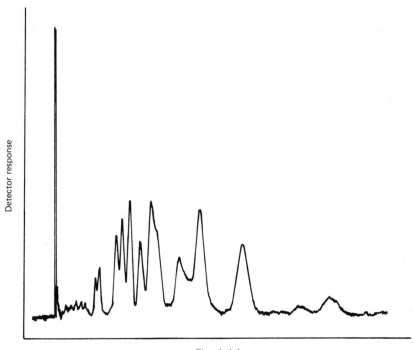

FIGURE 7   Gas chromatogram of PCB mixture (Aroclor 1260) using electron capture detector.

dieldrin, endrin, and other compounds, were also detected. Peaks of unknown origin that appeared on gas chromatograms were later identified as poly-chlorinated biphenyls, which initiated another phase of chemical epidemiology (Fig. 7).

The availability of these powerful analytical techniques made possible numerous studies on the storage of DDT and related compounds in humans. It was found that the general population contained about 10 ppm of DDT and related compounds in adipose tissue (Table 1). The levels of DDT stored in the fat of highly exposed persons was found to be 30–1000 times higher than for the general population (Table 2). Therefore, anxieties arose concerning the effects of storage of these materials on human health. These concerns set in motion a bioassay program to determine whether DDT and other pesticides and industrial chemicals were carcinogenic to mice (Innes et al., 1969). It was found that DDT was tumorigenic to two hybrid strains of mice with a confidence of $p = 0.01$. Based on these findings, the Report of the Secretary's Commission on Pesticides (Mrak Report, 1969) recommended that DDT be used only in applications where there was no suitable alternative.

Thus, analytical chemistry played a key role in the downfall of DDT. This compound is only mildly carcinogenic, and it is very doubtful if purely

TABLE 1   DDT and DDE Content of Body Fat of General Population
in the United States[a]

Year measured	No. of samples	DDT (ppm)	DDE (ppm)	Total as DDT (ppm)
1963	28	2.4	4.3	6.7
1964	282	2.9	8.2	11.1
1965	64	2.5	5.1	7.6
1965	25	2.3	8.0	10.3
1965	13	3.7	6.8	10.5

[a]From *Epidemiology of DDT*, Symposia Specialists, P.O. Box 610397, Miami, Florida 33161.

epidemiological surveys could have produced firm evidence that it is carcinogenic to humans. Almost all members of the human race contain it in their tissues so that there is no good control group. Also, if it caused an increase in incidence of cancer of only 0.01% in residents of the United States, this would represent 20,000 cases. This would be a serious health hazard, but still there would be no satisfactory epidemiologic way by which to measure it. Approximately 300,000 deaths/yr in the United States are caused by cancer. Since environmental exposures are estimated to be responsible for not less than 15% and as much as 80-90% of all cancer in human beings (Boyland, 1969), it was believed prudent by the Secretary's Commission to recommend restriction of the use of DDT on the basis of analytical and rodent bioassay data alone.

A Brief Review

Analytical chemistry has played a key role in studies of the chemical epidemiology of cancer. In the case of PNAs, cancer was observed first and the causative agent isolated and identified later. In the case of chlorinated hydrocarbon pesticides, analytical evidence provided the initial indication that

TABLE 2   DDT and DDE Content in Body Fat of Occupationally
Exposed Persons

Year measured	No. of persons	Occupation	DDT (ppm)	DDE (ppm)	Total as DDT (ppm)
1965	30	Applicators	14.0	21.1	35.1
1965	14	Applicators	10.7	24.1	34.8
1953	1	Formulator	122.0	141.0	263.0
1956	1	Formulator	648.0	434.0	1131.0
1956	6	Volunteers (35 mg/day)	234.0	24.0	258.0

compounds of this class are persistent and therefore might be injurious to human health.

Other analytical studies on causative agents of cancer in the environment are in progress, including the detection of PNAs in tobacco smoke (Hoffman et al., 1973) and the measurement of nitrosamines in tobacco smoke, meat, and fish (Sander et al., 1968; Johnson et al., 1968; Palframan et al., 1973; Panalaks et al., 1974).

Many carcinogens that have not been identified or for which analytical methods have not yet been developed might occur in the environment. For example, about 10% of all cattle in an isolated valley in Kenya develop cancer of the rumen, but this does not occur in an adjacent valley (Plowright et al., 1971). It is entirely possible that plants containing a naturally occurring carcinogen grow in this area. For example, the hepatocarcinogen cycasin is produced by *C. circinalis* L. and *C. revoluta* Thunb. This compound is hydrolyzed by β-glucosidase to yield methylazomethanol, which decomposes at pH 7 to yield a methylating agent (Laqueur, 1964; Matsumoto and Higa, 1966). Also, studies reported by IARC (1970) have shown that there is an east-west gradient in the occurence of esophageal cancer in the Caspian Littoral, the number of cases falling off (male/female average) from 142/100,000 per yr to 12/100,000 per yr, depending on location. This indicates that a strong carcinogen may be unevenly distributed in this region.

Although substantial progress has been made in identifying and monitoring environmental carcinogens, much more work remains to be done before the origin and distribution of these hazards to human health are fully understood, which is prerequisite to control of the disease.

ANALYTICAL CHEMISTRY IN CARCINOGENESIS BIOASSAY

The two principal roles of analytical chemistry in carcinogenesis studies are to isolate and identify potential carcinogens from environments in which incidence of cancer is high and to determine if persistent chemicals with widespread distribution in many environments are present that could cause cancer in humans but at rates too low for epidemiologic detection.

Once suspect compounds are identified, they must be bioassayed by assessing their capacities for inducing cancer in laboratory animals, including mice, rats, hamsters, and sometimes dogs. In these tests, analytical chemistry plays an essential although not dominant role.

The compounds to be bioassayed must be analyzed to determine if the active ingredients are the same as those represented on the suppliers' labels; moreover, impurities should be fingerprinted chemically in the event that information on these is required at some later date.

The chemicals under test may be applied to the animals by painting them on the skin, by gavage, by mixing them in feed, or, for volatile compounds, by mixing them with air. In all cases, the amount of compound present in the dosage form used must be measured to determine if mixing has been done correctly.

When compounds are mixed with feed, the feed is generally stored for various periods of time before offering it to the test animals. Analyses must be made throughout the projected storage period to determine if the compound is stable, since some chemicals are lost through volatilization, hydrolysis, or chemical reactions with feed components.

Contamination of feed and the environment of the test animals must be considered. Most animal chows contain small but variable amounts of pesticides, PCBs, and fungal toxins. Analysis of the basal feed will indicate whether these are present in large enough amounts to throw doubts on the results of the bioassay tests. Contamination of caging must also be considered. It has been found that plastic cages, when used over long periods of time, absorb test chemicals. These can be extracted and detected by the same analytical techniques used for their measurement in the environment. Thus, use of plastic cages for more than one compound should usually be avoided.

Contamination of the animal environment is not the only factor to be considered. Laboratory staff preparing the dosage forms are also exposed to carcinogenic and potentially carcinogenic compounds. Although the Occupational Safety and Health Administration's (OSHA) proposed standards will usually be followed in handling these materials, analyses of the air and washings from laboratory benches and equipment are needed to insure that maximum recommended levels of exposure are not exceeded.

Knowledge of excretion patterns and body burden are helpful in setting dose levels for chronic tests and for interpreting the results of bioassay experiments. When added to feed in increasing amounts, a saturation level is often reached, following which any additional compound added to feed is excreted entirely in the feces.

Measurement of body burden is also useful for setting dose levels and interpreting results. As the dose is increased, body burden will also increase, but eventually a dose level will be attained beyond which no further increase in body burden will occur.

When a dose level is reached beyond which body burden no longer increases and feces content of the compound increases linearally with dose, further increases in dose will have little toxicologic significance.

Measurement of body burden also provides reference points for comparing the toxicities of various compounds since it is conceded among pharmacologists that the amounts of compounds administered orally cannot be related to their biological activities, since compounds differ greatly in amounts in which they are absorbed from the GI tract. Thus, body burden rather than concentration of chemical in feed or air or the amount used for gavage is a much more realistic measure of the dose of the chemical assimilated.

Finally, almost all organic compounds are metabolized by the test animals. Sometimes it is the parent compound that is the carcinogen, in others it is a metabolite. Metabolic pathways may vary from species to species, both qualitatively and quantitatively. Also, chemicals are administered to experimental animals at levels that are several orders of magnitude greater than those encountered in the environment. Consequently, the relative amounts of metabolites that are produced and their distribution in tissues could differ greatly from that found for the same chemical administered at environmental levels. This, of course, could have profound effects on the biological responses of the test animals.

Thus, analytical chemistry provides information on the chemicals being tested, doses administered, and interactions with the test animals, information that is essential to establishing the validity of the carcinogenesis test results. Without this information, conclusions based on pathologic evidence alone could be disputed since it could not be demonstrated what levels of chemicals and/or metabolites produced the tissue changes observed.

Fingerprinting of Candidate Carcinogens

Early in the carcinogenesis bioassay program of the National Cancer Institute it was decided to evaluate technical-grade compounds rather than purify them. This was done for several reasons. Most important of these was that technical-grade 2,4,5-trichlorophenoxyacetic acid (2,4,5-T) (1) had recently been shown to be teratogenic (Courtney et al., 1970). Analysis of the material tested and subsequent bioassays showed that teratogenicity was caused by a series of chlorine-containing impurities in 2,4,5-T called dioxins, of which 2,3,7,8-tetrachlorodibenzo-*p*-dioxin (2) is an example. These compounds are also exceedingly toxic (Drill and Hiratzka, 1953; Rowe and

(1)   (2)

Hymas, 1954). Pure 2,4,5-T is not teratogenic. Therefore, if it had been purified prior to bioassay, this important piece of information would have been lost.

Another reason for testing technical-grade compounds is that large amounts of chemicals are required in 2-yr feeding studies. When a compound is tested on 400 animals at a level of 10,000 ppm, a total of about 20 kg is required. Preparation of analytical-grade chemicals in this quantity is time-consuming and costly. Preparation of a single pesticide metabolite that was not commercially available in sufficient quantity for bioassay cost $30,000. While this might be justified in advanced studies on compounds suspected to be carcinogenic, the expense is too high for preliminary screening in which the majority of compounds will probably be negative.

Total analysis of all technical-grade products prior to bioassay would be time-consuming and costly. Instead, a compromise was reached. It was decided to fingerprint each compound prior to bioassay by running a series of spectrometric and chromatographic tests on it. However, no attempt was made to isolate and identify individual components unless this information became essential at some future date because of positive bioassay test results.

As large a batch of compound as feasible is obtained so that analyses can be reduced to a minimum and uniform material is used throughout the bioassay test. Exceptions are made when the compounds are not stable in storage. A 100-g sample of each compound is stored for subsequent analysis should the bioassay results be positive. A sample of each batch and a sample of the chemically pure compound are then subjected to a battery of tests so that analytical results will be available on the compound both before and after storage.

Two classes of analyses are run: Tests designed to establish the identity of the principal component, and tests designed to detect the presence of impurities. Some tests accomplished both purposes. Analyses designed primarily for identifying the principal ingredient include elemental analysis, infrared spectrometry (ir), ultraviolet spectrometry (uv), and nuclear magnetic resonance spectrometry (nmr). Ir methods are primarily useful for the identification of functional groups such as hydroxyl, carbonyl, double bonds, C–Cl bonds, etc. Nmr methods are most useful for identifying the locations of protons with respect to each other in the molecules.

Tests designed primarily for the detection of impurities include glc and thin-layer chromatography (tlc) using a variety of stationary phases, mobile phases, and detection methods. Glc is also used as the primary method for determination of the percent of active ingredient (principal component) in the technical-grade product.

The most informative results are obtained from electron impact (eims) and chemical ionization mass spectrometry (cims), used alone and in combination with glc. Eims is of course a powerful tool for determining structure, and the results are used in combination with those obtained by ir and nmr for establishing the identity of the active ingredient. However, extensive fragmentation of the molecule occurs, and the fragments of the major constituent are difficult to sort out from those of impurities. This situation is improved by use of cims. Here the major ion produced is the parent compound that acquired a proton $(M + 1)^+$. Impurity peaks also form ions with mass $(M + 1)^+$ and may be detected by this method at a level of about 1% of the technical-grade product.

The most powerful technique is a combination of eims and cims with glc. Here the majority of the volatile compounds are resolved and several classes of ms data can be obtained on each peak. Care must be taken, however, in the interpretation of a cims analysis when the intent of such a procedure is to measure the level of impurities in a technical-grade chemical. If the sample is introduced via a direct probe, the cims result may vary during the time the sample is being vaporized and while repetitive scans are being made. Each component of the mixture must be assumed to have a different vapor pressure and hence vapor concentration at a given temperature and constant internal ms pressure. In any case, the more volatile components will vaporize first, and spectra taken immediately after sample introduction may be unrepresentative of the total composition of the sample. When no changes occur in the appearance of spectra taken at different times following sample introduction, the sample is either one pure compound or a mixture of compounds that have vaporized simultaneously.

Quantitative analyses of impurities in technical-grade mixtures by ms are best accomplished by combining the technique with glc. Here the majority of volatile compounds are resolved and both positive identification and quantity present can be obtained.

Results and methods used in specific cases are described below. The principal example used is the insecticide aldrin (3), although data obtained on other compounds are substituted when the analytical results obtained are most illustrative of the usefulness of the methods.

(3)

Melting point and elemental analysis. Elemental analyses and when applicable melting points are run on all technical-grade chemicals and analytical standards (Table 3). When possible the manufacturer's assay is also obtained. The batch of aldrin used in this investigation contained 85.5% aldrin (1,2,3,4,10,10-hexachloro-1, 4, 4a, 5, 8, 8a-hexahydro-1, 4-eno-exo-5, 8-dimethanonaphthylene, 4.5% insecticidally active related compounds, and 10% other compounds.

TABLE 3   Melting Point and Combustion Analysis of Aldrin
($C_{12}H_8Cl_6$, molecular weight = 364.9)

	mp (°C)	Combustion analysis		
		C (%)	H (%)	Cl (%)
Calculated	–	39.50	2.21	58.30
Analytical grade	98–99.5	39.50	2.23	58.30
Technical grade	92–99	39.29	2.24	58.51

As would be expected, the melting point of the technical-grade product had a wider range than that of the standard as measured on a Kofler hotstage melting-point apparatus. Elemental analyses indicate that the average compound in the mixture contains slightly more chlorine than pure aldrin.

Toxaphene, as described by one manufacturer, is a mixture of polychlorinated bicyclic compounds derived from camphene. The nominal molecular formula for the product is $C_{10}H_{10}Cl_8$, with chlorine specified to be 67–69% of the material by weight. Usual analytical methods (mp, ir, uv, tlc, glc, nmr, ms, etc.) are of limited value in confirming these data. The simple technique of elemental analysis by combustion provides the most useful guide to the purity of this pesticide by yielding the weight percentages of each element present. A batch of toxaphene proposed for use in the carcinogenesis screening program was analyzed for elemental composition and found to contain 68.84% Cl. In the absence of conflicting data from other analytical methods, this material was judged to be satisfactory for carcinogenesis bioassay.

Ultraviolet spectrum. Ultraviolet spectra are useful for characterizing compounds containing conjugated double bonds, aromatic rings, keto groups, etc., by measuring wavelengths of absorbance maxima and molecular extinction coefficients. For compounds that are not highly conjugated such as aldrin, uv measurements also have the potential of revealing the presence of conjugated or aromatic impurities. These were not observed in technical-grade aldrin (Fig. 8).

Infrared spectrum. Infrared spectra are of primary use in establishing the presence of functional groups such as OH, C=O, C–Cl, etc., in the major component of technical-grade products through measurement of the frequencies of the absorption maxima. It is not very useful for the detection of impurities since all organic compounds absorb in the ir, and the peaks are so numerous that it is difficult to detect small amounts of weakly absorbing compounds.

The infrared spectrum of chlordecone (4) is a good example of the value of ir spectroscopy for characterizing compounds (Fig. 9). Because of its unique structure, it should have absorbances corresponding to C–C, C–Cl, and C=O stretching and bending frequencies only. However, the C=O frequencies are absent from the spectrum and the 3,500–3,000 cm^{-1} region contains peaks that indicate the presence of hydroxyl groups. It must be concluded that the structure of chlordecone (4) as usually written is incorrect. The keto group should be replaced by two hydroxyl groups as is the case for chloral hydrate to yield the correct structure (5).

Nuclear magnetic resonance spectrum. Nuclear magnetic resonance is useful primarily for measuring the positions of protons in organic molecules

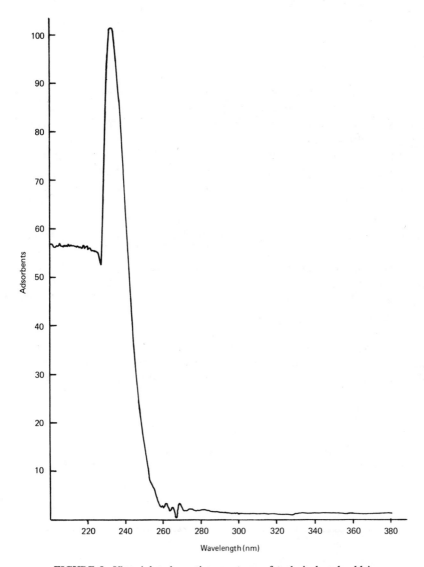

FIGURE 8 Ultraviolet absorption spectrum of technical-grade aldrin.

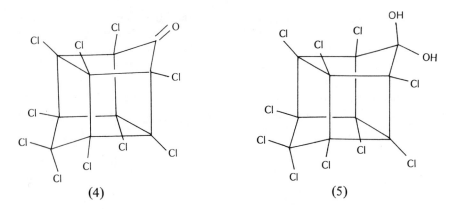

relative to each other and other atoms. The nmr peaks observed on analytical-grade aldrin (3) are summarized in Table 4. The nmr spectrum of technical-grade aldrin was identical except that two small impurity peaks were noted at $t = 3.98$ and $t = 6.65$.

Mass spectra. Mass spectra are useful for both the characterization of major components and for the detection of impurities. Electron impact fragmentation is most useful for the former since many ions are produced from which structure can be deduced. Chemical ionization fragmentation is most useful for the latter since fewer ions are produced, thus making assignments easier. The eims and cims spectra of the known carcinogen 2-acetylamino-fluorene are compared in Fig. 10.

The chemical ionization spectrum contains only five ions compared to 74 for the electron impact spectrum. The ions probably derived from the major components by cims have mass numbers of 447 and 224. The former is probably a dimer and the latter the molecule ion of the parent compound $(M + 1)^+$.

Gas–liquid chromatography (glc). Chromatography in the gas phase is of limited value for characterizing major constituents but very useful for detecting impurities. Its major drawback is that some impurities may

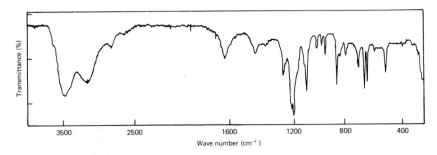

FIGURE 9 Infrared absorption spectrum of chlordecone.

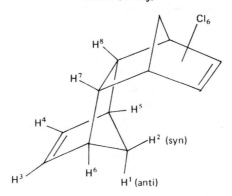

Chemical shift (τ)		Assignment
Doublet,	8.42	H^1 – anti ($J = 10.5$ Hz)
Doublet,	8.68	H^2 – syn ($J = 11.0$ Hz)
Triplet,	3.64	H^3 + H^4
Multiplet,	7.03	H^5 + H^6
Singlet,	7.20	H^7 + H^8, bridgehead

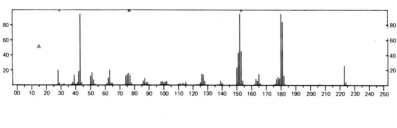

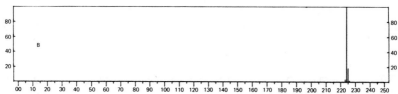

FIGURE 10 Mass spectra of *N*-2-fluorenylacetamide. (A) Electron impact ionization;
(B) isobutane chemical ionization.

decompose at the column temperature required to chromatograph the major constituent, while others may be insufficiently volatile to pass through the column. The electron capture detector (ECD), which is highly selective for polar compounds, and the flame ionization detector (FID), which is senstitive to all organic compounds, were used in the chromatography of aldrin (Table 5). Of the five sets of conditions evaluated for the chromatography of this compound, only one gave the resolution required. Four peaks were obtained using a DC-200 column at 230°C, and the major peak comprised 85% of the total area, which compares well with the value of 85.5% aldrin supplied by the manufacturer. The other columns failed to separate aldrin from the major impurities. However, one or more impurity peaks were observed on all columns; these do not necessarily correspond to those observed on the DC-200 column. For example, the peak that elutes at 7 min on the DC-200 column could conceivably be resolved into additional peaks on other columns.

Gas–liquid chromatography mass spectrometry (ms-glc). This combination is without doubt the most versatile technique for separating and identifying volatile and sparingly volatile compounds. The high resolving power of glc

TABLE 5   Gas Chromatography of Aldrin

Detector	Solid support	Liquid phase	Oven temp. (°C)	Injection size	Ret. time (min)	%
ECD	80–100 mesh Chromosorb W	6 ft 5% QF-1	170	56 pg	3.0	95.0
					3.5	3.0
					2.0	2.0
FID		6 ft 5% QF-1	190	7 µg	1.3	96.0
					2.0	4.0
FID		6 ft 5% QF-1	130	51 µg	15.0	97.0
					3.0	0.5
					7.5	0.5
					21.5	2.0
ECD	80–100 mesh Chromosorb W	6 ft 10% DC-200	230	3 ng	6.0	85.0
					3.5	2.5
					0.8	2.5
					7.0	10.0
FID	80–100 mesh Chromosorb W	6 ft 3% OV-1	150	32 µg	10.0	98.0
					2.0	1.5
					5.0	0.5
FID	80–100 mesh Gas Chrom Q	6 ft 3% HI-EFF-8 BP	170	43 µg	7.2	97.5
					4.0	0.5
					11.0	2.0

is used for making separations, which simplifies the interpretation of the mass spectra. However, even if the separations are not complete, the high resolving power of the spectrometer can be used to detect and identify the components of simple mixtures. Maximum information is obtained when both electron impact and chemical ionization are employed for fragmentation, for the reasons discussed previously.

The usefulness of ms-glc for obtaining information about chromatographable mixtures is well illustrated by data on technical-grade aldrin. The recorder traces shown in Fig. 11 were obtained from the gas chromatographic separation of the components of a mixture (technical-grade aldrin) with a rapid scanning quadrupole mass spectrometer operating in the chemical ionization mode (methane) functioning as the glc detector. The sum of all the ions detected per scan is plotted incrementally versus time by a computer-controlled data system to yield a mass chromatogram. This is quite similar in appearance to gas chromatograms obtained using more conventional detector systems. The mass chromatogram, TI (from *total-ion monitoring*), shows no special features (upper trace); however, the mass fragmentograms derived from single-ion monitoring, where the ms is sensitive to only one ion fragment of predetermined mass, are quite different (lower traces). The m/e values of 307, 303, 263, and 203 were chosen because of their high intensities during preliminary mass spectral scanning of the entire chromatographic effluent. They are the most stable ions derived from four compounds present in technical-grade aldrin and are not necessarily parent ions of these compounds.

Mass spectra taken at different times during the chromatography of technical-grade aldrin are shown in Fig. 12. The upper spectrum (no. 39) was taken during the elution of an impurity (ret. time = 1.5 min) and the lower one (no. 137) during the elution of aldrin itself (ret. time = 4.6 min). These spectra are indicative of the selectivity possible with highly sophisticated ms-glc/computer data systems.

Thin-layer chromatography (tlc). Thin-layer chromatography is used primarily for the detection of impurities; it has little value for the characterization of the principal components of technical-grade compounds. It is carried out on plates coated with silica gel that are developed with a variety of polar and nonpolar solvents (Table 6). The plates are then treated in a number of ways to visualize the compounds separated by chromatography. These include (1) viewing the plates under uv light to detect compounds that are fluorescent; (2) spraying the plates with 0.1 N $KMnO_4$ containing 5% sodium carbonate; (3) exposure of the plates to I_2 vapors in a sealed chamber followed by spraying with 1% starch in 1% aqueous boric acid solution; (4) spraying the plates with 5% palladous chloride in 10% HCl for the detection of thiophosphoric acid esters; and (5) spraying the plates with monoethanolamine and heating at 100°C for 20 min; the color that develops is intensified by respraying with a mixture of 10 volumes of 0.1 N $AgNO_3$ and 1 volume of concentrated HNO_3 following which they are exposed to uv light. Results

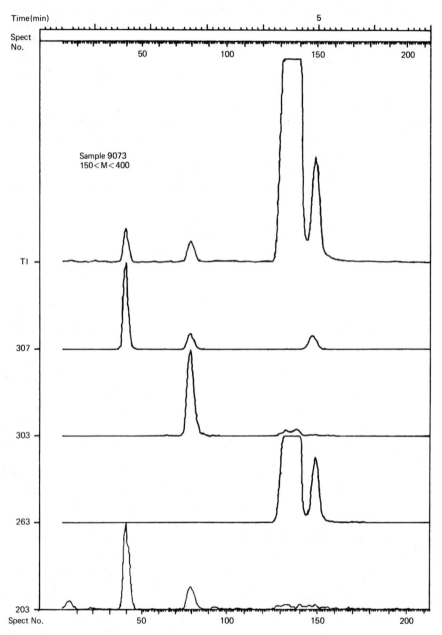

FIGURE 11 Gas chromatograms of technical-grade aldrin using mass spectrometric detection (mass chromatography).

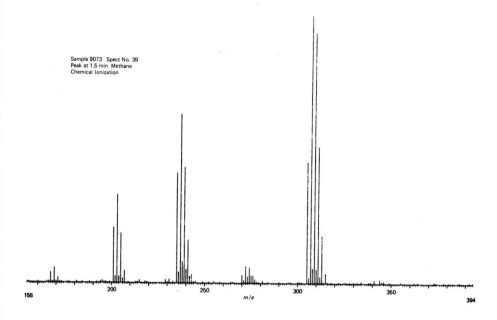

Sample 9073 Spect No. 39
Peak at 1.5 min Methane
Chemical Ionization

155

200

250

m/e

300

350

394

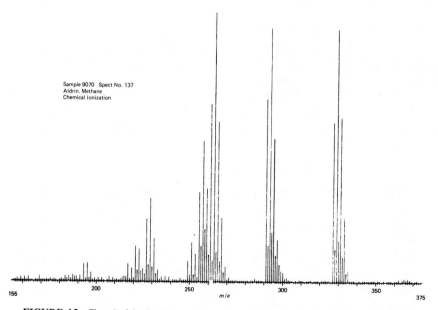

Sample 9070 Spect No. 137
Aldrin. Methane
Chemical Ionization

155

200

250

m/e

300

350

375

FIGURE 12 Chemical ionization mass spectra of technical-grade aldrin taken during mass chromatography.

195

TABLE 6   Thin-Layer Chromatographic Analyses of Safrole

Stationary phase	Mobile phase	R_f	% of total
Silica gel	Hexane:acetone (2:1)	0.72^a	20
		0.57	60
		$\left.\begin{array}{l}0.32^a\\0.00\end{array}\right\}$	20
Silica gel	C_6H_6:MeOH (85:15)	0.71	75
		0.54^a	10
		$\left.\begin{array}{l}0.45^a\\0.00^a\end{array}\right\}$	15
Silica gel	BuOH:AcOH:H_2O (4:1.5:1)	0.80	
Silica gel	95% EtOH:28% NH_4OH (4:1)	0.71	90
		0.84^a	10
Alumina	Hexane	0.77^a	30
		0.34	60
		0.00^a	10
Alumina	Hexane:acetone (4:1)	0.89^a	40
		0.77	60

[a]These spots could only be detected by method (3).

obtained on safrole, a known carcinogen, using methods (1)–(3) for visualizing compounds are shown in Table 6. From one to four compounds could be detected depending on the chromatographic system employed.

This procedure is a useful supplement to glc since many compounds cannot be chromatographed in the gas phase, and others can be chromatographed only after converting them to derivatives.

It is probable that hplc will eventually replace tlc as a method for performing chromatography with a liquid mobile phase because of its higher resolution. However, at present the number of detection techniques that can conveniently be applied with this method is very limited.

Control of Dosage Regimen

Amount and distribution of compound in vehicle. In all bioassay tests the principal objective is to relate the biological effect produced to the dose. After having decided on a dose or series of doses, it is necessary to make certain that this dosage regimen is followed. Therefore, the concentration of chemical in the vehicle must be determined by analyzing solutions, suspensions, emulsions, or feed for the active ingredient, depending on how the compound is administered.

Control of dosage in feed is most difficult since large batches must be prepared in advance and the compounds may deteriorate during storage. Therefore, it is necessary to analyze samples of fortified feed immediately after mixing to determine if they contain the correct amount of test compound and if the compound is distributed uniformly throughout the feed. If it is not uniformly distributed, animals on test will receive different doses than those scheduled and the dose-response curves will lose significance. Feed is mixed 104 times/2-yr test period for each compound under study; hence the analysis of all samples would be prohibitively expensive. As a compromise, every eighth batch is analyzed.

In general, the same analytical methods are employed that are used to determine residues of chemicals in the environment. Often cleanup steps can be reduced or eliminated since the concentration of chemical in feed is usually orders of magnitude higher than found in the environment. However, exceptions occur if the compound is highly toxic or for other reasons must be tested at a low dose. For example, a substance occurring in feed interfered in the measurement of 2-acetylaminofluorene by spectrophotofluorometry (M. C. Bowman, personal communication, 1974), and considerable research on cleanup methods was required to solve the problem. A similar situation occurred in our laboratory, in the analysis of a carcinogenic naphthylene derivative, 4-ethylsulfonylnaphthalene-l-sulfonamide, by hplc using a fluorescence detector. It was finally found that the compound and the fluorescing interference could be separated on a 60 cm X 2.2 mm i.d. column containing Sepcote 30PM40.

The most useful procedures for measuring candidate carcinogens in animal feed are glc using the electron capture, flame photometric, or electrical conductivity detectors, or hplc using a uv photometer or, where applicable, a spectrophotofluorometer for detection.

Many carcinogens are fluorescent and can be measured by their natural fluorescence or be converted to more highly fluorescent compounds by derivatization. As noted earlier, the PNAs can be measured by glc or hplc using a spectrophotofluorometric detector.

Seven of the 14 compounds listed by OSHA as being high-risk carcinogens are aromatic amines, and these are also fluorescent. They can be measured directly or following conversion to more highly fluorescent derivatives by causing them to react with fluorescamine (Udenfriend et al., 1972) or *o*-phthalaldehyde (Shore et al., 1959). The latter reagent is preferable since it does not by itself fluoresce.

Polychlorinated compounds including insecticides and PCBs are insensitive to fluorescence detectors; however, they yield very high responses to the electron capture, microcoulometric, and electrical conductivity detectors because of the presence of halogen atoms in the molecules. However, the ECD is nonspecific in its response while the coulometer and conductivity cells are highly selective for chlorine. Since the amounts of chlorinated compounds added to feed will be high compared to those found in environmental samples, the high senstitivity of the ECD is not ordinarily required. However, its high sensitivity can be utilized in some instances by diluting the extract sufficiently to attenuate impurity signals. If this does not give satisfactory results, the halogen-specific microcoulometer or the electrical conductivity detector should be used.

It should be possible to analyze for most carcinogens in feed using glc or hplc in combination with selective detectors. However, in refractory cases advantage can be taken of the fact that many carcinogens are biological alkylating agents and can be determined colorimetrically by causing them to react with organic bases. Compounds that are highly electronegative can be measured by causing them to react sequentially with pyridine and a strong base (Burchfield and Storrs, 1956a; Burchfield and Schuldt, 1958). These include compounds such as captan, dyrene, simazine, 1-fluoro-2,4-dinitrobenzene, and many others. Yellow to orange compounds are formed with absorbance maxima in the range of 440–550 nm. Less electronegative alkylating agents can be measured by causing them to react with 4-(4-nitrobenzyl)-pyridine (Schuldt et al., 1961). Absorbance is measured in the 560 nm region.

It is probable that analyses of alkylating agents that do not absorb or fluoresce in the ultraviolet region of the spectrum (β-propiolactone, for example) could be accomplished by first separating them from impurities by hplc followed by coupling this instrument with a Technicon autoanalyzer for introducing reagents and measuring the color produced. Of course, detection by measurement of alkylating power would not be applicable if the compound is a proximate carcinogen that is converted by metabolism to an alkylating agent.

Stability in the vehicle. In addition to insuring that the correct amount of test chemical has been added to the vehicle, the stability of the compound during storage must be determined. This problem is most serious when the compound is mixed with feed since the surface exposed is great and feed contains many chemically reactive constituents. In the interest of saving labor, it is desirable to mix chemicals with animal feed no more than once a week. Therefore, it is necessary to analyze feed samples daily for active ingredient before beginning bioassay tests to determine if it is stable for this long.

Difficulties have been encountered in several cases. The insecticide dichlorvos is used as a fumigant and has a vapor pressure of 0.032 mmHg at 32°C. When added to feed, 24% of it disappears within the first day. To overcome this problem, the feed was mixed weekly and stored at $-20°C$. Also, animals that were dosed with dichlorvos were housed in separate rooms to prevent exposure of other animals on test to vapors of this compound.

A more serious problem was encountered with the fungicide dyrene (6). When this compound was mixed with feed, 50% of it disappeared the first day as determined by glc.

Dyrene is a biological alkylating agent that reacts very rapidly with compounds containing amino and thiol groups such as cysteine, glutathione, proline, peptides, and proteins, which are normal constituents of feed (Burchfield and Storrs, 1956b, 1957, 1958).

The compounds that are formed (6a, 6b) contain ionized carboxyl and protonated amino groups in the R chains and are too polar to measure by glc, the procedure employed for the analysis of dyrene. Theoretically, the dyrene reaction products (6a, 6b) could combine with other metabolites to yield compounds in which both halogen atoms are replaced. However, when the first halogen is replaced by an electron-releasing group the remaining halogen becomes deactivated. Therefore, it is probable that the feed contains free dyrene, and a large group of compounds of types (6a) and (6b) possessing a single reactive halogen. These apparently retain biological activity since dyrene when administered to rats in feed inhibits liver carboxylesterase activity (Alley et al., 1973).

Dyrene undergoes further reactions in the GI tract and cannot be detected in the feces until the concentration reaches about 1% in the diet of the rat. At this point most of the nucleophilic compounds in the feces have probably reacted with dyrene since at higher doses the concentration of free dyrene in feces increases in proportion to the amount in the feed.

Although compounds of type (6a) and (6b) cannot be measured by glc, colorimetric methods are available based on reactions with pyridine and alkali that could be used for their measurement (Knüsli et al., 1964).

Measurement of contamination. Contamination must be avoided during carcinogenesis bioassay to avoid possible synergistic or antagonistic effects caused by the interactions of two or more chemicals. Fortunately, most compounds are assayed at far higher levels than those at which contaminants are found, so hopefully these effects are minimal.

Contaminants that are impossible to avoid in feeding studies using present methods are chlorinated hydrocarbon pesticides and PCBs found in animal chow (Table 7). In the past, these were analyzed routinely by glc, but this has now been discontinued since the levels are low and do not vary greatly from batch to batch. Also, there are no corrective measures that can

TABLE 7   Pesticide Residues in 10 Batches
of Wayne Rodent Chow[a]

Dieldrin	DDT family (DDT + DDD + DDE)(ppm)
0.002	0.014
ND[b]	0.019
0.004	0.019
ND	0.007
ND	0.021
ND	0.017
ND	0.018
ND	0.016
ND	0.016
ND	0.013

[a]Lindane, heptachlor, aldrin, heptachlor, epoxide, endrin, chlordane, toxaphene, organophosphates, or PCBs were not detected in these basal feed samples from 1973.
[b]ND = not detected.

be taken except use of artificial diets, and this is not feasible economically at the present time. Even though measures have been taken by government agencies to prevent distribution of these compounds in the environment, their persistence is so great that it may be years before they degrade to undetectable levels.

Contamination can result from the use of plastic cages, since these can absorb test compounds. This can be shown by washing them with solvents and analyzing the extracts. Absorption cannot be avoided. However, adverse effects can be minimized by always using the same cages for the same compounds and discarding them at the end of the test period.

One type of contamination that must be avoided is accidental exposure of personnel to carcinogenic chemicals. While not all compounds tested will be carcinogenic, they must be presumed to be carcinogenic until proven otherwise. The highest exposure group is the feed-mixing staff, where inhalation of compounds in addition to dermal contact is a possibility. Use of adequate hoods, face masks, and protective clothing are the best preventive measures. However, in case of spillage the area should be monitored analytically after cleanup to be certain that dangerous residues do not persist. This can be done by swabbing the area with cotton soaked with solvent, squeezing out the liquid, and analyzing it for the chemical that has been spilled by the appropriate residue analysis method.

Metabolism

Almost all carcinogens can be metabolized by humans and laboratory animals to yield other chemical species. Often metabolism is beneficial in that it detoxifies the compound by converting it to a derivative that is water-soluble and therefore readily excreted in urine. However metabolism is harmful if proximate carcinogens are converted to ultimate carcinogens. All compounds are metabolized differently, and sometimes the same compound is metabolized differently by different species. If the animal species used in carcinogenesis bioassay can metabolize a proximate carcinogen to an ultimate carcinogen, while human beings do not, the results of the bioassay obviously cannot be extrapolated to humans. False negative results could also be obtained if the test species does not produce the ultimate carcinogen, and this is formed in humans. Therefore, a knowledge of the comparative metabolism of candidate carcinogens is very useful in interpreting the results of bioassay tests.

Sophisticated metabolism studies of the type that can now be made would have been almost impossible using the analytical techniques of 30 yr ago. Huge quantities of urine and feces would have been required, and these would have had to be fractionated on pilot plant scale. During the ensuing years methods have been developed that have made it possible to measure compounds such as DDT and its metabolites rapidly and specifically using only a few grams of tissue. The principal metabolities of DDT (7) are DDE (8), DDD (9), and DDA (10).

The major metabolite that is ultimately excreted in urine, DDA, could not be measured in the same glc procedure used for DDT, DDE, and DDD because of the presence of the carboxyl group. However, when the carboxyl group is masked by methylation, it is possible to detect the methyl ester of DDA in a 20–50 ml urine specimen in amounts as low as 1 ppb by a combination of the parallel plate electron capture and the electrical conductivity detectors (Cranmer et al., 1972).

The combination of glc with ms has become an extremely powerful tool in studies on metabolism. It combines the high resolution of the gas chromatographic column with the ability of the mass spectrometer to detect and identify compounds at very low levels. This technique has been used to identify β-hexachlorocyclohexane (β-HCH) as an isomer of γ-hexachlorocyclohexane (lindane) in human tissues (Biros and Walker, 1970).

A glc peak was frequently observed in extracts of human tissues with the same relative retention as β-HCH but its identification as β-HCH was questionable since this compound is removed from lindane during manufacture because it imparts off-odors to some crops. However, ms-glc provided unequivocal evidence of identity. The presence of βHCH was finally explained by the finding that lindane is isomerized to its *alpha* and *beta* isomers by soil microorganisms (Benezet and Matsumura, 1973). This is ironic since considerable expense is incurred in separating these isomers from lindane during manufacture. These facts were unknown when bioassay studies were initiated on 99%+ lindane. Had they been known, it would have been preferable to evaluate crude HCH, which contains all of the isomers.

Even with modern analytical methods it would be an enormous task to detect all metabolites of all compounds bioassayed. However, the major metabolites should be measured, particularly if one of them is suspected of being the ultimate carcinogen.

The insecticides aldrin (3) and dieldrin (11), which are believed to be carcinogenic, are good examples of this. Both compounds are marketed as insecticides. Aldrin is oxidized to dieldrin in the factory with peracetic acid, and in humans, experimental animals, and plants by nonspecific epoxidases. We have never observed aldrin in human tissues, but dieldrin is almost always

(3)   (11)

present. Obviously, aldrin becomes oxidized to dieldrin at environmental levels. The same situation exists with respect to heptachlor. In human tissues it is found only as heptachlor epoxide.

Malathion (12) was fed to male rats at a level of 8000 ppm for 2 yr. At environmental levels malathion is oxidized to malaoxon (13), which is the biologically active compound. Following this, the malaoxon is hydrolyzed to other products. Carboxylase systems convert malathion and malaoxon to mono- and dicarboxylic acids, and phosphatases cleave the parent compounds and other metabolites to dialkylphosphorates (Krueger and O'Brien, 1959). Competition takes place between oxidation of malathion to malaoxon and hydrolysis of the ester linkages so that a variety of metabolic products are formed depending on age, sex, and species of the animal exposed to malathion (O'Brien, 1957; Knaak and O'Brien, 1960).

$$\underset{\text{(12)}}{(CH_3O)_2-\overset{\overset{\textstyle S}{\|}}{P}-S-\overset{\overset{\textstyle CO_2C_2H_5}{|}}{C}HCH_2CO_2C_2H_5} \qquad \underset{\text{(13)}}{(CH_3O)_2-\overset{\overset{\textstyle O}{\|}}{P}-S-\overset{\overset{\textstyle CO_2C_2H_5}{|}}{C}HCH_2CO_2C_2H_5}$$

Environmental exposure to malathion is probably low. However, at the dose levels used in bioassay the experimental animals might have been exposed to an abnormal dose of malathion if the oxidase systems responsible for converting it to malaoxon were swamped.

Modern analytical techniques have been of great assistance in following the conversion of proximate carcinogens to ultimate carcinogens. For example, they have been used to show that N-hydroxylation plays a key role in the conversion of most if not all carcinogenic aromatic amines and amides to ultimate carcinogens.

2-Acetylaminofluorene (14) is hydroxylated in the N-position to (15) and then esterified to yield (16). The esters can react rapidly and non-enzymatically with components of RNA and DNA at neutral pH, which probably accounts for their carcinogenicities (Miller, 1970; Kapuler and Michelson, 1971).

Even such apparently inert compounds as the PNAs can be metabolized. The rings are oxidized, which converts them to ultimate carcinogens that can alkylate macromolecules. Recently a method based on hplc has been developed to analyze these compounds.

Using BaP as a typical carcinogenic PNA, Selkirk et al. (1974) have demonstrated the usefulness of hplc in separating a number of oxygenated metabolites of BaP. Incubation of isotopically labeled BaP with liver microsomes prepared from rats that had been previously treated with another PNA (methylcholanthrene) resulted in the production of several hydroxylated and quinone derivatives of BaP. A chromatogram of these compounds is shown in Fig. 13.

Procarcinogen

(14)   Proximate Carcinogen   (15)

(16)

Without the aid of analytical chemistry, the concept of proximate and ultimate carcinogens would not have been developed.

Body Burden

Measurement of body burden and metabolites in test animals during bioassay are interrelated since body burden is the sum of the parent compound and the principal metabolites that are measured by the analytical method employed. Generally not all metabolites are measured because of the complexity of the task, although this would be desirable if feasible. Measurement of the amount of chemical in each organ would also be desirable, but again this is not practical. To simplify the task, body burden is measured on adipose tissues in which liposoluble compounds are stored, liver (which is the primary site of metabolism of xenobiotics), and all other soft tissues combined. Body burden can be expressed as $\mu g/g$ compound per tissue or $\mu g/g$ combined soft tissues.

Body burden is a key measurement in relating dose to biological response, particularly for compounds that are administered by gavage or in feed.

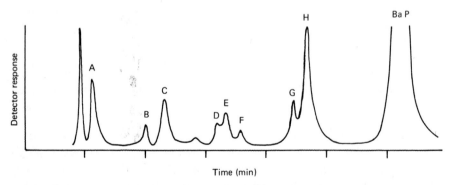

FIGURE 13 Hplc of benzo[a]pyrene (BaP) and its metabolites (Selkirk et al., 1974). (A) 9,10-dihydro-9,10-dihydroxy BaP; (B) 4,5-dihydro-4,5-dihydroxy BaP; (C) 7,8-dihydro-7,8-dihydroxy BaP; (D) BaP-1,6-dione; (E) BaP-3,6-dione; (F) BaP-6,12-dione (tentative); (G) 9-hydroxy BaP; (H) 3-hydroxy BaP.

Pharmacologists have long realized that oral doses of drugs are not reliable indications of therapeutic levels in plasma even for different dosage forms of the same drug. The same holds true for carcinogens.

If most of a compound that is administered orally is excreted unchanged in the feces, apparent carcinogenicity might be low even though the compound could be highly carcinogenic if applied dermally, by inhalation, or by injection into the peritoneum or circulatory system.

Also, some classes of compounds are stored in tissues in larger amounts and for longer periods of time than others, which greatly enhances their potential for carcinogenicity.

In a series of tests recently completed, the maximum tolerated dose for endrin in feed administered to male rats was 5 ppm. The maximum tolerated dose for amiben was 20,000 ppm. It is not known whether endrin is 4,000 times more toxic to mammalian cells or if this is caused in part by differences in absorption, metabolism, and storage of the two compounds. Information on this should tell whether other routes of administration should be considered, including dermal application and inhalation.

The differences between carcinogenic liposoluble compounds (chlorinated hydrocarbons), polar organic compounds (aromatic amines), metals such as beryllium, and completely inert materials like asbestos with respect to absorption, translocation, metabolism, and storage are enormous. Therefore, measurement of body burden is essential in carcinogenesis bioassay.

It is self-evident that for measurement of body burden, metabolites, dose levels, stability, and environmental exposure to carcinogens or potential carcinogens, analytical chemistry is essential.

REFERENCES

Alley, E. G., Dollar, D. A., Layton, B. R. and Minyard, J. P. 1973. *J. Agr. Food Chem.* 21:138.

Benezet, H. J. and Matsumura, F. 1973. *Nature (London)* 243(5408):480.

Biros, F. J. and Walker, A. C. 1970. *J. Agr. Food Chem.* 18:425.

Boyland, E. 1969. *Progr. Exp. Tumor Res.* 11:222.

Burchfield, H. P. and Schuldt, P. H. 1958. *J. Agr. Food Chem.* 6:106.

Burchfield, H. P. and Storrs, E. E. 1956a. *Contrib. Boyce Thompson Inst.* 18:319.

Burchfield, H. P. and Storrs, E. E. 1956b. *Contrib. Boyce Thompson Inst.* 18:395.

Burchfield, H. P. and Storrs, E. E. 1957. *Contrib. Boyce Thompson Inst.* 19:169.

Burchfield, H. P. and Storrs, E. E. 1958. *Contrib. Boyce Thompson Inst.* 19:417.

Burchfield, H. P., Wheeler, R. J. and Bernos, J. B. 1971. *Anal. Chem.* 43:1976.

Burchfield, H. P., Green, E. E., Wheeler, R. J. and Billedeau, S. M. 1974. *J. Chromatogr.* 99:697.

Butlin, H. J. 1892. *Brit. Med. J.* 1:1341; 2:1, 66.

Cook, J. W., Hewett, C. L. and Hieger, I. 1933. *J. Chem. Soc.* 395.

Coulson, D. M., Cavanagh, L. A., DeVries, J. E. and Walther, B. 1960. *J. Agr. Food Chem.* 8:399.

Courtney, K. D., Gaylor, D. M., Hogan, M. D. and Falk, H. L. 1970. *Science* 168:864.

Cranmer, M. F., Carroll, J. J. and Copeland, M. F. 1972. In *Epidemiology of DDT*, ed. J. E. Davies and W. F. Edmundson, app. 3, pp. 147-152. Mount Kisco, N.Y.: Futura.

Drill, V. A. and Hiratzka, T. 1953. *Arch. Ind. Hyg. Occup. Med.* 7:61.

Edmundson, W. F., Davies, J. E., Nachman, G. A. and Roeth, R. L. 1972. In *Epidemiology of DDT*, ed. J. E. Davies and W. F. Edmundson, chap. 7, pp. 57-65. Mount Kisco, N.Y.: Futura.

Hoffman, D., Rathkamp, G., Brunnemann, K. D. and Wynder, E. L. 1973. *Sci. Total Environ.* 2:157.

Innes, J. R. M., Ulland, B. M., Valerio, M. G., Petrucelli, L., Fishbein, L., Hart, E. R., Pallotta, A. J., Bates, R. R., Falk, H. L., Gart, J. R., Klein, M., Mitchell, I. and Peters, J. 1969. *J. Natl. Cancer Inst.* 42:1101.

International Agency for Research on Cancer (IARC). 1970. *Annual report. 1969.* 109 pp. Lyon: World Health Organization.

Johnson, D. E., Millar, J. D. and Rhoades, J. W. 1968. *Natl. Cancer Inst. Monogr.* 28, p. 181.

Kapuler, A. M. and Michelson, A. M. 1971. *Biochim. Biophys. Acta* 232:436.

Kennaway, E. L. and Hieger, I. 1930. *Brit. Med. J.* 1:1044.

Kmet, J. and Mahboubi, E. 1972. *Science* 175:846.

Knaak, J. B. and O'Brien, R. D. 1960. *J. Agr. Food Chem.* 8:198.

Knusli, E., Burchfield, H. P. and Storrs, E. E. 1964. In *Analytical methods for pesticides, plant growth regulators, and food additives*, ed. G. Zweig, vol. 4, pp. 213-233, New York: Academic Press.

Kruger, H. R. and O'Brien, R. D. 1959. *J. Econ. Entomol.* 52:1063.

Laqueur, G. L. 1964. *Fed. Proc.* 23:1386.

Lovelock, J. E. and Lipsky, S. R. 1960. *J. Amer. Chem. Soc.* 82:431.

Matsumoto, H. and Higa, H. H. 1966. *Biochem. J.* 98:200.

Miller, J. A. 1970. *Cancer Res.* 30:559.

Mrak Report. 1969. In *Report of the secretary's commission on pesticides and their relationship to environmental health*, pts. I and II, pp. 1-677. Washington, D.C.: Government Printing Office.

O'Brien, R. D. 1957. *J. Econ. Entomol.* 50:159.

Palframan, J. F., Macnab, J. and Crosby, N. T. 1973. *J. Chromatogr.* 76:307.

Panalaks, T., Iyengar, J. R., Donaldson, B. A., Miles, W. F. and Sen, N. P. 1974. *J. Assoc. Offic. Anal. Chem.* 57:806.

Plowright, W., Linsell, C. A. and Peers, F. G. 1971. *Brit. J. Cancer* 25:72.

Pott, P. 1775. (Reprinted in *Natl. Cancer Inst. Monogr.* 10, p. 7, 1963.)

Rowe, V. K. and Hymas, T. A. 1954. *Amer. J. Vet. Res.* 15:622.

Sander, J., Schweinsberg, F. and Menz, H. P. 1968. *Z. Physiol. Chem.* 349:1691.

Sawicki, E., Hauser, T. R. and Stanley, T. W. 1960. *Int. J. Air Pollut.* 2:253.

Schechter, M. S., Soloway, S. B., Hayes, R. A. and Haller, H. L. 1945. *Ind. Eng. Chem. Anal. Ed.* 17:704.

Schuldt, P. H., Burchfield, H. P., Stallard, D. E., Priddle, W. E. and Klein, S. 1961. *Contrib. Boyce Thompson Inst.* 21:163.

Selkirk, J. K., Croy, R. G. and Gelboin, H. V. 1974. *Science* 184:169.

Shore, P. A., Burkhalter, A. and Cohn, V. H., Jr. 1959. *J. Pharmacol. Exp. Ther.* 127:182.

Udenfriend, S., Stein, S., Böhlen, P., Dairman, W., Leimgruber, W. and Weigele, M. 1972. *Science* 178:871.

Yamagiwa, K. and Ichikawa, K. 1915. *Mitteil. Med. Facultät* 15:295.

Yamagiwa, K. and Ichikawa, K. 1918. *J. Cancer Res.* 3:1.

Chapter 6

INORGANIC AGENTS AS CARCINOGENS

Arthur Furst

Institute of Chemical Biology
University of San Francisco
San Francisco, California

INTRODUCTION

Background of Metal Carcinogenesis Studies

It is now believed that over 85% of all cancers are induced by exogenous chemicals. Ample evidence for this statement was available more than 100 yr ago but went unrecognized. The high incidence of lung cancer among the Scheenberg miners, for example, was ignored or not appreciated. The relationship between chemicals and cancer in man was dramatically pointed out by Percivall Pott in 1778; he explained that the high incidence of scrotal cancer among chimney sweeps was probably due to contact with soot. The greatest impetus to explore the relationship between chemicals and cancer came, however, after two Japanese workers (Yamagiwa and Ichikawa, 1915, 1918) discovered that they could obtain papillomas by painting coal tar on the ears of rabbits. Previously, Fischer (1906) had obtained the same tumor using scarlet red, an azo dye. As experimental animals became available, the search for the identification of chemical carcinogens progressed rapidly. Initially, most of the studies concentrated on hydrocarbons (these were the compounds implicated in the scrotal cancer noted by Pott); later, azo dyes became the focus of activity. But the compounds that commanded the greatest interest, from an experimental and theoretical point of view, were really not related to the human environment at all.

Metals, on the other hand, had been identified as primary carcinogens as early as 1942, by Schinz and Uehlinger, although this had very little impact on the field of chemical carcinogenesis. Thus, metals, which could be causative

In Memory of George Gallowhur.

agents for cancer in humans, were neglected for nearly 25 yr. Simple screening tests could be made in the laboratory; but still, little effort or energy was expended in the field of metal carcinogenesis. Hueper (1966) made a systematic study of several metals as potential carcinogens. He was able to compare the carcinogenic activity of metals and their compounds in different species and by different routes of administration, including inhalation and intrafemoral, subcutaneous, and intramuscular injection. He did extensive work with nickel and chromium. Also among the pioneer workers was Baetjer (1950), who studied chromium and chromates as they related to occupational hazards. Haddow (1958) was one of the first to recognize that metals might play a role in carcinogenesis.

Available Reviews

Hueper summarized most of his work in a book coauthored with Conway (1964). Suggesting a chelate hypothesis, Furst (1960) tried to relate both anticancer agent and carcinogenic agent with metals and metal binding. He later expanded his ideas in a monograph (1963), suggesting that platinum compounds should be synthesized as potential anticancer compounds. Almost a decade later, Rosenberg et al. (1969) did just that. A comprehensive review of platinum as an anticancer agent has been published recently (Cleare, 1974).

Furst and Haro (1969a) also compiled information from the literature on metal carcinogenesis and identified strict criteria to be met before a metal or, for that matter, any compound could be labeled a carcinogen. This was followed by a short review that included some laboratory procedures; Furst and Schlauder (1971) demonstrated that all metals are not carcinogenic when implanted intramuscularly using the same vehicle and the same strain of Fisher-344 rats.

Sunderman (1971) wrote an elegant review on the experimental details of those metals considered carcinogenic. Another comprehensive review was written by Kanisawa (1971); unfortunately, this review is in Japanese and is, therefore, not readily accessible. It is currently being translated into English.

In spite of the work done in this field to date, many reviewers of chemical carcinogenesis overlook the entire field of metals or treat them in only a cursory fashion. One of the exceptions is the review by Roe and Lancaster (1964). In terms of human hazard, however, many more people are exposed to metals, and their compounds and fumes, than to the more extensively investigated exotic dyes or aromatic amines or, for that matter, even to the hydrocarbons. In addition, it is interesting to note that minute amounts of trace elements, essential for life processes (Underwood, 1971), may also prove to be carcinogenic in large doses.

This review of metal carcinogenesis is not intended to be comprehensive, for that would take an entire book. Rather, the highlights of metal carcinogenesis are presented to give the reader an insight into this interesting aspect of the field.

COMPLICATIONS IN THE FIELD OF INORGANIC CARCINOGENESIS

Nonspecific Solid-State Carcinogenesis

Confusion still exists in the field of metal carcinogenesis. The phenomenon of nonspecific solid-state carcinogenesis is distinct from metal carcinogenesis, but it still clouds the issue. Oppenheimer et al. (1956) implanted subcutaneously various metal foils (among them silver) and later found local sarcomas surrounding these foils. Tin, which crumpled, did not seem to induce the fibrosarcomas. In a series of experiments, Nothdurft (1958) found more tumors in some cases but not in others. A variety of solids were tested by Becker et al. (1966), again with variable results.

A new field of chemical carcinogenesis is emerging. The term *foreign body carcinogenesis* is being used; however, since *foreign body* has classical connotations, the term *nonspecific solid-state carcinogenesis*, or *solid-state carcinogenesis*, is preferable. In other words, this new field should not be confused with metal carcinogenesis: some metals classified as carcinogenic may act via a foreign-body mechanism and the carcinogenic activity may not involve an ion at all.

Bischoff and Bryson (1964) reviewed the field of solid-state carcinogenesis. Later, it was demonstrated that many solids implanted under the skin of rats may produce local tumors; for example, dead bone chips, but not powder (Maatz and Palowsky, 1972). Furst (1971) suggested that these agents might work through an hypoxic mechanism; this hypothesis was not supported by Karp et al. (1973). Finally, Brand et al. (1975) reviewed the topic of *foreign-body tumorigenesis* from the aspects of etiology and the process of growth.

Plastics, Sheets, and Discs

In reevaluating foreign-body carcinogenesis, plastics must be considered. It must be recognized that pure substances are not being tested (Bischoff and Bryson, 1974). Plastics contain plasticizers, additives, and contaminants (van Esch, 1967); often, the monomer and catalysts are present too. Oppenheimer et al. (1955) studied a series of polymers for carcinogenicity and found some plastics active. Carter et al. (1971) tried to clarify the physiochemical nature of those plastics involved in inducing tumors when implanted under the skin of rats; cationic, anionic, and neutral films were evaluated. Animals carrying the cationic films had the greatest tumor yield. In this respect, it should be noted that carcinogenic metals liberate cations when dissolved; thus, the surface of the metal powders are, in actual fact, cationic, solid microspheres.

Moizhess and Prigozhina (1973) concluded that tumors start from cells that form a capsule in the early period, following implantation of the film. It is also important to note that Nothdurft (1958) failed to find tumors when powdered plastics were tested.

Asbestos and Fibers

Asbestos is described in this review in a brief fashion, but it deserves a review in itself. Asbestos is a depot of many metals that have been considered carcinogenic; among these are nickel and chromium. It must be recognized that there are a variety of asbestoses (crysolite, chrysotile, amphilbole, serpentine, etc.) and that each has its own composition of heavy metals. However, calcium and magnesium predominate in all (Cralley and Lainhart, 1973).

The use of asbestos in the building trades has resulted in the exposure of many workers to this material. Indeed, because of the technique used in applying asbestos to the frames of high-rise buildings, it has been estimated that as much as 50% of the applied fibers are blown off. Thus, large segments of any urban population have been exposed to asbestos.

Asbestosis is a recognized disease among workers employed in all aspects of asbestos manufacture, from mining to finished product. Lung cancer, especially mesothelioma (a cancer of the pleural lining), is a more recent finding.

Documentation of the human disease was first made by Lynch and Smith (1935), Lynch et al. (1937), and Gloyne (1935). Doll (1955) and later Selikoff and Churg (1965) also reported some cases. Much of the work has been summarized in these proceedings of the Conference of the New York Academy of Sciences and in the IARC monograph (1973).

A number of experimental attempts have been made to induce tumors with asbestos in a large variety of animal species. Practically every conceivable route of administration has been attempted. Smith et al. (1965) placed asbestos in the chest cavity of Golden Syrian hamsters and reported three pleural mesotheliomas. Wagner (1962) and Wagner and Berry (1969) conducted a similar experiment with rats, using silica and carbon black as control substances. Tumors were found only in the groups exposed to asbestos. Reeves et al. (1971), in a series of experiments in rats, administered asbestos by a number of routes but showed a very low tumor yield.

The IARC monograph (1973) describes the varieties of asbestos and reviews the dimensions of the various fibers. Stanton and Wrench (1972) believe that the major problem is not asbestos but a specific fiber dimension. They reported that the same type of tumor can be induced by aluminum oxide, if the dimensions of the needles are similar in length and diameter to those of the asbestos fibers.

Asbestos contains benzo[a]pyrene (Harington, 1962), but both Wagner and Berry (1969) and Wagner et al. (1969) ruled out the possibility of this hydrocarbon as the causative agent in their experiments. Roe et al. (1966) investigated the mineral oil associated with asbestos as a carcinogen, but this agent also cannot be considered as the primary cause of the tumors.

Mesotheliomas can be induced by other metals as well. Furst et al. (1973) reported the induction of this tumor when a mixture of cadium and zinc was introduced intrapleurally in rats.

Drawbacks to Subcutaneous Injection

Carcinogenesis studies in which materials are implanted or injected subcutaneously often give results that may be equivocal. It is not always easy to interpret the data when a few sarcomas appear at the site of injection. Grasso et al. (1971) varied their results when they modified the surface activity of the materials they injected; again, the variation seemed to depend on the concentration of the calcium ion in solution. Previously, Grasso and Golberg (1966) had studied this route of administration to see if the development of local sarcomas was an artifact of the method or if this route could be used as a means of assessing the carcinogenic potential of an agent.

Under similar conditions, Hueper (1965) tried to evaluate a report that sugar was carcinogenic. After testing 25% solutions of arabinose, galactose, and other sugars by injecting the solutions at the nape of the neck of almost 500 mice and 500 rats, he could not show that all sugars were innocuous. Nothdurft (1962) implanted the same material subcutaneously at the nape of the neck, the base of the tail, and the midline in a number of rats. The material, a silicone, had previously been found noncarcinogenic by other routes; but he observed that local tumors appeared at different times, depending on the site of implantation. According to his publication, in 15 months, four times as many tumors appeared at the nape of the neck as at the base of the tail. This work is very important and must be repeated; it has been more than a decade since this report was made.

INORGANIC CARCINOGENS

Animal Data Supported by Human Evidence

Nickel. The one element found carcinogenic in a variety of animal species and implicated in human cancer, supported by adequate epidemiological evidence, is nickel. The Mund process of refining nickel involves the conversion of nickel compounds into the gaseous nickel carbonyl, $Ni(CO)_4$. Many years ago, before the process became automated, some workers were exposed to the gaseous nickel compound. Nickel was held responsible for the induction of cancer in the nasal cavity (Sunderman, 1973) and in the lung (Baader, 1937). A series of papers on human exposure and lung cancer later appeared (Merewether, 1948; Doll, 1958; Sunderman, 1968), and a summary has been compiled (Mastromatteo, 1967).

Early experimental work was conducted on nickel by Hueper (1952, 1955, 1958), who implanted nickel subcutaneously, intramuscularly, intrafemorally, and intrathoracically. He obtained sarcomas in each case. In subsequent work, Hueper and Payne (1962) conducted inhalation experiments with nickel powder; they pretreated rats with SO_2 or limestone powder. The tumor yield was very low, showing only one sarcoma in the first pretreatment experiment and none in the second.

Sunderman and Donnelly (1965) did obtain lung squamous cell carcinoma when rats were exposed to gaseous nickel carbonyl. These tumors were similar to those found among nickel workers.

An extensive literature exists on the induction of local fibrosarcomas when nickel subsulfide (Ni_3S_2)—the nickel compound found in the ore—is implanted intramuscularly. Gilman (1962) injected ore dust and found it carcinogenic. Since then, others have repeated this experiment with similar results (Daniel et al., 1967; Mason, 1970; Maenza et al., 1971).

Pure nickel powder has also been used to induce fibrosarcomas in experimental animals. Heath and Daniel (1964) obtained 100% rhabdomyosarcomas with lymph node metastasis when Hooded rats were given nickel powder; Friedmann and Bird (1969) used random-bred Sprague-Dawley rats and obtained fewer tumors. Furst and Schlauder (1971) were able to induce fibrosarcomas in Syrian hamsters as well as Fischer rats with pure nickel powder. Hueper and Payne (1962) anticipated all of this work.

A variety of nickel compounds, including nickelocene, the pi-complex of nickel and dicyclopentadiene, and nickel acetate, were also active when administered intramuscularly (Haro et al., 1968). Payne (1964) related the carcinogenicity of nickel compounds to their solubility. Furst and Casetta (1973) found that nickel powder produced tumors in rats by all of the routes of administration tested. Sunderman (1973) has reviewed nickel carcinogenesis.

Chromium. Reports were published in the nineteenth century of the perforation of the nasal septum of workers using chromates (Pye, 1885); skin lesions were also noted. In 1932, lung cancer was reported in chromate-salt factory workers (Gross and Alwens, 1938). Baetjer (1950) compared the lung cancer rates among chromate workers and the population as a whole and found the former to be much higher.

In the main, the active agent is considered to be hexavalent chromate. However, Goldblatt (1956) studied the atmosphere in areas around the molten ore and tried to explain the different cancer rates in Great Britain and the United States. He concluded that trivalent chromium is also active. This idea is not supported by Grogan (1957). Dichromate is not as active as chromate (Gross and Alwens, 1938). There is some confusion; but until new research is conducted, it must be concluded that calcium chromate is the active material (i.e., any soluble chromate will become sparingly soluble calcium chromate in the body), dichromates are only slightly active, and chromium trivalent must be considered inactive.

Extensive laboratory work has been done with chromium compounds, but not many tumors have been induced in the experiments. Shimkin and Leiter (1940) administered powdered chromate ore intravenously to mice but did not succeed in producing tumors. Using an intratracheal technique, Baetjer et al. (1959) instilled potassium zinc chromate in rats; although some primary lesions developed, no squamous cell carcinoma was found. Hueper (1958) administered zinc potassium chromate intrathoracically and reported sarcomas. Hueper and Payne (1962) implanted a variety of chromates, either intramuscularly or into the chest wall, finding only a few tumors which were sarcomatous in nature. These slightly positive results led Steffee and Baetjer (1965) to claim that chromates might not be as active as previously believed; yet, Roe and Carter (1969) produced subcutaneous sarcomas by implanting calcium chromate. No squamous cell carcinomas were obtained by Nettesheim et al. (1971) after C57Bl mice were exposed to calcium chromate dust by inhalation; pulmonary adenomas were, however, reported.

Steffee and Baetjer (1965) had previously conducted an inhalation experiment with Wistar rats, using chromic trioxide. In addition, they administered roasted chromate dust intratracheally, with no observation of lung tumor incidence greater than in the controls. Payne (1960) also studied roasted chromate ores. Khachatryan (1964) studied the role of chromium compounds on the formation of primary lung cancers.

Kanisawa and Schroeder (1969) studied the administration of chromium (III) acetate, at a dose of 5 ppm in drinking water, over the life span of rats and concluded that no great differences were found in the treated rats as opposed to the controls.

Furst (1971) compared a series of metals for carcinogenicity by suspending pure powders in trioctanoin and injecting the material intramuscularly. Chromium produced few fibrosarcomas at the site of injection in contrast to nickel, which produced an incidence of over 70%. These results are similar to those obtained by Schinz and Uehlinger (1942). The different histological types of bronchogenic carcinomas are described, and chromium is listed as one of the etiological agents.

Metals Active in Animals with No Supporting Human Evidence

Cadmium. There is no conclusive epidemiological evidence that cadmium is carcinogenic in humans (Kipling and Waterhouse, 1967). It is quite toxic and is responsible for Itai disease in Japan (Riihimäki, 1972). It has also been implicated as a factor in the etiology of hypertension in humans; in animals, this physiologic state can be induced by the feeding of low oral doses of cadmium to rats (Kanisawa and Schroeder, 1969).

In rats, cadmium was found to be more active than nickel as a carcinogen (A. Furst, unpublished data). In a comparative study, fibrosarcomas were induced in 50% of Fischer-344 rats when a trioctanoin suspension of 3 mg cadmium powder was injected intramuscularly once; to achieve the same percentage of response with nickel powder, it took five monthly injections of 5 mg nickel powder per rat. Heath et al. (1962) were among the first to find this element to be carcinogenic in rats. Kipling and Waterhouse (1967), in a preliminary report, found a slightly higher percentage of prostatic cancers in workers exposed to cadmium oxide than in the male population as a whole. Malcolm (1972) discussed cadmium as a potential carcinogen in animals and humans.

Soluble salts of cadmium are also active. Gunn et al. (1963) injected cadmium chloride subcutaneously and found interstitial cell tumors in the testes of rats; the simultaneous injection of zinc ion somewhat negated this activity. It must be recognized that many rat strains develop Ledig cell tumors in the testes as a spontaneous event (Jacobs and Huseby, 1967). Local subcutaneous tumors were noted by Haddow et al. (1964a,b), Kazantzis (1963), and Kazantzis and Hanbury (1966) in mice after treatment with cadmium chloride. Guthrie (1964) injected cadmium chloride into the testes of Leghorn fowl and reported teratoma formation. Kanisawa and Schroeder (1969) kept rodents on 5 ppm cadmium in the drinking water and found no statistically significant total tumor incidence over controls, although there were a few more mammary gland and adrenal tumors in the treated groups.

Furst and Casetta (1972) were unable to negate the local appearance of fibrosarcomas when cadmium powder was injected intramuscularly in one leg and zinc powder was administered in the opposite leg. Lucis et al. (1972) reviewed this field recently; there is extensive documentation of the experiments with cadmium as a rodent carcinogen (Roe and Lancaster, 1964; Gunn et al., 1964, 1967; Nazari et al., 1967). Cadmium can induce sarcoma of the skin in rats (Knorre, 1970). Friberg et al. (1971) have a chapter on this topic.

Lead. A few recent experiments show that some lead compounds can induce tumors, particularly in the kidney. Zollinger (1953) administered lead phosphate subcutaneously to rats and reported renal adenomas and carcinomas, but Roe et al. (1965a) failed to find carcinomas after injecting rats with lead acetate. Given orally, basic lead acetate (van Esch et al., 1962) and lead acetate (Zawirska and Medras, 1968) resulted in renal tumors, including carcinomas. Van Esch and Kroes (1969) repeated these experiments with Swiss mice and found the same renal tumors. Kanisawa and Schroeder (1969), however, exposed mice over their life span to 5 ppm lead acetate in their drinking water; it appeared that the incidence of spontaneous tumors was lower in the treated than in the control groups.

Epstein and Mantel's 1968 experiment needs repeating; they treated newborn Swiss mice with subcutaneous doses of lead tetraethyl and found an incidence of lymphomas greater than in the controls. Further evaluation of lead compounds as they relate to carcinogenesis is necessary.

Beryllium. Berylliosis, a disease entity appearing in animals or humans after exposure to beryllium compounds for varying periods of time, is characterized by the occurrence of granulomas in the skin or the subcutaneous tissue, if the chemical penetrates beneath the skin. After chronic inhalation of some beryllium compounds, a granulomatous fibrosis of the lungs may appear. Gardner and Heslington (1946) reported induction of osteosarcoma in rabbits following repeated intravenous injection of beryllium oxide. These results were confirmed by Hoagland et al. (1950), Barnes et al. (1950), Dutra and Largent (1950), and Yamaguchi (1963), among others.

Beryllium sulfate was administered by inhalation to Sherman rats (Schepers, 1964) and to Sprague-Dawley rats (Reeves et al., 1967); in both cases, pulmonary neoplasms were found. Dutra et al. (1951) also used beryllium oxide in inhalation studies with positive results.

Schepers (1964) found one neoplasm in a *Macacus mulatta* species of subhuman primate after exposure to beryllium phosphate (BeHPO$_4$); this may have been a spontaneous tumor.

Vorwald et al. (1966) induced pulmonary tumors in Rhesus monkeys after exposing these primates to beryllium sulfate aerosol. Wagner et al. (1969) reported no tumors in hamsters but noted possible preneoplastic lesions following exposure to beryl ore.

No cancer has been found in humans exposed to beryllium compounds (Stokinger, 1966); however, this possibility is not ruled out. Neither Hardy et al. (1967), Stoeckle et al. (1969), nor Mancuso and El-Attar (1969) could conclude from available case studies that workers exposed to beryllium compounds developed lung cancer.

Claims without Sufficient Supporting Evidence to Date

Zinc. Zinc has been reported to be carcinogenic, but this was demonstrated only by injecting zinc salts directly into the gonads. After necrosis of the testes, teratomas developed in both rats and fowl (Anissimowa, 1939; Falin and Gromzewa, 1939; Smith and Powell, 1957; Rivière et al., 1960). Guthrie (1964) also noted that zinc chloride induced teratomas in fowl, whereas both zinc acetate and zinc stearate failed to do so. Zinc powder, administered intramuscularly in rats, failed to produce sarcomas (Heath et al., 1962).

Zinc is essential for many enzymes (Underwood, 1971), for cell division and for DNA synthesis (Chesters, 1974). Although less work has been done on zinc carcinogenesis itself, a number of studies have been made to determine what effect the addition or restriction of zinc might have on the formation of tumors induced by other carcinogenics. For example, administration of dietary zinc sulfate retarded the expected development of tumors when DMBA was painted on the cheek pouch of hamsters (Poswillo and Cohen, 1971); similar results were found by Ciapparelli et al. (1972) in the rat. On the other hand, DeWys et al. (1970) found that the growth of transplanted Walker-256 rat tumor was inhibited when the rats were kept on a zinc-deficient diet; further experiments were done with other tumors (DeWys and Pories, 1972). Similar results were obtained by Barr and Harris (1973), who transplanted the mouse leukemia, P-388. Although zinc has been reported to negate the induction of cadmium-induced, interstitial cell tumors of the testes of rodents (Gunn et al., 1963), it failed to prevent the formation of sarcomas at the site of application of cadmium powder (Furst and Casetta, 1972).

It is obvious that the function and role of zinc in cancer must be explored further.

Cobalt. Heath (1956) found cobalt to produce rhabdomyosarcomas in Hooded rats 5–12 months following intramuscular implantation of the pure powder. This finding was confirmed by Gilman (1962b), who also investigated cobalt oxide and sulfide and noted that mice were less susceptible than rats to the induction of local fibrosarcomas (Gilman and Ruckerbauer, 1962).

Previously, Vollman (1940) and Schinz and Uehlinger (1942) had been able to produce sarcomas in rabbits by administering cobalt either intraosseously or subcutaneously.

As the metal portion of vitamin B_{12}, cobalt is known for its antipernicious anemia action; it is also a necessary cofactor for some enzymes. It is, therefore, of interest to note that excess amounts of an essential trace element can induce tumors.

Much more work needs to be done with cobalt, especially with the pure soluble salts. It must also be borne in mind that many dusts are not pure but are mixtures of other metals and their compounds; this is noted by many investigators but is sometimes overlooked in summary reports of the literature.

Iron. The epidemiological evidence would seem to indicate carcinogenicity for iron, or at least its oxide, although not much substantiating experimental data are available. Gurevich (1967) reported that underground hematite miners in the USSR had a higher rate of lung cancer than those who transported the ore or worked in the smelter. That miners of iron ore are susceptible to lung cancer has been known for some time (Faulds and Stewart, 1956; Braun et al., 1960). Among the earliest to report this was Dreyfus (1936).

Boyd et al. (1970) made an extensive study of the death certificates of nearly 6,000 males who lived near an iron ore mine in England. They found a greater incidence of lung cancer among the miners than in the population at large.

Hematite is not a simple compound and because it contains a proportion of silica material, silicosis may be a complicating factor in the interpretation of the pathology observed among miners. Monlibert and Ronbille (1960) noted this, as did Faulds and Stewart (1956). The observation of a high rate of lung cancer among iron ore miners has been made in a number of countries; this topic is summarized in vol. 1 of the IARC monograph (1972).

Kraus et al. (1957) suggested that the incidence of gastric cancer was greater in males exposed to iron ore than in the normal population; this needs verification. Muller and Erhardt (1956) have questioned the statistics.

In animal studies, neither conclusive nor negative results were obtained when rodents were exposed to ferrous oxide. Campbell (1942) subjected mice to dusts of a variety of oxides, including ferrous oxide, and claimed a higher frequency of lung tumors in mice; however, his actual number of tumors was low. Muller and Erhardt (1956) obtained no greater number of tumors using mice. Saffiotti et al. (1968) and Ho and Furst (1973) administered pure ferrous oxide intratracheally to hamsters and mice, respectively. No tumors developed, although both studies demonstrated that the ferrous oxide remained in the lungs for many months. Similar results had been found earlier by Hueper (1966). Exposure to hematite dust failed to produce lung tumors in hamsters (Vorwald and Karr, 1937).

A different picture is presented when iron carbohydrate complexes are injected subcutaneously in rodents (see the section Drawbacks to Subcutaneous Injections, above). Various iron dextran compounds, injected subcutaneously in rats (Haddow et al., 1964a; Golberg et al., 1960) or mice (Fielding, 1962), produced local tumors. Other iron complexes are also active under the conditions of the experiments. These include the glyconate and glucoside (Carter et al., 1968); sorbital was not as active (Lundin, 1961) or failed to be active (Roe and Haddow, 1965).

There seems to be a species difference in response to the iron carbohydrate complexes; neither rabbits (Haddow and Horning, 1960) nor dogs (Golberg et al., 1960) produced tumors when injected. Carter et al. (1968) failed to induce tumors when they tested squirrel monkeys. To date, only one report lists a sarcoma at the site of injection of iron dextran, in a 74-yr-old woman (Robinson et al., 1960).

Dilemmas

Arsenic. As early as 1888, Hutchinson reported skin cancer among miners and attributed this to arsenic. At present, good epidemiological evidence exists to implicate arsenic as a causative agent for skin cancer (Lee and Fraumeni, 1969; Ott et al., 1974). The described sequelae include keratosis of the hands and feet (Tseng et al., 1968) and hyperpigmentation. Bowen's disease is associated with arsenic poisoning. Arsenicism and invasive carcinomas of the skin have also been documented (Sommers and McManus, 1953; Sanderson, 1963). In addition, multiple tumors have been seen where arsenic is the suspected etiological agent. Chronic arsenicism has been associated with lung cancer (Robson and Jelliffe, 1963), but the IARC monograph (1973) states that this may be coincidental.

The dilemma in this field is the complete absence of a valid biological model for experimental arsenic-induced cancer. It is interesting how often arsenic is singled out as *the carcinogen* when metals or metaloids are discussed. Yet, repeated attempts to induce any type of neoplasm in any strain or species of animal have been made without success.

Leitch and Kennaway (1922) painted over 100 mice with an alcoholic potassium arsenite solution and found one tumor in 33 surviving mice. Neubauer (1947) documents a number of unsuccessful attempts to repeat this experiment. No positive results were found with any arsenic compound in the drinking water of mice (Hueper and Payne, 1962; Kanisawa and Schroeder, 1967). Rats fed lead arsenate failed to develop any malignancy (Fairhǎll and Miller, 1941). Similar negative results were obtained in rats by Byron et al. (1967).

Arsenic compounds have also been evaluated as possible cocarcinogens. Baroni et al. (1963) tested sodium arsenate in conjunction with croton oil, urethane, and dimethylbenzanthracene, with no positive results. Boutwell (1963) was also unsuccessful in showing any cocarcinogenicity of arsenic. Kroes et al. (1974) failed to show any effect of arsenic on diethylnitrosamine activity in rats.

Frost (1967) has suggested a reassessment of the toxicity of arsenic; he believes that arsenic is not carcinogenic.

Thus, the question of arsenic and carcinogenicity remains unresolved. A body of literature exists on the antineoplastic properties of this element, but a review of this property is not part of this discussion. Unfortunately, arsenic will remain in the controversial category until a really exhaustive study is made of this element, using a variety of routes (including intratracheal); but funds for such a study are not forthcoming.

Selenium. Selenium is another element for which definitive information on its ability to induce tumors is lacking. Indeed, conflicting results exist. A major factor may be the diet given to the experimental animals.

Prior to the finding that selenium was an essential element for fowl and mammals (Schwarz and Foltz, 1957), Nelson et al. (1943) reported that rats maintained on a diet of 12% protein, incorporated with 10 ppm potassium ammonium sulfoselenide, developed cirrhosis and subsequent adenomas of the liver. Similar results were reported by Tscherkes et al. (1963) and Volgarev and Tscherkes (1967), who claimed a 35% incidence of liver tumors in rats fed 10 mg sodium selenite/kg food containing 12% casein. Seifter et al. (1946) found multiple thyroid adenomas in rats receiving acetoaminophenyl selenium dihydroxide (Seifter did not publish a follow-up report). Clayton and Baumann (1949) studied the cocarcinogenic action of selenium and an azo dye; they found more hepatomas in the animals when selenium was given with the dye.

Harr et al. (1967) found no liver tumors in over 1,000 rats fed between 0.5 ppm and 16 ppm of selenite; they doubted the carcinogenicity of selenium. On the other hand, Frost (1967) suggested that selenium might actually be the agent that caused the toxic reactions attributed to arsenic; by inference, this would include the carcinogenic action. Scott (1973) tried to explain the variable results by attributing the difference to diet and the difficulty of diagnosis.

Schroeder et al. (1970) found no greater incidence of spontaneous tumors in mice given selenite or selenate in the drinking water over their life span; however, they found more tumors in rats given selenate than in the controls. Shapiro (1972) has summarized much of this work.

Studies have also been made of selenium compounds as antitumorigenic agents. Weisberger and Suhrland (1956) successfully treated transplanted leukemia with selenocystine; and Shamberger (1970) administered selenide orally, thus reducing the incidence of papillomas on mouse skin following painting with the hydrocarbon 7, 11-DMBA.

The diagnosis of the nature of an hepatic lesion is not always clear in the literature. The term *hepatoma* is often used but may not be too useful; more descriptive terms should be utilized.

Miscellaneous Metal Studies

A number of metals have been evaluated as potential carcinogens. Either totally negative results were obtained or, if local sarcomas were induced, they were, in all probability, the result of an Oppenheimer effect.

Negative results were obtained with copper (Gilman, 1962; Furst, 1971) and aluminum (Furst, 1971). On the other hand, O'Gara and Brown (1967) tested aluminum foil subcutaneously and obtained both fibrosarcomas and rhabdomyosarcomas; this may have been a smooth-surface effect. Similar statements can be made about the positive results with mercury (Druckrey et al., 1957); silver should also be in this class (Oppenheimer et al., 1956). Manganese chloride was administered subcutaneously and intraperitoneally in mice at weekly intervals for 6 months; more lymphosarcomas were found in the treated mice than in the controls (DiPaolo, 1964). A more complete study of manganese compounds, and especially the various oxides, is necessary; yet, 10 yr later, no further work has been done. An organic titanium compound, titanocene dichloride, at very high levels (about 500 mg), seemed to produce more lymphomas in Fischer-344 rats than did the vehicle in the controls (Furst, 1971). (Furst has requested the National Cancer Institute to repeat this work.) Roe et al. (1965b) tested tin compounds and found them negative.

With the increased use of coal as a fuel, more heavy metals will be liberated into the atmosphere; at the same time, more and different alloys are being introduced. It is essential to test these as potential carcinogens. Human beings are exposed to these metals by ingestion and/or inhalation, but most of the experimental work has involved the intramuscular or subcutaneous routes. Much of this work should be repeated, administering the materials orally, either by gavage or by mixing the metal or its compound in the food, and by inhalation. Where inhalation is not possible, the animal should be exposed to a quantitative amount of the agent intratracheally.

Schroeder (1963) used the drinking water to convey the agents to the animals. Much of his work should be repeated at the *maximum tolerated dose*. The levels he used were those to which humans are exposed; this was a first, essential step, but not the final one. Ho and Furst (1973) have described a useful technique. They also suggest that mice have the advantage over all other rodents, because more is known about their viral profile, their genetics, and their biochemical responses.

EFFECTS OF METALS ON OTHER CARCINOGENS

An entire review is necessary to cover this subject. The highlights, however, have been given in good detail by Kanisawa (1971). This review will also not attempt to describe metal compounds as anticancer agents; again, this subject deserves to be a topic in its own right.

Enhancement

Copper seemed to accelerate the appearance of skin papillomas induced by a dimethylbenzanthracene compound (Fare, 1965). Recently, Furst (unpublished data) found more tumors in Fischer-344 rats when nickel was administered with cadmium than when an equal amount of cadmium was given alone.

Cobalt enhanced the induction of skin tumors by 3-methylcholanthrene (Finogenova, 1973).

Inhibition

The addition of a copper salt to the diet delayed the onset of liver tumors by the well-known p-dimethylaminoazobenzene (Sharpless, 1946); this was a partial confirmation of Pedrero and Kozelka's work (1951) with the 3'-methyl derivative of the azo dye. The copper salt may enhance the azo-dye metabolizing enzyme (Yamane et al., 1969) or hasten the destruction of the dye by oxidation; thus, the animals may not be consuming as much dye as expected.

Aluminum, in various forms and by different routes of administration, lowered the usual incidence of pulmonary tumors induced by 4-nitroquinoline N-oxide (Kobayashi et al., 1970).

Sodium cobaltinitrite and cobaltous chloride somewhat negated the carcinogenic activity of 3-methylcholanthrene (Orzechowski et al., 1964; Kasirsky et al., 1965).

Zinc, as an enhancer or inhibitor, has already been discussed, as has selenium.

THEORIES OF ACTION

Metals have not been studied as extensively as other carcinogens. The mechanisms of metal action have apparently been relegated to an area of low priority. Furst and Haro (1969b) attempted to give some background for mechanistic studies, but no experimental data were presented. In most reviews on mechanisms, metals are mentioned only in a cursory fashion with all-inclusive statements, such as, chemicals that induce cancer go through a cation form, and metal ions are already cations (Miller and Miller, 1971). This ignores the fact that many metallic cations are not carcinogenic and that chromium is active only as a hexavalent anion.

Weinzierl (1972) studied the rapid solution of metals in body tissues and fluids; he produced ample evidence to show that metals are not inert in the animal body but are reactive and dissolve rapidly. By some means or other, they also enter into cells and are distributed in an orderly fashion. For example, over half of the nickel that induces rhabdomyosarcomas localizes in the nucleus, especially the nucleolar fraction (Webb et al., 1972; Webb and Weinzierl, 1972).

The majority of the work on the mechanism of metal carcinogenesis has been done with nickel. Sunderman (1971, 1973) has written the best reviews on the subject. He summarized the various ways in which nickel may modify, and hence alter, the growth of cells, including the inhibition of RNA-polymerase activity in hepatocytes, the binding of nickel to various nucleic acids and nucleoproteins, the inhibition of antiviral proteins, the interference with cell division by nickel, and the alteration of energy metabolism by nickel (1973). Thus, he followed Miller and Miller's (1971) suggestion on how chemicals may initiate neoplastic growth. Specific data on the biochemical alterations caused by nickel carbonyl are given in Sunderman's 1971 review. These two reviews ought to be considered required reading for those interested in metal carcinogenesis.

SUGGESTED RESEARCH

Much more work needs to be done on the investigation of metals as primary carcinogens. Testing of new metals and their alloys should attempt to duplicate the ways in which humans are exposed to these agents. Thus, oral applications and drinking water solutions must be tested at different dose levels, including maximum tolerated doses. Airborne metals must be tested by inhalation and also by intratracheal instillation (in mice, if possible). Alloys that will be used as prosthesis or suture materials, intrauterine contraceptive devices, and dental castings must be tested in that manner. More work on the solubility of metals and their alloys by body fluids, especially serum, should be conducted.

Is there a preferred oxidation state of the inorganic carcinogens? Does a carcinogenic metal displace an essential metal from an enzyme or tissue?

REFERENCES

Anissimowa, W. W. 1939. *Amer. J. Cancer* 36:229–232.

Baader, W. W. 1937. In *Neuere Ergebnisse auf dem Gebiete der Krebskrankheiten*, ed. C. Adam and D. Auler, pp. 116–117. Leipzig: Hirzel Verlag.

Baetjer, A. M. 1950. *Arch. Industr. Hyg. Occup. Med.* 2:487–504.

Baetjer, A. M., Lowney, J. F., Steffee, H. and Budacz, V. 1959. *Arch. Industr. Health* 20:124–135.

Barnes, J. M., Denz, F. A. and Sissons, H. A. 1950. *Brit. J. Cancer* 4:212–222.

Baroni, C., van Esch, G. J. and Soffiotti, V. 1963. *Arch. Environ. Health* 7:668–674.

Barr, D. H. and Harris, J. W. 1973. *Proc. Soc. Exp. Biol. Med.* 144:284–287.

Becker, T., Markgraf, E., Oswald, H., Schyra, B. and Winnefeld, K. 1966. *Wiss Chir.-Tag, 6th Symp.* 2:1722–1727.

Bischoff, F. and Bryson, G. 1964. *Prog. Exp. Tumor Res.* 5:85–133.

Bischoff, F. and Bryson, G. 1974. *J. Natl. Cancer Inst.* 52:1383.

Boutwell, R. K. 1963. *J. Agr. Food Chem.* 11:381–385.

Boyd, J. T., Doll, R., Faulds, J. S. and Leiper, J. 1970. *Brit. J. Industr. Med.* 27:97–105.

Brand, K. G., Buoen, L. C., Johnson, K. H. and Brand, I. 1975. *Cancer Res.* 35:279–286.
Braun, P., Guillerm, J., Pierson, B., Lacoste, J. and Sadoul, P. 1960. *Rev. Med. (Nancy)* 85:702–708.
Bryson, G. and Bischoff, F. 1969. *Prog. Exp. Tumor Res.* 11:100–133.
Byron, W. R., Bierbower, G. W., Brouwer, J. B. and Hansen, W. H. 1967. *Toxicol. Appl. Pharmacol.* 10:132–147.
Campbell, J. A. 1942. *Brit. Med. J.* 1:217–221.
Carter, R. L., Mitchley, B. C. V. and Roe, F. J. C. 1968. *Brit. J. Cancer* 22:521–526.
Carter, R. L., Roe, F. J. C. and Peto, R. 1971. *J. Natl. Cancer Inst.* 46:1277–1289.
Chesters, J. K. 1974. In *Biochemical functions of zinc with emphasis on nucleic acid metabolism and cell division in trace element metabolism in animals*, ed. W. G. Huekstra, J. W. Suttie, H. E. Janther and W. Mertz, vol. II, pp. 39–50. Baltimore, Md.: University Park Press.
Ciapparelli, L., Retief, D. H. and Fatti, L. P. 1972. *S. African J. Med. Sci.* 37:85–90.
Clayton, C. C. and Baumann, C. A. 1949. *Cancer Res.* 9:575–582.
Cleare, M. J. 1974. *Coordination Chem. Rev.* 12:349–405.
Cralley, L. J. and Lainhart, W. S. 1973. *J. Occup. Med.* 15:262–266.
Daniel, M. R., Heath, J. C. and Webb, M. 1967. *Brit. J. Cancer* 21:780–786.
DeWys, W. and Pories, W. 1972. *J. Natl. Cancer Inst.* 48:375–382.
DeWys, W., Pories, W. J., Richter, M. C. and Strain, W. H. 1970. *Proc. Soc. Exp. Biol. Med.* 135:17–22.
DiPaolo, J. A. 1964. *Fed. Proc.* 23:393.
Doll, R. 1955. *Brit. J. Industr. Med.* 12:81–86.
Doll, R. 1958. *Brit. J. Industr. Med.* 15:217–223.
Dreyfus, J. R. 1936. *Z. Klin. Med.* 130:256–260.
Druckrey, H., Hamperl, H. and Schmahl, D. 1957. *Z. Krebsforsch.* 61:511–519.
Dutra, F. R. and Largent, E. J. 1950. *Amer. J. Pathol.* 26:197–202.
Dutra, F. R., Largent, E. J. and Roth, J. L. 1951. *AMA Arch. Path.* 51:473–479.
Epstein, S. S. and Mantel, N. 1968. *Experientia* 24:580–581.
Fairhall, L. T. and Miller, J. W. 1941. *Publ. Health Rep. (Wash.)* 56:1610–1625.
Falin, L. I. and Gromzewa, K. E. 1939. *Amer. J. Cancer* 36:233–236.
Fare, G. 1965. *Experientia* 21:415–416.
Faulds, J. S. and Stewart, M. J. 1956. *J. Pathol. Bact.* 72:353–366.
Fielding, J. 1962. *Brit. Med. J.* 1:1800–1803.
Finogenova, M. A. 1973. *Byull Eksp. Biol. Med.* 75:73–75.
Fischer, B. 1906. *München Med. Wochenschr.* 53:2041–2047.
Friberg, L., Piscator, M. and Nordberg, G. 1971. In *Cadmium in the environment*, pp. 107–110. Cleveland, Ohio: Chemical Rubber Co. Press.
Friedmann, I. and Bird, E. S. 1969. *J. Pathol.* 97:379–382.
Frost, D. C. 1967. *Fed. Proc.* 26:194–208.
Furst, A. 1960. In *Chelation and cancer—A speculative review in metal binding in medicine*, ed. M. J. Seven and L. A. Johnson, pp. 336–344. Philadelphia: Lippincott.
Furst, A. 1963. *Chemistry of chelation in cancer*, pp. 17–18: Springfield, Ill.: Thomas.

Furst, A. 1971. In *Environmental geochemistry*, ed. H. L. Cannon and H. C. Hopps, pp. 109–130.Memoir 123. Boulder, Colo.: Geological Society of America.

Furst, A. and Casetta, D. 1972. *Proc. Amer. Assoc. Cancer Res.* 13:62.

Furst, A. and Casetta, D. 1973. *Proc. Amer. Assoc. Cancer Res.* 14:31.

Furst, A. and Haro, R. T. 1969a. In *Possible mechanism of metal ion carcinogenesis. Jerusalem symposia on quantum chemistry and biochemistry*, ed. E. D. Bergmann and P. Pullman, vol. 1, pp. 310–320. Jerusalem: Israel Academy of Sciences and Humanities.

Furst, A. and Haro, R. T. 1969b. *Prog. Exp. Tumor Res.* 12:102–133.

Furst, A. and Schlauder, M. C. 1971. *Proc. West. Pharmacol. Soc.* 14:68–71.

Furst, A., Casetta, D. M. and Sasmore, D. P. 1973. *Proc. West. Pharmacol. Soc.* 16:150–153.

Gardner, L. V. and Heslington, H. F. 1946. *Fed. Proc.* 5:221.

Gilman, J. P. W. 1962. *Cancer Res.* 22:158–162.

Gilman, J. P. W. and Ruckerbauer, G. M. 1962. *Cancer Res.* 22:152–157.

Gloyne, S. R. 1935. *Tubercle* 17:5–10.

Golberg, L., Martin. L. E. and Smith, J. P. 1960. *Toxicol. Appl. Pharmacol.* 2:683–707.

Goldblatt, M. W. 1956. *Industrial medicine and hygiene*, vol. III. London: Butterworths.

Grasso, P. and Golberg, L. 1966. *Fed. Cosmet. Toxicol.* 4:297–320.

Grasso, P., Gangolli, S. D., Golberg, L. and Hooson, J. 1971. *Fed. Cosmet. Toxicol.* 9:463–478.

Grogan, C. H. 1957. *Cancer* 10:625–638.

Gross, E. and Alwens, D. 1938. *VIII Intern. Kongr. Unfall Med. Berufskrank.* Leipzig.

Gross, P., de Treville, R. T. P., Tolker, E. B., Kaschak, M. and Babyak, M. A. 1967. *Arch. Environ. Health* 15:343–355.

Gunn, S. A., Gould, T. C. and Anderson, W. A. 1963. *J. Natl. Cancer Inst.* 31:745–753.

Gunn, S. A., Gould, T. C. and Anderson, W. A. D. 1964. *Proc. Soc. Exp. Biol. Med.* 115:653–657.

Gunn, S. A., Gould, T. C. and Anderson, W. A. 1967. *Arch. Pathol.* 83:493–499.

Gurevich, M. A. 1967. *Arkh. Pat.* 29:19–23.

Guthrie, J. 1964. *Brit. J. Cancer* 18:255–260.

Haddow, A. 1958. In *The possible role of metals and metal chelation in the carcinogenic process in carcinogenesis*, ed. G. E. W. Wolstenholme and M. O'Connor, pp. 300–307. Boston: Little, Brown.

Haddow, A. and Horning, E. S. 1960. *J. Natl. Cancer Inst.* 24:109–147.

Haddow, A., Roe, F. J. C. and Mitchley, B. C. V. 1964a. *Brit. Med. J.* 1:1593–1594.

Haddow, A., Roe, F. J. C., Dukes, C. E. and Mitchley, B. C. V. 1964b. *Brit. J. Cancer* 18:667–673.

Hardy, H. L., Rabe, E. W. and Lorch, S. 1967. *J. Occup. Med.* 9:271–276.

Harington, J. S. 1962. *Nature (London)* 193:43–45.

Haro, R. T., Furst, A., Payne, W. W. and Falk, H. 1968. *Proc. Amer. Assoc. Cancer Res.* 9:28.

Harr, J. R., Bone, J. F., Tinsley, J. J., Tinsley, I. J., Weswig, P. H. and Yamamoto, R. S. 1967. In *Selenium in biomedicine*, ed. O. H. Muth, p. 153. Westport, Conn.: Avi.

Harris, C. C. 1973. *Cancer Chemother. Rept.* 4:59–61.
Heath, J. C. 1956. *Brit. J. Cancer* 10:668–673.
Heath, J. C. and Daniel, M. R. 1964. *Brit. J. Cancer* 18:251–264.
Heath, J. C., Daniel, M. R., Dingle, J. T. and Webb, M. 1962. *Nature (London)* 193:592–593.
Ho, W. and Furst, A. 1973. *Oncology* 27:385–393.
Hoagland, M. B., Grier, R. S. and Hood, M. B. 1950. *Cancer Res.* 10:629–635.
Hueper, W. C. 1952. *Tex. Rept. Biol. Med.* 10:167–186.
Hueper, W. C. 1955. *J. Natl. Cancer Inst.* 16:55–73.
Hueper, W. C. 1958. *Arch. Pathol.* 65:600–607.
Hueper, W. C. 1965. *Cancer Res.* 25:440–443.
Hueper, W. C. 1966. *Recent results in cancer research. 3. Occupational and environmental cancers of the respiratory system.* New York: Springer-Verlag.
Hueper, W. C. and Conway, W. D. 1964. *Chemical carcinogenesis and cancer.* Springfield, Ill.: Thomas.
Hueper, W. C. and Payne, W. W. 1962. *Arch. Environ. Health* 5:445–462.
IARC. 1972. *Monographs on the evaluation of carcinogenic risk of chemicals to man,* vol. I, pp. 17–28. Lyon: International Agency for Research on Cancer.
IARC. 1973. *Monographs on the evaluation of carcinogenic risk of chemicals to man. Some inorganic and metalorganic compounds,* vol. II, pp. 5–47. Lyon: International Agency for Research on Cancer.
Jacobs, B. B. and Huseby, R. A. 1967. *J. Natl. Cancer Inst.* 39:303–309.
Kanisawa, M. 1971. *Ann. Rept. Inst. Food Microbiol. (Chiba University)* 24:1–35.
Kanisawa, M. and Schroeder, H. A. 1967. *Cancer Res.* 27:1192–1195.
Kanisawa, M. and Schroeder, H. A. 1969. *Cancer Res.* 29:892–895.
Karp, R. D., Johnson, K. H., Buoen, L. C., Brand, I. and Brand, K. G. 1973. *J. Natl. Cancer Inst.* 50:1403–1405.
Kasirsky, G., Gantieri, R. F. and Mann, D. E., Jr. 1965. *J. Pharmacol. Sci.* 54:491–493.
Kazantzis, G. 1963. *Nature (London)* 198:1213–1214.
Kazantzis, G. and Hanbury, W. J. 1966. *Brit. J. Cancer* 20:190–199.
Khachatryan, E. A. 1964. *Zh. Eksp. Klin. Med.* 4:119–129.
Kipling, M. D. and Waterhouse, J. A. 1967. *Lancet* 1:730–731.
Knorre, D. 1970. *Arch. Geschwulst. Jorsch* 36:119–126.
Kohayashi, N., Katsuki, H. and Yamane, Y. 1970. *Gann* 61:239–244.
Kraus, A. S., Levin, M. L. and Gerhardt, P. R. 1957. *Amer. J. Publ. Health* 47:961–970.
Kroes, R., Van Logten, J. M., Berkvens, J. M., de Vries, T. and van Esch, G. J. 1974. *Fed. Cosmet. Toxicol.* 12:671–679.
Kuratsune, M., Tonudome, S., Shirakusa, T., Yoshida, M., Tokumitsu, Y., Hayano, T. and Seita, M. 1974. *Int. J. Cancer* 13:552–558.
Lee, A. M. and Fraumeni, J. F., Jr. 1969. *J. Natl. Cancer Inst.* 42:1045–1052.
Leitch, A. and Kennaway, E. L. 1922. *Brit. Med. J.* ii:1107–1108.
Lucis, O. J., Lucis, R. and Sterman, K. 1972. *Oncology* 26:53–67.
Lundin, P. M. 1961. *Brit. J. Cancer* 15:838–847.
Lynch, K. M. and Smith, D. A. 1935. *Amer. J. Cancer* 24:56–64.
Lynch, K. M., McIver, F. A. and Cain, J. R. 1937. *Arch. Indust. Health* 15:207–214.
Maatz, R. and Palowsky, G. 1972. *Bruns Beitr. Klin. Chir.* 219:276–287.

Maenza, R. M., Pradham, A. M. and Sunderman, F. W., Jr. 1971. *Cancer Res.* 31:2067–2071.
Malcolm, D. 1972. *Ann. Occup. Hyg.* 15:33–36.
Mancuso, T. F. and El-Attar, A. A. 1969. *J. Occup. Med.* 11:422–434.
Mason, M. M. 1972. Nickel sulfide, a model carcinogen. *Environ. Physiol. Biochem.* 2:137–141.
Mastromatteo, E. 1967. *J. Occup. Med.* 9:127–136.
Merewether, E. R. 1948. *Annual report, chief inspector of factories, for the year 1948.* London: Her Majesty's Stationery Office.
Miller, J. A. and Miller, E. C. 1971. *J. Natl. Cancer Inst.* 47:5–14.
Moizhess, T. G. and Prigozhina, E. L. 1973. *Byull. Eksp. Biol. Med.* 76:92–94.
Monlibert, L. and Ronbille, R. 1960. *J. Franc. Med. Chir. Thor.* 14:435–439.
Muller, E. and Erhardt. W. 1956. *Z. Krebsforsch.* 61:65–77.
Nazari, G., Favino, A. and Pozzi, U. 1967. *Riv. Anat. Pathol. Oncol.* 31:251–270.
Nelson, A. A., Fitzhugh, O. G. and Calvery, H. O. 1943. *Cancer Res.* 3:230–236.
Nelson, W. C., Lykins, M. H., Mackey, J., Newill, V. A., Finklea, J. F. and Hammer, D. I. 1973. *J. Chron. Dis.* 26:105–118.
Nettesheim, P., Hanna, M. G., Jr., Doherty, D. G., Newell, R. F. and Hellman, A. 1971. *J. Natl. Cancer Inst.* 47:1129–1144.
Neubauer, O. 1947. *Brit. J. Cancer* 1:192–251.
Nothdurft, H. 1958. *Naturwissenschaften* 45:549–550.
Nothdurft, H. 1962. *Naturwissenschaften* 49:18–19.
O'Gara, R. W. and Brown, J. M. 1967. *J. Natl. Cancer Inst.* 38:947–957.
Oppenheimer, B. S., Oppenheimer, E. T. and Danishefsky, I. I. 1955. *Cancer Res.* 15:333–340.
Oppenheimer, B. S., Oppenheimer, E. T., Danishefsky, I. I. and Stout, A. P. 1956. *Cancer Res.* 16:439–441.
Orzechowski, R. F., Gantieri, R. F. and Mann, D. E., Jr. 1964. *J. Pharmacol. Sci.* 53:388–391.
Ott, M. C., Holder, B. B. and Gordon, H. L. 1974. *Arch. Environ. Health* 29:250–255.
Payne, W. W. 1964. *Proc. Amer. Assoc. Cancer Res.* 5:50.
Payne, W. W. 1960. *Arch. Environ. Health* 1:20–26.
Pedrero, E., Jr. and Kozelka, F. L. 1951. *Arch. Path.* 52:455–457.
Poswillo, D. E. and Cohen, B. 1971. *Nature* 231:447–448.
Pott, P. 1778. Cancer scroti. In *Chirurgical works of Percivall Pott,* pp. 403–406. Dublin: James Williams.
Pye, W. 1885. *Ann. Surg.* 1:303–308.
Reeves, A. L., Deitch, D. and Vorwarld, A. J. 1967. *Cancer Res.* 27:439–445.
Reeves, A. L., Puro, H. E., Smith, R. G. and Vorwald, A. J. 1971. *Environ. Res.* 4:496–511.
Riihimäki, V. 1972. *Work-Environ.-Health* 9:91–101.
Rivière, M. R., Chonroulonkov, I. and Guérin, M. 1960. *Bull. Assoc. Franc. Cancer* 47:55–87.
Robinson, C. E. G., Bell, D. N. and Sturdy, J. J. 1960. *Brit. Med. J.* ii:648–650.
Robson, A. O. and Jelliffe, A. M. 1963. *Brit. Med. J.* ii:207–209.
Rockstroh, H. 1959. *Arch. Geschwulstforsch.* 14:151–162.
Roe, F. J. C. and Carter, R. L. 1969. *Brit. J. Cancer* 23:172–176.
Roe, F. J. C. and Haddow, A. 1965. *Brit. J. Cancer* 19:855–859.

A. Furst

Roe, F. J. C. and Lancaster, M. C. 1964. *Brit. Med. Bull.* 20:127–133.
Roe, F. J. C., Dukes, C. E., Cameron, K. M., Pugh, R. C. B. and Mitchley, B. C. V. 1964. *Brit. J. Cancer* 18:674–681.
Roe, F. J. C., Boyland, E., Dukes, C. E. and Mitchley, C. V. 1965a. *Brit. J. Cancer* 19:860–866.
Roe, F. J. C., Boyland, E. and Millican, K. 1965b. *Fed. Cosmet. Toxicol.* 3:277–280.
Roe, F. J. C., Walters, M. A. and Harington, J. S. 1966. *Int. J. Cancer* 1:491–492.
Rosenberg, B., Van Camp, L., Trosko, J. E. and Mansour, V. H. 1969. *Nature* 222:385–386.
Saffiotti, U., Cefis, F. and Kolb, L. H. 1968. *Cancer Res.* 28:104–113.
Sanderson, K. V. 1963. *Trans. St. John Hosp. Derm. Soc.* 49:115–122.
Schepers, G. W. H. 1964. *Indust. Med. Surg.* 33:1–16.
Schinz, H. R. U. and Uehlinger, E. 1942. *Z. Krebsforsch.* 52:425–437.
Schroeder, H. A. 1963. In *Essays in toxicology*, ed. W. J. Hayes, Jr., vol. IV, pp. 107–199. New York: Academic Press.
Schroeder, H. A., Frost, D. V. and Balassa, J. J. 1970. *J. Chron. Dis.* 23:227–243.
Schwarz, K. and Foltz, C. M. 1957. *J. Amer. Chem. Soc.* 79:3292–3293.
Scott, M. L. 1973. *Amer. J. Clin. Nutr.* 26:803–810.
Seifter, J., Ehrich, W. E., Hudyma, G. and Mueller, G. 1946. *Science* 103:762.
Selikoff, I. J. and Churg, J., eds. 1965. Biological effects of asbestos. *Ann. N.Y. Acad. Sci.* 132.
Shamberger, R. J. 1970. *J. Natl. Cancer Inst.* 44:931–936.
Shapiro, J. R. 1972. *Ann. N.Y. Acad. Sci.* 192:215–219.
Sharpless, G. R. 1946. *Fed. Proc.* 5:239–240.
Shimkin, M. B. and Leiter, J. 1940. *J. Natl. Cancer Inst.* 1:241–254.
Smith, A. G. and Powell, L. 1957. *Amer. J. Pathol.* 33:653–669.
Smith, W. E., Miller, L., Elsasser, R. E. and Hubert, D. D. 1965. *Ann. N.Y. Acad. Sci.* 132:456–488.
Sommers, S. C. and McManus, R. G. 1953. *Cancer* 6:347–359.
Stanton, M. F. and Wrench, C. 1972. *J. Natl. Cancer Inst.* 48:797–821.
Steffee, C. H. and Baetjer, A. M. 1965. *Arch. Environ. Health* 11:66–75.
Stoeckle, J. D., Hardy, H. L. and Weber, A. L. 1969. *Amer. J. Med.* 46:545–561.
Stokinger, H. E., ed. 1966. *Beryllium: Its industrial hygiene aspects.* New York: Academic Press.
Sunderman, F. W. and Donnelly, A. J. 1965. *Amer. J. Pathol.* 46:1027–1041.
Sunderman, F. W., Jr. 1968. *Dis. Chest* 54:527–534.
Sunderman, F. W., Jr. 1971. *Fed. Cosmet. Toxicol.* 9:105–120.
Sunderman, F. W., Jr. 1973. *Ann. Clin. Lab. Sci.* 3:156–180.
Tscherkes, L. A., Volgarev, M. N. and Aptekar, S. G. 1963. *Acta Unio Intern. Contra Cancrum* 19:632–633.
Tseng, W. P., Chu, H. M., How, S. W., Fong, J. M., Lin, C. S. and Yeh, S. 1968. *J. Natl. Cancer Inst.* 40:453–463.
Underwood, E. J. 1971. *Trace elements in human and animal nutrition*, 3rd ed. New York: Academic Press.
van Esch, G. J. 1967. *Plastic carcinogenesis: Suggestions for the use of plastics in surgery, orthopedics, etc.*, vol. 7, pp. 196–201. UICC Monograph Series. Berlin: Springer-Verlag.
van Esch, G. J. and Kroes, R. 1969. *Brit. J. Cancer* 23:765–771.

van Esch, G. J., van Genderen, H. and Vink, H. H. 1962. *Brit. J. Cancer* 16:289–297.

Volgarev, M. N. and Tscherkes, L. A. 1967. In *Selenium in biomedicine*, ed. O. M. Muth, pp. 179–184. Westport, Conn.: Avi.

Vollmann, J. 1940. *Schweiz. Allg. Path. Bakt.* 1:440.

Vorwald, A. J. and Karr, J. W. 1937. *Amer. J. Pathol.* 13:654–655.

Vorwald, A. J., Reeves, A. L. and Urban, E. C. J. 1966. In *Beryllium: Its industrial hygiene aspects*, ed. H. E. Stokinger, pp. 201–234. New York: Academic Press.

Wagner, J. C. 1962. *Nature* 196:180–181.

Wagner, J. C. and Berry, G. 1969. *Brit. J. Cancer* 23:567–581.

Wagner, W. D., Groth, D. H., Holtz, J. L., Madden, G. E. and Stokinger, H. E. 1969. *Toxicol. Appl. Pharmacol.* 15:10–29.

Webb, M. and Weinzierl, S. M. 1972. *Brit. J. Cancer* 26:292–298.

Webb, M., Heath, J. C. and Hopkins, T. 1972. *Brit. J. Cancer* 26:274–278.

Weinzierl, S. M. and Webb, M. 1972. *Brit. J. Cancer* 26:279–291.

Weisberger, A. S. and Suhrland, L. G. 1956. *Blood* 11:11–18.

Yamagiwa, K. and Ichikawa, K. 1915. *Tokyo Igakkai Zasshi* 15:295.

Yamagiwa, K. and Ichikawa, K. 1918. *J. Cancer Res.* 3:1–29.

Yamaguchi, S. 1963. *Nagasaki Igakkai Zasshi* 38:127.

Yamane, Y., Sakai, K., Uchiyama, I., Tabata, M., Taga, N. and Hamaki, A. 1969. *Chem. Pharmacol. Bull.* 17:2488–2493.

Zawirska, B. and Medras, K. 1968. *Zentbl. Allg. Path. Anct.* 111:1–12.

Zollinger, H. V. 1953. *Virchows Arch. Abt. A Path. Anat.* 323:694–710.

Chapter 7

ONCOGENICITY OF CYCADS AND ITS IMPLICATIONS

G. L. Laqueur

Laboratory of Experimental Pathology
National Institute of Arthritis, Metabolism and Digestive Diseases
National Institutes of Health
Bethesda, Maryland

INTRODUCTION

Oncogenic properties of a crude meal prepared from the starchy components in seeds of cycads were uncovered incident to an investigation of the possibility that these plants might contain a substance with neurotoxic properties (Laqueur et al., 1963). Clinical observations on Guam had demonstrated unusually high rates in morbidity and mortality among the Chamorros, who are native to this island, from amyotrophic lateral sclerosis (ALS) (Kurland and Mulder, 1954; Kurland, 1964; Hirano et al., 1966; Hirano, 1973). In the search for possible etiologic factors, exposure to a readily accessible, environmental agent with toxic effects was one of several possibilities considered. Whiting, who has had wide experience in population nutrition and food practices among natives in the Pacific area, on her visit to Guam called attention to cycads as a possible environmental agent. Her suggestion was based on evidence collected from published reports on poisons in cycads and on her knowledge of the folklore related to these plants. Particularly impressive was the information that cattle grazing on land where cycads grew frequently developed gait disturbances that progressed through states of motor weakness to paralysis of the hindquarters. It was widely believed, moreover, that ingestion of cycad leaves by cattle was responsible for the disease, which at times caused severe economic losses in affected geographic areas. A review paper dealing with the toxicity of cycads by Whiting (1963) remains an important source of information. It contains descriptions of the manifold nutritional uses of cycads, their preparation as a source of food for humans and fodder for animals, as well as their reported ill effects on both animals and humans.

An exploration of the nature of the toxin in seeds of cycads started in 1961. Evidence of neurotoxicity resulting in lesions akin to ALS was not detected in small laboratory animals dying of tumors or in those surviving for 2 yr after initial exposure to cycads. Brains and spinal cords in nearly all the animals were examined with histopathology methods. However, exposure of several animal species to cycad toxins at specific periods during fetal development and immediately after birth produced acute lesions in the central nervous system, resulting in various malformations or structural disorganizations. They are reviewed in the section Teratogenic Effects. It is possible that small laboratory animals such as rats, mice, guinea pigs, and hamsters are unsuitable for an investigation that has the creation of an animal model for demyelinating diseases such as ALS as one of its goals. It is of interest, therefore, that recent studies by Hall and McGavin (1968) from Queensland, Australia, and by Mason and Whiting (1968), who studied the disease in the Dominican Republic, have found loss of myelin and evidence of myelin degeneration in spinal cords of afflicted cattle. In view of the rather complex situation when working with cattle and the technical and monetary difficulties in attempting to demonstrate neurologic lesions in them with the isolated, chemically pure compounds, it would seem prudent to withhold final judgment as to the etiologic importance of cycads in the development of cattle and human diseases.

The recent development of an active program in cycad research, occasioned by the detection of oncogenic properties, led to several conferences over the years, two of which are published in *Federation Proceedings* (vol. 23, pp. 1337-1388, 1964, and vol. 31, pp. 1465-1546, 1972). Papers contributed to these conferences are listed under the individual author's name in this article. Review papers dealing with cycad toxicity have been published by Laqueur and Spatz (1968), Yang and Mickelsen (1969), Spatz (1969), and Jones et al. (1973), in addition to the paper by Whiting (1963) already cited.

DISTRIBUTION AND USES OF CYCADS

Cycads are ancient gymnospermous plants and are considered intermediate forms in the evolution from ferns to flowering plants. They were widely distributed throughout the world in the mesozoic period, about 200 million yr ago. The cycads living today are essentially limited to the tropical and subtropical zones around the globe but occasionally extend to the temperate zones, such as in Florida, Japan, and Australia. Nine genera of living cycads, several with many species, have been identified, and together with the places in which they are found, are as follows: the most widely distributed is *Cycas*, which extends from East Africa and Madagascar across the Indian Ocean to Japan and the Mariana Islands. Important species are *C. circinalis* L. and *C. revoluta* Thunb. The second most widely distributed cycad is *Zamia*, found in Florida, the Caribbean Islands, Mexico, and the northern parts of South America. Two genera are located in Australia, namely, *Macrozamia* and *Bowenia,* the latter mainly in Queensland. The two African genera are

Encephalartos in central and southern Africa and *Stangeria* in southeast Africa. *Microcycas* is found in Cuba and *Dioon* and *Ceratozamia* in Mexico (Fosberg, 1964; Birdsey, 1972).

Cycads are used in many parts of the world as a source for medicines and for food, as reviewed in detail by Whiting (1963). The size and depth of the roots of cycads probably account for the fact that they survive periods of drought as well as heavy storms with high winds such as hurricanes or typhoons and thus can provide food when other agricultural products are destroyed. The peoples who use cycads as food know that the seeds, stems, and tubers contain, besides an eatable starch, poisonous substances that need to be removed prior to use. The preparation of poison-free cycad starch requires time, and it is thought that the reported accidental poisonings may have occurred when cycad flour was prepared in haste at times of natural disasters.

The procedures for detoxification developed by the early and present users of cycads are remarkably similar and vary only slightly in often widely separated geographic areas. They consist of cutting the crude, white starchy parts of seeds, stems, or tubers into small pieces, followed by prolonged and repeated soaking in fresh water, and discarding the wash water each time. The pieces are then dried in the sun (sometimes accompanied by evidence of fermentation), and finally the remaining chunks are ground in a mortar, resulting in a flour that can be stored and used as needed. The most important step, which also requires much time, involves the washing of the starch-containing parts. To do this properly several days are normally needed. Shortcuts in the preparation of cycad flour taken at times of emergency may have resulted in incomplete removal of the poison. Although detailed clinical descriptions and pathologic findings in cases of presumed human poisoning are entirely lacking, the symptoms of cycad intoxication as described by Whiting (1963), Mugera and Nderito (1968a,b), and Hirono et al. (1970) are similar and point to an enteric involvement leading terminally to signs of generalized intoxication. Thus, nausea and vomiting are the first symptoms, followed by headache, abdominal pain, swollen liver, convulsions, unconsciousness, and death usually within 2 or 3 days. Of some importance is the fact that jaundice has been observed in one case surviving the acute poisoning (Hirono et al., 1970) and in adults who died several days after the onset of the intoxication (Mugera and Nderito, 1968b). The appearance of clinical jaundice, suggesting hepatic involvement, is consistent with all the observations in animals exposed to the toxin, and its being observed in human beings indicates that cycads are hepatotoxic for humans as well.

Thus far no studies have been reported that would indicate that populations eating cycad material have an increased incidence of neoplastic disease. Mugera and Nderito (1968a) have suggested that the ingestion of cycad meal might play some contributory role in the etiology of liver cancer in parts of Africa where cycads are eaten. Hirono et al. (1970), searching for evidence of cycad toxicity and increases in neoplastic disease, found none among the inhabitants of the Myako Islands, who subsisted on cycads during a period of repeated, strong typhoons late in 1959. Apparently the natives properly prepared the cycad flour and thus escaped the effects of the toxin. In one study in which cycad flour prepared in several households on Guam was fed to rats in the diet over prolonged periods of time, tumors were not induced, indicating that most if not all the toxic and oncogenic material had been removed (Yang et al., 1966).

CHEMISTRY

Isolation of Azoxyglycosides

Cooper (1941) from Australia is credited with having first isolated from seeds of *Macrozamia spiralis* a crystalline toxic substance that she named macrozamin. The substance was toxic to guinea pigs when given by mouth but nontoxic when injected subcutaneously. The carbohydrate component in macrozamin was identified by Lythgoe and Riggs (1949) as primeverose, a glucose xylose disaccharide, which is attached to the aglycone in a β-glucosidic linkage. Two years later, the aglycone part of macrozamin was shown to have an aliphatic azoxy structure (Langley et al., 1951). Macrozamin was subsequently reported by Riggs (1954) to be present in seeds of cycads growing in Queensland, Australia, and, according to a footnote by Lythgoe in this paper, in an African cycad, *Encephalartos barkeri*. It was also found in *Encephalartos hildebrandtii* by Dossaji and Herbin (1972). Toxic properties of seeds of several species of *Encephalartos* had previously been recognized and described by Steyn et al. (1948).

The isolation of a glycoside from seeds of *C. revoluta* and the determination of its chemical structure was accomplished by Nishida and collaborators (1955a). The compound was named cycasin to indicate its original plant source. It is closely related to macrozamin except for its sugar moiety, which is D-glucose in cycasin. Its chemical name is therefore β-glucosyloxyazoxymethane.

$$CH_3 - N = N - CH_2 - O - C_6H_{11}O_5$$
$$\downarrow$$
$$O$$

Cycasin like macrozamin is toxic for mice and guinea pigs only when enterically administered, whereas parenteral injections fail to produce toxicity. It is also nontoxic in cold-blooded animals (Nishida et al., 1956a). Methods for quantitative determinations of cycasin in cycad seeds are described by Nishida et al. (1956b), Palekar and Dastur (1965), and Wells et al. (1968). Cycasin was also identified in seeds of *Cycas circinalis,* the principal cycad genus on

Guam, by Riggs (1956) and Matsumoto and Strong (1963). Nagahama et al. (1964) confirmed this but noted that in the outer shell of such seeds macrozamin is the main azoxyglycoside and cycasin only a minor component.

Nishida and his group at Kagoshima University, Japan, reported over the years on several additional azoxyglycosides they found in seeds of *C. revoluta* growing in southern Japan; they named them neocycasins. Their isolation, nature, and evidence of reciprocal conversions have been described in detailed papers written originally in Japanese but available in English translations (Nishida, 1959; Nagahama, 1964). The aglycone of all azoxyglycosides, including the neocycasins, is identical and is methylazoxymethanol. Toxicologic and oncogenic activities depend on the hydrolysis to the common aglycone.

It is thus apparent that azoxyglycosides have been isolated from several species of four of the nine living genera of cycads. The remaining five genera have apparently not been examined for the presence of azoxyglycosides. This remains to be done.

The Aglycone Methylazoxymethanol (MAM)

The observations of Cooper (1941) and Nishida et al. (1956a) indicate that macrozamin and cycasin exert their toxic effects in animals after enteric administration but not after parenteral injection. Moreover, both authors note that signs of toxicity begin to appear several hours after the glycosides are fed to animals. This symptom-free interval suggested to them that a metabolite of the azoxyglycosides might be the toxic component. It became important, therefore, to investigate the factors that would lead to the degradation of these compounds. It was demonstrated first that cycasin could be hydrolyzed with a cycad emulsion prepared from the seeds of *Cycas revoluta* and that the end products of this reaction are formaldehyde, nitrogen gas, methanol, and glucose (Nishida et al., 1955b). The aglycone was not isolated at that time probably because of methodological difficulties. These were largely overcome several years later, and free aglycone was demonstrated after hydrolysis of crystalline cycasin with purified cycad β-glucosidase (Kobayashi, 1962). The importance of the aglycone became even more evident when Matsumoto and Strong (1963) obtained chemical and toxicologic evidence for cycasin in two fractions as well as for the aglycone of cycasin, methylazoxymethanol (MAM), in one separate fraction. The aglycone fraction was highly toxic when compared with milliequivalent amounts of pure cycasin as tested in rats. Matsumoto and Strong presented the first evidence that the aglycone of cycasin was a constituent of cycad seeds, together with cycasin and the enzymatically active cycasin emulsion. Still to be clarified in detail is the internal structural compartmentalization that allows substrate, enzyme, and product to coexist in one tissue of a plant. Several observations pertaining to this problem are cited in the section Mutagenic Effects. The mechanisms by which hydrolysis of azoxyglycosides occurs *in vivo* in animals are discussed in the next section.

Synthesis of the Aglycone Methylazoxymethyl
Acetate (MAM Acetate)

As the interest in cycasin and its aglycone, MAM, increased, the need for a synthetic compound to allow continuation of research became apparent. Cycasin, which had been isolated from seeds of cycads by several investigators for research purposes, had become scarce and attempts to interest commercial enterprises in obtaining cycasin from plant sources had failed. The synthesis of the aglycone as reported by Matsumoto et al. (1965) was accomplished by the oxydation of 1,2-dimethylhydrazine to azomethane to azoxymethane followed by bromination of azoxymethane in the allylic position by the Wohl-Ziegler reaction and subsequent conversion into the acetate. Azoxymethane and 1,2-dimethylhydrazine have since become well-established carcinogens for the colon and rectum in many animals (Druckrey et al., 1967a; Druckrey, 1970, 1973). The synthesis has made it also possible to prepare labeled azoxy compounds (Horisberger and Matsumoto, 1968). MAM acetate, which is now commercially available, has since been used in oncologic as well as in metabolic studies. It can be administered by any parenteral route in addition to the oral one and thus is not subject to all the variables that complicate the *in vivo* hydrolysis of the glycosides.

HYDROLYSIS OF AZOXYGLYCOSIDES *IN VIVO*

This section covers observations that indicate that the toxicologic and oncogenic effects of cycad glycosides in animals only occur when these glycosides are hydrolyzed. Because the sources for enzymatic hydrolysis are different in mature and very young rats, they are separately discussed, using cycasin as the best studied example of these glycosides.

Mature Animals

In animals older than 28 days, the hydrolysis of cycasin only occurs when it is given orally, either as part of the diet or by stomach tube. The observations of Cooper (1941) and of Nishida et al. (1956a) indicate this, as do observations by Kobayashi and Matsumoto (1965), who were the first to publish quantitative data for the recovery of cycasin after oral and intraperitoneal administrations. Whereas urinary recovery after intraperitoneal injection of cycasin is nearly quantitative, that after intragastric intubation varies from 30 to 63% over a 2-day period, the bulk of it being excreted during the first 24 hr. This means that from 23 to 70% has been metabolized and that the intestinal tract probably plays an important role in this process.

Further support for this assumption comes from several long-term studies in rats concerned with the oncogenicity of cycasin in which a small but recurring percentage of the animals did not develop tumors after oral administration. They also were free of hepatic changes, which would have indicated liver injury usually seen after sufficiently large doses of cycasin. It was postulated, therefore, that differences might exist between rats in their ability to hydrolyze cycasin in the intestinal tract, and several studies were undertaken to determine the cause for the observed difference. Using germfree and conventional Sprague-Dawley rats and large amounts of cycasin (200 mg%) in the diet for 20 days, germfree rats gained weight and were alive and well at 20 days, whereas the majority of the conventional rats had died or were moribund at that time. Moreover, the livers of the germfree rats were normal in contrast to the livers of conventional rats, which exhibited evidence of severe, diffuse, centrilobular liver cell necrosis often accompanied by hemorrhage (Laqueur, 1964). A group of germfree rats identically treated and maintained thereafter in the germfree state for 2 additional yr were free of those tumors that might have resulted from the administration of excessively large amounts of cycasin over a 20-day period, 2 yr previously (Laqueur et al., 1967).

The findings once more emphasized the importance of the intestinal tract for the hydrolysis. The literature contained evidence that mucosal enzymes with the activity of a β-glucosidase existed in the small intestine and might possibly contribute to cycasin hydrolysis (Dahlquist et al., 1965). To examine this possibility, quantitative measurements of the fate of orally given cycasin to germfree and conventional rats were done; germfree rats excreted 97% of the intake in urine and feces, whereas the corresponding figure in conventional rats was 20% (Spatz et al. 1966). Apparently, mucosal enzymes played no or only a minor role in cycasin hydrolysis. Spatz et al. also indicated that a substantial part of the cycasin was excreted in the feces by germfree but not by conventional rats. The bacterial flora absent in germfree rats was then considered as the likely source of the hydrolytic enzyme, and hydrolysis of cycasin by monocontamination of germfree rats with organisms known to produce β-glucosidase was subsequently reported (Spatz et al., 1967a). There was good agreement between the enzymatic activity of the microorganisms as measured before use, by the difference between cycasin intake and excretion, the severity of liver damage, and the survival times of the animals. Conversely, monocontamination with microorganisms that did not have β-glucosidase activity also did not alter the pattern of cycasin excretion from that found in germfree rats.

In summary, the toxicity and oncogenicity of cycasin in mature animals depended on its enteric administration and on its subsequent hydrolysis by enzymes with the activity of a β-glucosidase supplied by certain micro-organisms of the intestinal bacterial flora. In retrospect, it would seem possible, therefore, that variations in the intestinal bacterial flora could explain those isolated cases in which mature rats exposed to tumor-inducing amounts of cycasin by the enteric route failed to develop evidence of hepatotoxicity and, subsequently, neoplasms.

Postnatal Period

The observation by P. N. Magee (personal communication) that sub-cutaneously administered cycasin to newborn rats resulted in kidney tumors presented the first indication that the hydrolysis of cycasin might proceed differently in neonatal animals and presumably in the absence of a bacteria-derived β-glucosidase. Repeating the experiment, the observation by Magee was confirmed in rats of the Fischer strain that had received a single injection of 2.5 mg cycasin under the skin of the neck within 24 hr after birth. Of 55 rats thus treated, 46 (or 84%) were found to have tumors at various sites such as kidneys, liver, intestinal tract, lung, and brain. Multiplicity of primary tumors was common, indicating that the oncogen had been absorbed from the site of injection and entered the circulation (Hirono et al., 1968). The question arose, therefore, as to possible sites at which cycasin might have been hydrolyzed. The hydrolysis could have occurred locally at the site of injection or at distant organ sites after absorption of the intact glucoside and its transport. Evidence is cited below for both possibilities, indicating activity of hydrolytic enzymes both locally in the skin and at distant sites.

Spatz (1968) examined the subcutaneous tissue for β-glucosidase activity in fetal and newborn rats of the Fischer and Sprague-Dawley strains and of germfree newborn Sprague-Dawley rats and found about equal activity in both strains and in the germfree Sprague-Dawley rats. The peak in activity was observed for several days before and after birth, decreasing sharply by the 6th postnatal day and remaining low from then on. The activity of the enzyme was measured using cycasin and two synthetic glucosides as substrates. A similar though more extensive study was reported by Matsumoto et al. (1972a), who investigated the activity of β-glucosidase in tissues of various organs of preweanling Wistar rats. In a concommitant study, the tumor incidence was determined in groups of rats into which cycasin had been parenterally injected on postnatal days corresponding to the days at which the determinations of β-glucosidase activity had been performed. Matsumoto et al. (1972a) found the greatest activity in the small intestine at about the 15th postnatal day, after which it steeply decreased to a plateau at a measurable level that was maintained from the 28th to the 90th days after birth. In contrast, determinations in skin, pancreas, liver, muscle, and stomach uni-formly and persistently gave low levels of activity. Enzyme activity in kidney tissue remained low but increased after weaning to a level comparable to that which prevailed in the small intestine at that time. There was good positive correlation between levels of activity in the small intestine and the tumor yield when the results between the two parallel experiments were compared. No tumors were found in rats that had parenterally received cycasin on the 25th postnatal day. We have recently repeated in germfree rats the part of the experiment that concerned postnatal tumor induction with cycasin (1 mg/g body weight) when given parenterally and have observed successful tumor induction as late as the 25th to 35th days after birth in 14 of 34 germfree rats (41%) (Laqueur and Spatz, 1975). It would seem possible that the lowered but persistent levels of β-glucosidase activity in small intestine and kidney described by Matsumoto et al. (1972a) were sufficient for hydrolysis of the injected cycasin. It would seem possible also that the hydrolytic enzyme was supplied by some other as yet unrecognized source, such as the large intestine in which five of the 14 neoplasms developed. Lastly, the distribution and pattern of mucosal glucosidases may differ in some detail between germfree and conventional rats, although this appears to be more true for the α- than for the β-glucosidases, according to Dahlquist et al. (1965).

ACUTE TOXIC EFFECTS

The acute toxic effects of crude cycad meal prepared from seeds of *C. circinalis* in animals have been described (Laqueur et al., 1963). The toxic manifestations roughly paralleled the concentrations of the meal in basal animal diet, which in turn depended on the concentration of cycasin in the crude meal. This concentration varied from 1.2 to 3.0% depending in part at least on the ripeness of the cycad seeds at the time of collection and on the age of the stored, prepared meal (Dastur and Palekar, 1966). Analysis of the cycad meal showed that its composition was in general similar to white flour except for the absence of cycasin in the latter (Campbell et al., 1966). In subsequent studies in which cycasin and MAM, the aglycone of cycasin, or the synthetic MAM acetate were used, the acute toxic manifestations were essentially identical although at widely different amounts, as seen from the data on LD_{50} reported by several investigators. The LD_{50} of cycasin given by stomach tube to male Osborne-Mendel rats was 562 mg/kg body weight (Hirono et al., 1968), whereas the LD_{50} of MAM acetate when intraperitoneally injected into Osborne-Mendel rats was 90 mg/kg body weight (Ganote and Rosenthal, 1968).

Structural Evidence

The acute toxic manifestations of cycad materials were seen first in the liver, and the severity of the hepatic alterations appeared to determine subsequent events. Using a crude cycad meal containing 2.3% cycasin, the earliest changes were recognizable by light microscopy within 24 hr and consisted of loss of cytoplasmic basophilia and glycogen from isolated liver cells around the central vein. Focal cellular necrosis, pyknosis of nuclei, and cytoplasmic eosinophilia were well established within 48 hr. These alterations progressed to involve uniformly all lobules in the liver and centrilobular necrosis, usually with a hemorrhagic component apparent by the 5th day. The central veins remained unaltered even after prolonged exposure of rats to the experimental diet. Surviving midzonal and peripheral cells in the liver lobule were often enlarged and the cytoplasm filled with glycogen and basophilic material. Rats that died within a few days were found at autopsy to have accumulations of free, slightly yellowish fluid in the serosal cavities, occasionally a mild degree of subcutaneous edema, and often a marked edema of the perilobular pancreatic connective tissue. Small punctate hemorrhages were seen beneath the serosal surfaces, sometimes at many sites. There were no other pathologic changes, and examination of the bone marrow in many rats revealed only a generally hyperplastic cellular marrow with precursors of all cellular elements. Smaller concentrations of the toxic material produced milder effects, consisting of loss of cytoplasmic basophilia from centrilobular regions and prolonged survival times (Laqueur et al., 1963).

Rats developing severe liver cell necrosis were observed to become progressively more aggressive and sensitive to noise and motion even when handled daily by the same person who had attended them prior to the onset of the experiment.

Ultrastructural studies of liver cells by Ganote and Rosenthal (1968) showed that changes occurred sooner when MAM acetate was used. Within 2 hr nuclear changes and loss of cytoplasmic polysomal aggregates were noted. The nuclear changes consisted of segregation of the nucleolar components into zonal arrangements without formation of nuclear caps. With time, depletion of the granular component of the nucleolus was noted, whereas the fibrillar component was seen in a clumped pattern. The nucleolar changes were seen in most centrilobular cells after 24 hr. Loss of free and membrane-associated polysomes was accompanied by loss of cytoplasmic ribosomes. Membrane whorls were seen in many cells and were in continuity with those of the endoplasmic reticulum, which was increased. Because centrilobular hemorrhage is a common occurrence in the acute phase of liver damage, the EM studies revealed after 6 hr a widening of the fenestrae in the sinusoidal endothelium and after 24 hr an increase in the width of the space of Disse with resulting hemorrhage into the liver cell cords. The ultrastructural observations were regarded as evidence of altered nucleolar ribonucleic acid synthesis and the loss of polysomal aggregates as evidence of a decrease in the protein-synthesizing capability of the liver cells. The marked hypertrophy of the smooth endoplasmic reticulum was interpreted as indicating increases in the activities of drug-metabolizing enzymes. Ganote and Rosenthal (1968) suggested that the primary site of interaction between MAM and the cell was the nucleolus and that the observed cytoplasmic changes were dependent on an altered nucleolar function.

These ultrastructural observations were confirmed and extended by Zedeck et al. (1970). Following intravenous injections of MAM acetate, Zedeck et al. noted nucleolar changes in liver cells as early as 15 min after MAM acetate administration. The nucleolar changes consisted of the appearance of nucleolar plaques (round electron-dense bodies composed of fibrillar and granular material) and were reported to be the only change at 30 min. An irregular separation of nucleolar components was seen at 1 hr and was complete 6 hr after the injection of MAM acetate. By light microscopy, nuclear debris was noted in the duodenum and colon. The biochemical changes associated with the structural alterations are discussed below.

Biochemical Evidence

Loss of cytoplasmic basophilia from liver cells during the prenecrotic phase was supported by evidence of more profound biochemical alterations. Significant dose-dependent decreases in liver RNA and phospholipids without affecting DNA concentration were reported by Williams (1964) and Williams and Laqueur (1965). The changes were accompanied by increases in cholesterol and neutral glycerides. In the same livers a marked reduction in liver catalase activity was described (Rechcigl, 1964), which was shown to have resulted from a reduced rate of enzyme synthesis accompanied by a reduced rate in degradation (Rechcigl and Laqueur, 1968). Determinations of plasma cholinesterase (pseudo-cholinesterase) in the blood of such animals revealed an elevation in the enzyme level within 24 hr after cycasin feeding had begun and remained so for the next 10 days when titration of the plasma became technically uncertain due to its coloration in cycasin-treated rats (Orgell and Laqueur, 1964). Alterations in phosphatases and nonspecific esterases by histochemical procedures were described by Spatz (1964a). The changes were dose-dependent to some extent. Large doses of cycasin in the diet (200–400 mg%) caused decreases in glucose-6-phosphatase and in 5-nucleotidase; adenosine triphosphatase was decreased in centrilobular areas and increased in the periportal zones. Smaller doses (25–100 mg%) caused only a reduction in glucose-6-phosphatase activity, whereas no effects were noted on histochemically demonstrable phosphatases with still smaller doses of cycasin (5 and 10 mg%). Esterase activity was examined with a variety of ester substrates, but the effects were less clear cut. The hepatocellular distribution of esterase activities was altered to some degree in all rats fed cycasin in a dietary concentration of 75 mg%. Within 24 hr a loss of uniformity of the peribiliary granular esterase reaction was described, followed by slight decreases in activity in central and periportal zones after the diet had been fed for 48 hr.

Methylation of nucleic acids *in vitro* by MAM was reported by Matsumoto and Higa (1966) and *in vivo* by Shank and Magee (1967) and by Nagata and Matsumoto (1969). The methylated purine base in hydrolysates of RNA and DNA was identified as 7-methylguanine in both studies. According to Shank and Magee (1967), liver RNA was methylated to a greater extent than the RNA from kidney and small intestine. Also, guanine in liver DNA was methylated to a greater extent than that in RNA.

Protein synthesis was inhibited in the liver, but not in the kidney, spleen, and ileum as measured by labeled leucine incorporation into the protein (Shank and Magee, 1967). The inhibition was demonstrable 5 hr after giving cycasin by stomach tube and the delay in demonstrable protein inhibition when compared with that in rats treated with dimethylnitrosamine (DMN) was interpreted by Shank and Magee (1967) to have been due to the time interval necessary for hydrolysis of cycasin to MAM by the gut bacteria. This interpretation appears to be correct inasmuch as inhibition of protein synthesis was subsequently observed within 1 hr after intravenous administration of MAM acetate by Zedeck et al. (1970), who also found no evidence for inhibition of protein synthesis in the kidney or small intestine. In addition to inhibiting protein synthesis, Zedeck et al. (1970) and Goerttler et al. (1970) reported that the incorporation of nucleotide precursors into RNA and DNA was inhibited, becoming demonstrable within 1 hr in liver DNA and within 3 hr in liver RNA. A less pronounced inhibition of RNA and DNA synthesis was noted with MAM acetate in the small intestine of weanling rats.

Inhibition of protein synthesis was demonstrated in liver microsomal preparations from young rats that had received an intraperitoneal injection of MAM acetate. The inhibition was noticeable 1 hr after MAM administration and reached its peak in 2 hr, after which protein synthesis returned to normal control values (generally within 24 hr after the start of the experiment). There was additional evidence that MAM acetate also reduced microsomal function as shown by a 50% inhibition of the activity of two drug-metabolizing enzymes, ethyl morphine-N-demethylase where the inhibition was dose-dependent, and O-dealkylation of norcodeine (Lundeen at al., 1971).

The methylation of nucleic acids as described above raised the question as to the nature of the decomposition of MAM that would provide the methyl donor. Early in the study of the metabolism of cycasin the possibility was considered that diazomethane may be the intermediate product of decomposition of MAM providing the methyl donor (Miller, 1964). Subsequent studies by Nagasawa et al. (1972) in which the decomposition of MAM in D_2O was examined have shown no evidence that diazomethane formed as the intermediate. The studies, however, indicated that methyl diazonium hydroxide may be the intermediate providing the methyl donor analogous to the metabolism of DMN as proposed by Druckrey (1970) and Miller (1970) as the ultimate alkylating agent and carcinogen in both MAM and DMN.

ONCOGENIC EFFECTS

The development of neoplastic lesions at various organ sites such as the liver, kidney, colon, and lung was first observed in rats that were fed crude cycad meal in various concentrations as part of the diet (Laqueur et al., 1963). The nature of the acute lesion in the liver and the subsequently observed tumors in the liver and kidneys strikingly resembled those that had previously been described with dimethylnitrosamine (DMN) by Barnes and Magee (1954) and by Magee and Barnes (1956, 1959, 1962). The question arose, therefore, whether the crude cycad material contained a chemical similar to DMN. The literature on cycads indicated that an azoxyglycoside, which was named cycasin, had been isolated from cycads by Nishida et al. (1955a). The historical aspects of the isolation of cycasin are reviewed in the chemistry section above.

Pursuing this lead, oncogenic effects of cycasin extracted from seeds of *C. circinalis* from Guam were subsequently reported by Laqueur (1964), of MAM by Matsumoto and Strong (1963) and Laqueur and Matsumoto (1966), and of MAM and MAM acetate in germfree rats by Laqueur et al. (1967). The studies collectively indicated that cycasin, the compound isolated from crude cycad meal, was the oncogen responsible for tumor induction and, furthermore, that the aglycone MAM was the proximate carcinogen of cycasin, inducing neoplasms irrespective of the route of administration (Laqueur et al., 1967). In the ensuing descriptions, the oncogenic effects are cited independent of whether they were induced with crude cycad meal, cycasin, or MAM, because in the last analysis they all are due to the activity of MAM. Attention is called to the possible importance of age and sex and the route of administration in instances in which these factors contributed to the localization of the neoplasms.

Rats

Rats have been used most widely in studies in oncogenesis with cycads, and tumor induction has been successful in all strains used thus far. The most frequently reported tumors are observed in the liver, kidneys, colon, lung, brain, and duodenum. Occasional neoplasms are found in small intestines, ear canal, or arising from peripheral nerves, renal pelvis, and urinary bladder.

Analogous to the observations with DMN (Magee and Barnes, 1962), primary cancer of the liver generally resulted from chronic feeding whereas tumors of the kidneys were most frequently observed after short-term or single exposures to cycads. Colonic neoplasm, which ranked third in frequency among all tumors, developed independently of the length of exposure. Tumors in lungs and brain, although occasionally seen in mature animals, were more readily inducible during the period surrounding birth. Duodenal neoplasms were observed in rats that had received multiple intraperitoneal injections of MAM or the synthetic MAM acetate. The interval between first exposure and the appearance of neoplasms was generally in the neighborhood of 6 months, and age at the onset of treatment appeared to have little influence on the length of the induction period.

The tumors in the *liver* as judged on the basis of personal observations were for the most part hepatocellular carcinomas arising from single or multiple foci. The liver parenchyma immediately surrounding the carcinomas was commonly invaded by neoplastic liver cells, which on occasion were also found in small groups in branches of the hepatic vein. Islands of extramedullary hemopoiesis were found in the carcinoma and in the nontumorous part of the liver in several animals. Massive hemorrhage into the carcinomas with rupture of the overlying Glisson's capsule was relatively common and when present often resulted in intraabdominal hemorrhage, from which the animals died. These hepatocellular carcinomas readily metastasized to the lung by way of the bloodstream; it was common to find in addition to nodular metastases, tumor cell emboli within the lumens of the pulmonary vascular system. When the carcinomas occurred multiply, some variation in the degree of anaplasia was common and it was not unusual to find in the cases of multiple primary liver cancers an associated cirrhosis. In contrast, solitary liver carcinomas usually were found in livers without cirrhosis. In retrospect it would seem possible that this difference was due to the severity of the acute injury produced by varying concentrations of cycasin in the crude material. In addition to liver cell tumors, cystic and papillary cystic adenomas presumably arising from intrahepatic biliary tracts were described, but they were more frequently observed after intraperitoneal administration of MAM or the synthetic MAM acetate than after feeding crude cycad meal or cycasin.

Tumors of the *kidneys* were commonly found bilaterally. They were histogenetically derived either from epithelial cells lining the nephrons or from mesenchymal elements occupying the spaces between the tubules. The majority of the renal epithelial tumors were considered benign as solid or intracystic adenomas. Evidence of metastasis was lacking. The individual adenomas were composed of epithelial cells in which the cytoplasm was clear, amphophilic, or eosinophilic. The mesenchymal tumors, originally called interstitial tumors to indicate their cellular origin and considered benign neoplasms, have been renamed mesenchymal tumors (Hard and Butler, 1970, 1971) after a study of comparable tumors induced with DMN. Renal sarcomas that had metastasized to the lung were occasionally seen, as were angiosarcomas. The latter were more frequently observed in rats that had received MAM. A tumor which we called nephroblastoma, was probably overdiagnosed as such, although several of these large renal tumors seem to fit this diagnosis because they exhibited evidence of multiple differentiation in the direction toward epithelial and mesenchymal components. Detailed light microscopic and electron microscopic investigations of cycasin-induced renal neoplasms have been published and cover both the epithelial growths (Gusek, 1972, 1975; Gusek and Mestwerdt, 1969) and the mesenchymal tumors (Gusek et al., 1967; Gusek, 1968; Buss and Gusek, 1968).

Tumors of the *colon,* the third most frequently observed neoplasm, were derived from the epithelium of the colon. These tumors ranged from benign sessile and polypoid adenomas to papillary and infiltrating carcinomas. Production of mucus by the tumor cells was more frequently observed in the distal than in the proximal colon. The mucous carcinomas commonly metastasized to regional lymph nodes and also spread by continuity throughout the abdominal cavity after having infiltrated the bowel wall and reached the serosal covering. In such cases, the pancreas, splenic hilum, and the peritoneal surface of the diaphragm were seeded by mucin-producing carcinoma cells. As the colonic neoplasms grew, they frequently caused intussusception with resulting bleeding and ulceration of the intusussceptum. Details of the colonic neo-plasms induced by feeding crude cycad meal or cycasin have been published (Laqueur, 1965).

Whereas these colonic tumors developed exclusively in the proximal colon in feeding experiments, parenteral injections of MAM and MAM acetate resulted in a wider distribution, and carcinomas of the lower colon and rectum and of the small intestine were more frequently observed (Laqueur and Matsumoto, 1966; Laqueur et al., 1967). There were no tumors in the esophagus and stomach or in the anal region. MAM acetate instilled daily intrarectally for 7–26 days into Donryn rats has been reported to induce a very high incidence of carcinomas in the large bowel from cecum to rectum (Narisawa and Nakano, 1973).

Tumors of the *lung* were alveolar cell adenomas often with squamous metaplasia occurring as solitary or multiple whitish nodules usually situated beneath the pleura. They and tumors of the *brain,* while occasionally observed in young animals that had received crude cycad meal or cycasin in the diet, were much more commonly found in rats that had been exposed to MAM shortly before birth or to cycasin given subcutaneously within 24 hr after birth. The majority of experimentally induced brain tumors resembled oligo-dendrogliomas such as seen in humans, though a few had astrocytic admix-tures or resembled astrocytomas (Spatz and Laqueur, 1967; Hirono et al., 1968; Laqueur and Spatz, 1973).

Tumors of the *duodenum* with one exception were found only in rats that had received repeated parenteral injections of MAM or MAM acetate. The tumors were usually located in the middle third of the duodenum and were adenocarcinomas sometimes producing abundant amounts of mucus (Laqueur, 1965; Laqueur and Matsumoto, 1966). They were also found in germfree rats after intraperitoneal injections of MAM acetate (Laqueur et al., 1967).

Tumors did not develop at sites of injections. Other neoplasms often seen in aging rats such as those of the endocrine organs and of the mammary glands in female rats were not found earlier or in greater numbers in carcinogen-treated rats when compared with those that had presumably developed inde-pendent of cycasin administration in control animals of the same age, sex, and strain.

Oncogenic effects were also demonstrated in rats fed ground fresh or dried husks of cycads from Guam. Husks are the covering parts enclosing the seed kernel. According to Hoch-Ligeti et al., (1968), malignant tumors of liver and kidneys developed in nearly all rats when ground, dried, or fresh husk was added to the diet; a footnote in their paper indicates that the dried husk contained macrozamin at a concentration of 1.5% whereas an azoxycompound not further identified as to its original sugar moiety was found at a concentra-tion of 1.15% in the fresh husk. Similar observations were independently reported by Yang et al. (1968), who described benign and malignant tumors of liver and kidneys in rats fed a diet containing ground dried husk in low concentrations of 0.5 and 1.0%, respectively, for many months. Because fresh cycad husks are used to relieve thirst and dried husks as sweets by Guamanians and their children (Whiting, 1963), the demonstration of oncogenic activity of the husks of cycad seeds is important.

Although the studies in rats just summarized were conducted mainly with cycasin, the glycoside of *Cycas*, tumor induction in rats has been reported with crude seeds of *Encephalartos hildebrandtii* from Kenya, one of the African genera of cycads (Mugera and Nderito, 1968c). The azoxyglycoside in this cycad is macrozamin (Dossaji and Herbin, 1972). The changes observed in acute toxicity studies were similar to those described with cycasin, as were the tumors in the liver, kidney, and lung in rats fed the experimental diet for 6-10 months.

A sample of tubers of *Z. floridana,* belonging to the genus *Zamia,* was used in my laboratory in 1963 and found to be oncogenic for rats. The chemical structure of the azoxyglycoside was not further identified but probably was cycasin. Among 25 male Osborne-Mendel rats fed 2% ground *Zamia* tubers in the diet, only three rats (or 12%) had tumors, of which two were found in the kidney and one in the liver. The overall tumor incidence rose to 60% when the percentage of ground *Zamia* tubers was increased to 3%. Of these, seven were found in the kidney, six in the liver, three in the colon, and one, an undifferentiated sarcoma, in the omentum. Histologically, these tumors differed in no way from those observed with cycasin from the genus *Cycas* (G. L. Laqueur, unpublished observation).

Thus in rats, oncogenic properties have been demonstrated from four species belonging to three genera of cycads. The four species are *Cycas circinalis* L., *Cycas revoluta* Thunb., *Zamia floridana,* and *Encephalartos hildebrandtii.*

One of the remarkable features of oncogenesis with cycad compounds in the rat is its effectiveness in simultaneously inducing tumors at different sites. This results in many instances of multiple primary neoplasms. The material of the past 12 yr has recently been reviewed, and it was found that among 439 rats with tumors, 227 had single neoplasms. These were located in the kidney (47%), the liver (24%), and in the colon (15%). The remaining 212 rats had two or more primaries. Of them 168 rats (38%) had two, 40 rats (9%) had three, and four rats (1%) had four independent primary tumors. The most frequently observed combinations were liver and kidney, noted in 41%, and kidney and colon, noted in 33% of the rats with two primaries, whereas 52% of the rats with three primaries had neoplasms in the liver, kidney, and colon. Pulmonary and intracerebral tumors were found predominantly in rats exposed to cycads shortly before birth or during the 1st day after birth. When the sites of multiple primary neoplasms in this group were compared with those of weanling rats (28 days old), lung and a second primary ranked in first place among the rats with two primaries in the "perinatal" group, whereas tumors of the liver and kidney were the most commonly observed multiple primary tumor sites in the group of weanling rats. A similar although less striking situation was noted with respect to the simultaneous occurrence of intracerebral tumors together with another primary. Obviously, age at exposure influenced, at least in part, tumor sites and also the sites for multiple primary neoplasms.

Mice

Oncogenic effects of cycads in mice were first described by O'Gara et al. (1964), who noted tumors in the liver or kidney in male C57 Bl mice after repeated topical application of an aqueous emulsion from seeds of *C. circinalis* to skin ulcers artificially induced with 10% croton oil in mineral oil. The mice that died during the 1st wk had severe hemorrhagic centrilobular liver cell necrosis, a lesion identical to that observed in rats given acutely toxic amounts of cycads. Three of 11 surviving mice were found to have tumors of the liver or kidney or both 12–14 months later. One of the three mice had a hepato-cellular carcinoma, adenomas in each kidney, and a subcutaneous hemangioma at the site of injection. A second mouse had a large adenoma in one kidney and a multilocular cyst in the liver while the third mouse had a large hemangiosarcoma of the liver. This was the first and until now the only observation that described the development of a tumor at the site of local application to an artificially induced skin ulcer. These exploratory studies, which unfortunately could not be continued by the late Dr. O'Gara, are of special interest in view of the reports of medicinal applications of cycad pastes for the treatment of skin ulcers (Whiting, 1963).

Oncogenic effects in mice after subcutaneous injection of cycasin into C57 Bl/6 mice were also reported by Hirono et al. (1969a). These authors described a marked difference in relative tumor incidence between newborn mice, in which 62% later developed liver and reticulum cell neoplasms, and mature mice, which had a tumor incidence of only 12% involving the liver, kidney, and lung. They noted, moreover, that liver tumors had developed and metastasized more frequently in mice treated as newborns than as adults. In a later study (Shibuya and Hirono, 1973), it was shown that the tumor incidence in postnatally injected mice progressively dropped from 100% in mice treated at birth to 16% in mice when treated with a comparable dose at the 14th postnatal day. The ability to hydrolyze cycasin after its parenteral administration apparently decreased in mice as the postnatal length increased, which is compatible with the observations made in rats (Matsumoto et al., 1972b). A high incidence of pulmonary tumors in two groups of mice of the dd strain, amounting to 83 and 88% respectively, was reported by Hirono and Shibuya (1970). The mice had received single subcutaneous injections of cycasin at two dose levels at birth. In addition to the neoplasms observed in mice of these two strains, neurotoxic effects were noted in many mice of both strains (see the section Other Biological Effects).

Hamsters

Studies in hamsters have shown that cycasin and MAM are oncogenic for this species as well. When cycasin was given subcutaneously to newborn hamsters or by stomach tube to adult hamsters, the most extensive changes involved the intranepatic bile ducts. In addition to proliferative and cystic changes of the ducts, 21 intrahepatic bile duct carcinomas were recorded among 151 hamsters, and several were subsequently established as transplantable tumor lines (Hirono et al., 1971). These authors also described a carcinoma of the gallbladder and several hepatocellular carcinomas and hemangioendothelial sarcomas of the liver in hamsters treated as newborns whereas such tumors rarely developed in adult hamsters who had received cycasin by stomach tube. In addition to the hepatic neoplasms a few colonic tumors, pulmonary adenomas, and an occasional renal tumor were observed (Hirono et al., 1971). The successful induction of hepatic and colonic carcinomas and of two gallbladder carcinomas in hamsters was also reported by Spatz (1970); her then preliminary data were recently brought up to date (Laqueur and Spatz, 1975). Methylazoxymethanol was used and administered either by the intravenous or intraperitoneal routes as single or multiple injections and at three different doses varying from 10 to 20 mg/kg body weight. In addition to benign and malignant hepatic lesions involving both liver cells and bile duct epithelium, many adenomas and adenocarcinomas were found in the colon. All hamsters that received four to five intraperitoneal injections of MAM had colonic carcinomas, often at multiple sites, whereas the relative incidence of colonic carcinomas in hamsters that received a single intravenous dose was only 42%. Metastases from the colonic carcinomas were found in 25% of the hamsters receiving multiple doses. Gallbladder carcinomas were observed in two hamsters 32 and 37 wk after they had received three intraperitoneal injections of MAM. Their individual total doses varied from 5.06 to 6.16 mg of MAM. Tumors were not found in kidneys, lungs, or small intestine, and 56 saline-treated or uninjected hamsters serving as controls were free of tumors.

Guinea Pigs

The first successful tumor induction in the liver of guinea pigs with cycads was published by Spatz (1964b), who in the course of dietary studies used crude cycad meal as a hepatotoxic agent. The experiment was begun when hepatotoxicity of cycads was known but before their oncogenic properties had become established. Confirming the acute toxic effects of crude cycad meal on the liver of guinea pigs, nine of 27 guinea pigs, subsequently sacrificed between 44 and 62 wk after first exposure to the crude cycad meal, had liver tumors. Five of the tumors were of bile duct origin and four were hepatocellular carcinomas. They were multicentric and found in the right and left lobes of the liver. The possibility that the dietary manipulations might have contributed in some way to the induction of liver tumors in guinea pigs was undeniable, and the study was subsequently repeated with pigs on a standard guinea pig diet and with MAM and MAM acetate in the place of crude cycad meal.

Repeated intraperitoneal or subcutaneous injection of MAM and MAM acetate alike produced results; hepatocellular carcinomas were found in 30 of 45 guinea pigs so treated. Metastases were observed in 23 guinea pigs with liver cell cancer. Two additional bile duct carcinomas and 17 tumors of vascular nature were noted in the liver. Among the extrahepatic neoplasms, one jejunal adenocarcinoma, two pulmonary adenomas, one hemangiosarcoma of the nose, one carcinoma of the breast, and three squamous cell carcinomas apparently arising in the anterior nasal cavities were observed. No tumors were found among 59 control guinea pigs (47 males and 12 females) that had served as saline-injected controls. The experiments with guinea pigs have recently been reviewed (Laqueur and Spatz, 1975).

Fishes

There is only one report that describes the development of liver tumors in an aquarium fish, *Brachydanio rerio,* after initial subtotal destruction of the liver parenchyma by cycasin (Stanton, 1966).

Transplacental Oncogenesis

The widespread uses of cycads by people in areas where cycads grow, the solubility of the isolated glycosides in aqueous solutions, and the oncogenicity of these glycosides after hydrolysis prompted an early inquiry into the transplacental passage of the active compound and its possible effects on the development of embryos and fetuses. We cite here the experimental induction of tumors by the transplacental route; the teratologic effects are discussed in the next section.

The experiment demonstrating that transplacental induction of tumors was possible was done in Sprague-Dawley rats fed cycad meal that contained 3% cycasin (Spatz and Laqueur, 1967). This paper contains the detailed data covering the fate of the various pregnancies as well as that of the litters obtained from them. Of 81 rats born from mothers that had been exposed to various concentrations of cycad meal in the diet and surviving for 6 months or longer, 15, or 18.5%, had tumors at various sites. They included mesenchymal tumors in the jejunum of four litter mates and gliomas in five rats. Several additional neoplasms were found, including one carcinoma of the colon with metastases.

Although the experimental results indicated that transplacental induction of tumors with cycad was possible, it remained to be proven that the oncogen was present in the fetuses before it could be classified as a true transplacental oncogen. Cycasin and MAM were subsequently demonstrated in fetal tissue and in mammary glands of the maternal lactating rats (Spatz and Laqueur, 1968a). Using tritium-labeled MAM acetate, it was shown that MAM had not only crossed the placenta but had also reacted with fetal nucleic acids and proteins by finding guanine methylated in the seventh position in both DNA and RNA. The protein reaction products were not identified, although some radioactivity was incorporated into the protein (Nagata and Matsumoto, 1969).

The study on transplacental tumor induction was repeated in Fischer rats with a single dose of parenterally injected MAM (20 mg/kg body weight) to avoid variations in hydrolysis of cycasin *in vivo* when fed in a diet. Although the total number of tumors was smaller than in the previous study, amounting to only 12%, there was a noticeable preponderance of pulmonary and intracerebral tumors among the rats that had become exposed to MAM late in fetal development. Thus, 10 of 16 rats with pulmonary adenomas and six of seven rats with gliomas had been exposed *in utero* on the 21st day of fetal development, that is, approximately 24–36 hr before birth. Although no definite explanation can be given for the increased tumor incidence in lungs and brain, it seems reasonable to assume that the metabolic situation around the day of birth must have been unusually suitable for an interaction between the ultimate carcinogen of MAM and the cellular constituents in these two sites (Laqueur and Spatz, 1973).

Taken together, the results of these studies in transplacental oncogenesis indicated that the azoxyglycoside of cycads as well as its aglycone, MAM, crossed the placental barrier and were chemically demonstrable in the fetal tissues where MAM reacted with cellular constituents of the fetus. Cycasin and MAM were also found in the mammary gland, giving rise to the possibility that the active oncogen can be transmitted through the milk to the offspring, as previously postulated by Mickelsen et al. (1964) and Yang et al. (1969).

OTHER BIOLOGICAL EFFECTS

Teratogenic Effects

The evidence that MAM was teratogenic was supplied by Spatz et al. (1967b). When MAM was injected intravenously into pregnant female hamsters on the 8th day of gestation, malformations of the brain, eyes, and extremities resulted that could be seen by the 12th day. The method developed by Ferm (1965) for rapid detection of substances suspected of possessing teratogenic properties was used. Among the malformations observed were cranioschisis, rachischisis, and exencephaly, suggesting that the effect of MAM on embryonic development was rapid since the neural tube closes by the 9th day. The optimal dose of MAM that would produce the highest incidence of malformation in fetuses alive on the 12th day as evidenced by a regularly beating heart was 20 mg/kg body weight. Only slightly larger doses resulted in a high percentage of fetal death and many sites of fetal resorption, whereas smaller doses failed to induce malformations in the majority of living fetuses.

No attempt was made to observe malformed fetuses until parturition, and it seems doubtful that many would have survived as judged from the severity of the malformations. Detailed descriptions of the underlying pathologic lesions resulting in the cerebral malformations have not been reported, although a preliminary personal study of several hamster fetuses indicated necrosis of cells in the region that is involved in the closure of the neural tube. It will become apparent from the following description that focal necrosis of undifferentiated cells in cerebrum, retina, and cerebellum was an important pathologic feature common to the acute lesions.

Cerebellar malformations. The first experimental production of a neurologic disorder induced with cycasin, consisting of gait disturbances and in the most severely afflicted mice, paralysis of the hind legs, was reported by Hirono and Shibuya (1967). It was observed in mice of the C57 B1/6 strain that had received a single subcutaneous injection of 0.5 mg of cycasin/g body weight at birth. Similar effects were also produced in the dd strain of mice and in hamsters under the same experimental conditions (Hirono et al., 1969b). The development of this neurologic disorder in newborn mice and hamsters was accompanied by early histologic evidence of cellular necrosis in the cerebellar external granular layer, resulting in a scarcity of cells in the molecular and granule cell layers of the cerebellum. Purkinje cells were irregularly scattered between surviving cells of the granule cell layer but lacked their normal alignment between molecular and granule cell layers. The changes persisted throughout the remainder of the life and were demonstrable in histologic sections of cerebella of afflicted mice as late as 260 days after birth.

Shimada and Langman (1970) confirmed these observations in newborn hamsters. Injections of MAM acetate when given from the 2nd to 4th postnatal days produced severe necrosis of the cells in the external granular cell layer. This resulted in a marked diminution of cells in the granule cell layer, cellular disorganization, and a striking diminution in the size of the cerebellum when examined on the 10th postnatal day. When MAM acetate was administered from the 4th to 6th days of postnatal life, a quantitative difference between the anterior and posterior lobes in the extent of cellular necrosis in the external granular cell layer was noted; the necrosis was more severe in the anterior lobes. In such cerebella examined 20 days postnatally, it was found that rows of cells resembling those of the internal granule cell layer occupied a zone midway through the molecular layer in the anterior regions. They were considered evidence of the regeneration of cells of the external granular cell layer that, however, had failed to complete their migration. I have seen rows of cells in the middle of the molecular layer in rats treated postnatally with MAM acetate (G. L. Laqueur, unpublished observations) and Sanger et al. (1972) have described focal accumulations of similar cells in the cerebellar molecular layer of pups treated with MAM acetate within 24 hr after birth. Jones et al. (1972), using Swiss albino mice, and Sanger et al. (1972), using C57 B1/6j mice and mongrel pups, also confirmed the effect of postnatally administered MAM on cerebellar maturation. Jones et al. (1972), moreover, noted that the cerebellar changes were more uniform and severe with MAM than with cycasin and that they required less time with MAM to become apparent. The difference is probably explained by the fact that cycasin first requires hydrolysis before its toxicity is expressed.

Effects of MAM on normal cerebellar maturation have also been reported in rats, hamsters, rabbits, ferrets, cats, and dogs by Haddad et al. (1972). In the Long-Evans strain of rats the degree of cerebellar hypoplasia was shown to be dose-dependent.

Retinal malformations. A severe atrophy of the retina by the 20th postnatal day was observed in hamsters that had received injections of MAM acetate between the 4th and 6th days of life (Shimada and Langman, 1970). The atrophy was most conspicuous in the retinal nuclear layers and was accompanied by formation of rosettes. The ganglion cell layer was, however, uninvolved. Similar observations were described by Hirono (1972) in the retina of mice and rats treated neonatally with cycasin and by Goerttler et al. (1970) in Sprague-Dawley rats after intraperitoneal administration of MAM acetate. Studies that included the acute lesions showed extensive necrosis of the undifferentiated retinoblast layers (Hirono, 1972).

Cerebral malformations. Evidence that MAM could affect transplacentally the development of the cerebrum was obtained incident to studies in transplacental oncogenesis. It was first noted in four litters of rats of the Fischer strain, about 13–14 months old, whose mothers had received MAM (20 mg/kg body weight) in divided doses on days 14, 15, and 16 of pregnancy. During the postmortem examination, it was found that the brains of all litter mates were abnormally small. Although the diminution in brain size varied between the four litters, it was uniform within each litter. One of the small brains had a tumor nodule in the forebrain that on histologic examination proved to be an oligodendroglioma. The reduction in brain size and weight appeared mainly to be due to a uniform reduction in the size of both hemispheres. Except for a variable degree of ventricular dilatation, the remainder of the brain, including the cerebellum, was essentially normal. Nor was there gross evidence of a deformed skull. This microencephaly was readily reproducible in Fischer and Osborne-Mendel strains of rats, and the earliest recognizable lesion leading to microencephaly was visible within 24 hr after MAM had been injected. The acute changes consisted of extensive cellular necrosis in the undifferentiated subependymal matrix zone destined to produce the final cerebral cortex. A single injection of MAM (20 mg/kg body weight) on days 14 or 15 of gestation was shown to result in the identical cerebral malformation (Spatz and Laqueur, 1968b; Spatz, 1969). Successful induction of microencephaly with MAM acetate administered on days 14 or 15 of gestation was also reported by Fischer et al. (1972), who noted an additional generalized growth retardation in rats of the Long-Evans strain, involving the weights of body, brain, kidneys, liver, spleen, and testes. This more general effect became discernible at 35 days of age when data on organ and body weights were given.

An estimate of the cellular loss from the hemispheres of MAM-treated rats was obtained by comparing the quantitative changes with age in DNA content of microencephalic brains with those from controls (Matsumoto et al., 1972a). The difference in the DNA content between normal and MAM-treated whole brain amounted to about 25% at birth and persisted into maturity. Analyzing hemispheres and the remainder of the brain separately, the hemispheres of a 7-day-old MAM-treated rat contained about one-half (53%) of the DNA content of the hemisphere of a control rat whereas no difference was noted in the remaining brain.

The studies of Haddad et al. (1972, 1975) indicated that the ferret, among the animals tested, proved most suitable for the study of induced malformations of cerebrum and cerebellum. The ferret, in contrast to the rat, normally has cerebral convolutions visible by external inspection. Therefore the ferret offers the opportunity to look for additional disturbances involving their formation, such as lissencephaly.

The observed effects depended on the prenatal and postnatal age when MAM acetate was parenterally administered to either the pregnant ferret at timed days of gestation or to the newborn ferrets. Injections of MAM acetate into pregnant ferrets on days 27–32 of gestation resulted in young with severe degrees of microencephaly and other malformations of the cerebral hemispheres, whereas similar treatment in later periods of pregnancy beginning at the gestational age of 38 days until immediately after birth (42 days) produced severe cerebellar alterations comparable to those seen in newborn mice, rats, and hamsters. In general, the most severely malformed brains were induced when MAM was given relatively early in pregnancy, that is, at about the 27th to 32nd days of gestation, or the beginning of the third trimester. Various degrees of microencephaly, dose-dependent degrees of lissencephaly, hydrocephaly, hydranencephaly, and cerebellar dysplasia resembling the Dandy-Walker syndrome were the most remarkable malformations observed in these young (Haddad et al., 1975).

The separation into neonatally (cerebellar) and prenatally (cerebral) induced brain alterations appears in general to be fairly distinct except in the ferret, in which moderate degrees of cerebellar and cerebral involvement were simultaneously observed when MAM acetate was injected on the 38th day of gestation (Haddad et al., 1972). The combination of severe microencephaly and cerebellar hypoplasia apparently was also inducible in Long-Evans rats but only by giving one injection at day 15 of gestation and a second injection at day of birth (R. K. Haddad, personal communication, 1974). The neurotoxicity of MAM has recently been reviewed by Jones et al. (1973).

The reduction in the number of cells in the hemispheres by nearly 50% as judged from the DNA values (Matsumoto et al., 1972a) was accompanied by structural disorganization of the cerebral cortices in the MAM-treated brains.

Cerebral cortical laminas were indistinct or focally absent and foci of ectopic islands composed of small undifferentiated cells were found in the narrow cortices overlying dilated ventricular spaces. In spite of these marked changes, the rats did not show any grossly recognizable deficiencies. They exhibited normal activity in locomotion and their longevity did not appear to be significantly shortened although the period of observation was limited by termination of the study when the animals were 18–21 months old. Sister-brother matings between microencephalic rats as a rule were successful, resulting in physically normal litters except in a few instances of very severe microencephaly where matings were unsuccessful. There remained the possibility, however, that microencephalic rats might differ from their controls when properly tested for behavioral and intellectual performance. These studies are briefly summarized in the next paragraphs.

When microencephalic rats of the Fischer strain were tested in a Hebb-Williams maze, a method devised for testing intellectual functions in the rat, their performance was substantially and significantly inferior to that of normal rats (Haddad et al., 1969). It was also noted that the error rate was considerably greater for females than males in the group of microencephalic rats but this difference was absent among the control rats. On repeating the tests, the microencephalic rats decreased their error rate in a manner similar to the controls, suggesting that both groups of rats were learning how to learn.

The observations originally made in Fischer rats were confirmed in rats of the Osborne-Mendel strain and subsequently in rats of the Long-Evans strain, in which a dose-dependent degree of microencephaly was, moreover, demonstrated that also correlated well with the deficits in performance. A summary of these experiments indicated that the various aspects of behavior were not uniformly affected in the rats (Rabe and Haddad, 1972). They noted deficiencies in solving tasks in maze problems but not in operant conditioning schedules nor in acquiring a discrimination learning set. They also found that an enriched environmental condition during rearing considerably improved the performance of microencephalic-impaired rats in a problem-solving task.

The studies cited thus far have shown that cycasin and MAM are toxic for nervous tissue during the period that the brain and its constituent parts develop. In each of the three sites (cerebrum, cerebellum, and retina), the initial changes observable with the light microscope are similar and consist of necrosis of undifferentiated cells resulting in substantial losses of precursor cells from which normally the structures are formed.

Other Neurotoxic Effects

Cycasin and its aglycone MAM were not the only toxic substances identified in cycads. A new basic amino acid, α-amino-β-methylamino propionic acid, was discovered and isolated by Vega and Bell (1967) from seeds of *C. circinalis*. It was synthesized and the compound was reported to be markedly neurotoxic to chicks and rats. The natural compound was found only in seeds and leaves of the genus *Cycas* but not in seeds of the other genera. However, leaf extracts of *Dioon, Zamia, Bowenia, Macrozamia, Lepidozamia,* and *Encephalartos* contained a compound similar to α-amino-β-methylamino propionic acid (Polsky et al., 1972; Dossaji and Bell, 1973).

Although doubts have been expressed that this or a related compound may be responsible for the human disease ALS, chronic toxicity studies including pathological examinations of the tissues should be conducted before a final decision is made with respect to the neurologic disease in cattle.

Mutagenic Effects

According to Smith (1966), the aglycone of cycasin, MAM, was found to be a good mutagen in the bacterium *Salmonella* typhimurium. The effect was demonstrated by measuring the frequency of reversion to histidine independence of several histidine-requiring mutants of *Salmonella.* Cycasin was ineffective, suggesting that the *Salmonella* lacked the necessary hydrolytic enzyme, whereas MAM caused the majority to revert. In a different system used by Teas and Dyson (1967), mutagenicity was tested in *Drosophila melanogaster* using the induction of sex-linked recessive lethals in males from feeding cycasin, MAM, and MAM acetate. Whereas cycasin was not mutagenic, MAM and MAM acetate were significantly mutagenic. Testing homogenates of *Drosophila* and the yeast strain used in the medium for enzyme activity, they noted substantial esterase activity whereas β-glucosidase activity was absent or very low, probably accounting for the activity of the MAM acetate and its absence in the tests with cycasin. Cycasin however, was found to be mutagenic in those plants that contain emulsins capable of hydrolyzing the glycosides to the respective aglycones. Using seeds of the common bean (*Phaseolus vulgaris* L.), which on testing were found to have β-glucosidase activity, a high mutation frequency was found to have resulted from treatment of such seeds with cycasin (Moh, 1970).

Cycasin was also reported to have radiomimetic effects; it induced chromosomal aberrations in the root-tip cells of *Allium cepa* comparable to those brought about by exposure to 200 roentgens of gamma irradiation (Teas et al., 1965). The chromosomal aberrations included dot deletions, rod deletions, and chromatid and chromosome bridges.

The finding of chromosomal aberrations raised the more general question of the nature of resistance of cycad plants to the action of cycasin, to the cycad emulsin (β-glucosidase), and particularly to MAM, the reaction product resulting from the interaction of cycasin and β-glucosidase. These three compounds had been biochemically identified in seeds of *C. circinalis* by Matsumoto and Strong (1963). Following the observations made with *Allium cepa,* chromosome studies were extended to a representative member of the cycad family, namely *Z. integrifolia,* and observations were compared with those obtained with roots of *Allium cepa,* a noncycad plant. Root tips of both plants were treated with cycasin, emulsin, a mixture of cycasin and emulsin, MAM, and X-rays. The incidence of anaphase bridges was used as an index for comparison. It was found that cycasin and emulsin when administered separately to *Zamia* roots produced chromosome damage; this damage was more severe when cycasin and emulsin were incubated first, producing MAM. *Allium* roots when placed in cycasin for several hours produced a β-glucosidase, and chromosome damage was greater in *Allium* under these conditions than in *Zamia* (Porter and Teas, 1971). The conclusion was that some protective mechanism, either compartmentalization or chemical inhibition, was operative in the intact cycad plant under normal conditions.

The observation that larvae of the arctiid moth, *Seirarctia echo* Abbot and Smith, fed on cycad plants without apparent ill effects opened the possibility of exploring the nature of the detoxification in a different system. According to Teas et al. (1966), when analyzed for azoxyglycosides and β-glycosidases, extracts of larvae feeding on cycas leaves have relatively large amounts of cycasin in the tissues and cycasin was carried over into the pupa, adult, and egg. It was also observed that all stages of *Seirarctia* except the egg contained an emulsin-like enzyme although free MAM, which should have resulted from their interaction, was not detected in undamaged insects or in the plant tissue. In a subsequent study reported by Teas (1967), larvae of *S. echo* were fed an artificial diet to which MAM had been added for 24 hr prior to analysis. The larvae were dissected and assays for cycasin and β-glucosidase activity were performed separately on the gut, hemolymph, Malpighian tubules, fat body, and body wall. The hemolymph contained the largest amount of cycasin followed by the Malpighian tubules and only relatively small amounts were found in the gut and other tissue. In contrast, enzymatic activity determined as β-glucosidase activity was greatest in the gut and absent from the other sites. Apparently the MAM fed to the larvae had been glucosylated to cycasin and was retained in part in the hemolymph and in part excreted by the Malpighian tubules, thus protecting the larvae from the potentially hazardous effects of MAM.

COMMENTS AND IMPLICATIONS

It is somewhat surprising in retrospect that the oncogenic nature of the cycad toxin escaped detection for so many years. The time-consuming procedures in removing the poison as practiced by the people who use cycad starch as food nevertheless indicated their general awareness of the danger to their lives when the cycad starch was improperly prepared. Most likely, the need for chronic toxicity studies was not fully appreciated even after the chemical identification of the principal component, namely the azoxyglycosides, was accomplished and their acute toxicity established.

Once the oncogenic properties of crude cycad meal were recognized, however, the characterization of the oncogen was greatly facilitated by prior chemical and biochemical explorations that had resulted in the isolation of several azoxyglycosides, of β-glucosidase, and of the aglycone common to all azoxyglycosides.

It was recognized early in the studies with cycads that the glycoside cycasin and its aglycone, MAM, shared many of their biologic effects with DMN. The rapid advances made at that time in the study of the carcinogenic *n*-nitroso compounds (Magee and Barnes, 1967; Druckrey et al., 1967b) also significantly contributed to the progress of work with cycasin and MAM, and many additional similarities in the biochemical effects of MAM and DMN became apparent over the years. It is now believed that these similarities are due to a common metabolite thought to be most likely methyl carbonium hydroxide, which forms as a highly reactive intermediate in the process of decomposition of both MAM and DMN and which serves as the methyl donor, ultimate carcinogen, mutagen, and teratogen (Druckrey, 1970; Miller, 1970). In this sense, cycasin and MAM can, therefore, be regarded as naturally occurring representatives of the synthetic, carcinogenic *n*-nitroso compounds.

Cycasin and MAM, although well-established as oncogenic agents in small laboratory animals, are thus far not known to have produced comparable effects in wild rodents in their natural settings. Thus no information is available that tumors occur more frequently among animals from areas where cycads grow. In fact there is no indication that this question has even been asked. The possibility exists, moreover, that wild rats or mice might avoid eating unprocessed seeds of cycads because of their intense sweet-bitter taste. Similarly, no definite observations have been reported that eating cycad-containing food has been associated with an increase in the incidence of neoplastic disease in man.

The situation is not very different when the experimentally induced malformations are assessed in terms of their significance for human beings. Satisfactory answers to these questions simply do not at present exist. It will depend on future clinicopathological and epidemiologic observations to clarify the potential etiologic role of cycad toxins or other compounds of similar structure on the incidence of neoplasia and malformations in human beings.

The mechanisms by which cycasin as a representative of the azoxyglycosides is hydrolzyed *in vivo* to the aglycone methylazoxymethanol has been emphasized in this review. The demonstration that the hydrolysis in the gut results from and is dependent on an intestinal microflora has been important for understanding toxicity and oncogenicity of cycasin. These effects are absent in germfree animals and in those into which cycasin is administered by parenteral routes. The observations have provided a stimulus for further exploring the general role of intestinal microflora in the *in vivo* metabolism of other exogenous or endogenous substances that potentially may act or are suspected of acting as carcinogens, cocarcinogens, promoters, or initiators in the carcinogenetic process. The reverse can be imagined as well, namely that enzymes of intestinal microflora may assist in the detoxification of carcinogenic compounds such as has been observed by Teas (1967) in the conversion of the toxic and carcinogenic MAM to cycasin with the help of a β-glucosidase in the intestines of *S. echo*.

Lastly, it is of some historical interest that the detection of oncogenic properties of cycad plants occurred as awareness of a widespread presence of carcinogenic substances in nature was stimulated by the observations that certain species of *Aspergillus flavus* produced a toxin that would induce cancer of the liver in animals (Lancaster et al., 1961; Sargeant et al., 1961). The potential importance of aflatoxins (as they became known) for human disease was immediately apparent; this subject is separately reviewed elsewhere in this book. Recognizing the importance of aflatoxins, the possibility was considered that a substance like aflatoxin might be responsible for the oncogenic effects of crude cycad meal. The possibility was explored by Forgacs and Carll (1964), who found a large number of fungi, including *Aspergillus flavus*, in various parts of cycad seeds used for the preparation of cycad meal. Although these studies were discontinued when cycasin was shown to be the carcinogen in cycad meal, it is possible that some of the metabolic differences noted between rats fed crude cycad meal and those fed cycasin (Williams and Laqueur, 1965) may have been due to a toxic fungal contaminant in the crude meal.

REFERENCES

Barnes, J. M. and Magee, P. N. 1954. *Brit. J. Industr. Med.* 11:167–174.
Birdsey, M. R. 1972. *Fed. Proc.* 31:1467–1469.
Buss, H. and Gusek, W. 1968. *Virchows Arch. Abt. B* 1:251–268.
Campbell, M. E., Mickelsen, O., Yang, M. G., Laqueur, G. L. and Keresztesy, J. C. 1966. *J. Nutr.* 88:115–124.
Cooper, J. M. 1941. *Proc. Roy. Soc. New South Wales* 74:450–454.
Dahlquist, A., Bull, B. and Gustafson, B. E. 1965. *Arch. Biochem. Biophys.* 109:150–158.
Dastur, D. K. and Palekar, R. S. 1966. *Nature* 210:841–843.
Dossaji, S. F. and Herbin, G. A. 1972. *Fed. Proc.* 31:1470–1472.
Dossaji, S. F. and Bell, E. A. 1973. *Phytochemistry* 12:143–144.
Druckrey, H. 1970. In *Carcinoma of the colon and antecedent epithelium*, ed. W. J. Burdette, pp. 267–279. Springfield, Ill.: Charles C Thomas.
Druckrey, H. 1973. *Xenobiotica* 3:271–303.
Druckrey, H., Preussmann, R., Matzkies, F. and Ivankovic, S. 1967a. *Naturwissenschaften* 54:285–286.
Druckrey, H., Preussmann, R., Ivankovic, S. and Schmähl, D. Untermitarbeit von Afkham, J., Blum, G., Mennel, H. D., Müller, M., Petropoulos, P. and Schneider, H. 1967b. *Z. Krebsforsch.* 69:103–201.
Ferm, V. H. 1965. *Lab. Invest.* 14:1500–1505.
Fischer, M. H., Welker, C. and Waisman, H. A. 1972. *Teratology* 5:223–232.
Forgacs, F. and Carll, W. T. 1964. *Fed. Proc.* 23:1370–1372.
Fosberg, F. R. 1964. *Fed. Proc.* 23:1340–1342.
Ganote, C. E. and Rosenthal, A. S. 1968. *Lab. Invest.* 19:382–398.
Goerttler, K., Arnold, H. P. and Michalk, D. V. 1970. *Z. Krebsforsch.* 74:396–411.

Gusek, W. 1968. *Verh. Dtsch. Ges. Path.* 52:410–415.
Gusek, W. 1972. *Verh. Dtsch. Ges. Path.* 56:625. (Abstr.)
Gusek, W. 1975. *Virchows Arch. Abt. A Path. Anat. Histol.* 365:221–237.
Gusek, W. and Mestwerdt, W. 1969. *Beitr. Path. Anat.* 139:199–218.
Gusek, W., Buss, H. and Laqueur, G. L. 1967. *Beitr. Path. Anat.* 135:53–74.
Haddad, R. K., Rabe, A., Laqueur, G. L., Spatz, M. and Valsamis, M. P. 1969. *Science* 163:88–90.
Haddad, R. K., Rabe, A. and Dumas, R. 1972. *Fed. Proc.* 31:1520–1523.
Haddad, R. K., Rabe, A. and Dumas, R. 1975. *Comp. Path. Bull.* 7:2–4.
Hall, W. T. and McGavin, M. D. 1968. *Pathol. Vet.* 5:26–34.
Hard, C. C. and Butler, W. H. 1970. *Cancer Res.* 30:2806–2815.
Hard, C. C. and Butler, W. H. 1971. *Cancer Res.* 31:337–347.
Hirano, A. 1973. In *Progress in neuropathology*, ed. H. M. Zimmerman, vol. II, pp. 181–215. New York: Grune & Stratton.
Hirano, A., Malamud, N., Elizan, T. S. and Kurland, L. T. 1966. *Arch. Neurol.* 15:35–51.
Hirono, I. 1972. *Fed. Proc.* 31:1493–1497.
Hirono, I. and Shibuya, C. 1967. *Nature* 216:1311–1312.
Hirono, I. and Shibuya, C. 1970. *Gann* 61:403–407.
Hirono, I., Laqueur, G. L. and Spatz, M. 1968. *J. Natl. Cancer Inst.* 40:1003–1010.
Hirono, I., Shibuya, C. and Fushimi, K. 1969a. *Cancer Res.* 29:1658–1662.
Hirono, I., Shibuya, C. and Hayashi, K. 1969b. *Proc. Soc. Exp. Biol. Med.* 131:593–599.
Hirono, I., Kachi, H. and Kato, T. 1970. *Acta Pathol. Japan* 20:327–337.
Hirono, I., Hayashi, K., Mori, H. and Miwa, T. 1971. *Cancer Res.* 31:283–287.
Hoch-Ligeti, C., Stutzman, E. and Arvin, J. M. 1968. *J. Natl. Cancer Inst.* 41:605–614.
Horisberger, M. and Matsumoto, H. 1968. *J. Label. Compounds* 4:164–170.
Jones, M., Yang, M. and Mickelsen, O. 1972. *Fed. Proc.* 31:1508–1511.
Jones, M., Mickelsen, O. and Yang, M. G. 1973. In *Progress in neuropathology*, ed. H. M. Zimmerman, vol. II, pp. 91–114. New York: Grune & Stratton.
Kobayashi, A. 1962. *Agr. Biol. Chem.* 26:203–207, 208–212.
Kobayashi, A. and Matsumoto, H. 1965. *Arch. Biochem. Biophys.* 110:373–380.
Kurland, L. T. 1964. *Fed. Proc.* 23:1337–1339.
Kurland, L. T. and Mulder, D. W. 1954. *Neurology* 4:355–378, 438–448.
Lancaster, M. C., Jenkins, F. P. and Philp, J. McL. 1961. *Nature* 192:1095–1096.
Langley, B. W., Lythgoe, B. and Riggs, N. V. 1951. *J. Chem. Soc.* 46:2309–2316.
Laqueur, G. L. 1964. *Fed. Proc.* 23:1386–1387.
Laqueur, G. L. 1965. *Arch. Pathol. Anat. Physiol.* 340:151–163.
Laqueur, G. L. and Matsumoto, H. 1966. *J. Natl. Cancer Inst.* 37:217–232.
Laqueur, G. L. and Spatz, M. 1968. *Cancer Res.* 28:2262–2267.
Laqueur, G. L. and Spatz, M. 1973. In *Transplacental carcinogenesis*, ed. L. Tomatis and U. Mohr, IARC Scientific Publication no. 4, pp. 59–64. Lyon: International Agency for Research on Cancer.
Laqueur, G. L. and Spatz, M. 1975. In *Recent topics in chemical carcinogenesis*, ed. S. Odashima, H. Sato and S. Takayama, Gann Monograph on Cancer Research, vol. 17, pp. 189–204. Tokyo: University of Tokyo Press.

Laqueur, G. L., Mickelsen, O., Whiting, M. G. and Kurland, L. T. 1963. *J. Natl. Cancer Inst.* 31:919–951.

Laqueur, G. L., McDaniel, E. G. and Matsumoto, H. 1967. *J. Natl. Cancer Inst.* 39:355–371.

Lundeen, P. B., Banks, G. S. and Ruddon, R. W. 1971. *Biochem. Pharmacol.* 20:2522–2527.

Lythgoe, B. and Riggs, N. V. 1949. *J. Chem. Soc.* 4:2716–2718.

Magee, P. N. and Barnes, J. M. 1956. *Brit. J. Cancer* 10:114–122.

Magee, P. N. and Barnes, J. M. 1959. *Acta Unio Intern. Contra Cancrum* 15:187–190.

Magee, P. N. and Barnes, J. M. 1962. *J. Path. Bact.* 64:19–31.

Magee, P. N. and Barnes, J. M. 1967. *Adv. Cancer Res.* 10:163–246.

Mason, M. M. and Whiting, M. G. 1968. *Cornell Veterinarian* 58:541–554.

Matsumoto, H. and Higa, H. H. 1966. *Biochem. J.* 98:20c–22c.

Matsumoto, H. and Strong, F. M. 1963. *Arch. Biochem. Biophys.* 101:299–310.

Matsumoto, H., Nagahama, T. and Larson, H. O. 1965. *Biochem. J.* 95:13c–14c.

Matsumoto, H., Spatz, M. and Laqueur, G. L. 1972a. *J. Neurochem.* 19:297–306.

Matsumoto, H., Nagata, Y., Nishimura, E. T., Bristol, R. and Haber, M. 1972b. *J. Natl. Cancer Inst.* 49:423–433.

Mickelsen, O., Campbell, E., Yang, M., Mugera, G. and Whitehair, C. K. 1964. *Fed. Proc.* 23:1363–1365.

Miller, J. A. 1964. *Fed. Proc.* 23:1361–1362.

Miller, J. A. 1970. *Cancer Res.* 30:559–576.

Moh, C. C. 1970. *Mutation Res.* 10:251–253.

Mugera, G. M. and Nderito, P. 1968a. *E. Afr. Med. J.* In *Cancer in Africa*, ed. P. Cliffor, C. A. Linsell, and G. L. Timms, pp. 323–326. Nairobi, Kenya.

Mugera, G. M. and Nderito, P. 1968b. *E. Afr. Med. J.* 45:732–741.

Mugera, G. M. and Nderito, P. 1968c. *Brit. J. Cancer* 22:563–568.

Nagahama, T. 1964. *Bull. Fac. Agr. Kagoshima University* no. 14:1–50 (in Japanese with English summary).

Nagahama, T., Ijuin, I. and Watabe, T. 1964. *Agr. Biol. Chem.* 28:573–574.

Nagasawa, Y., Shirota, F. N. and Matsumoto, H. 1972. *Nature* 236:234–235.

Nagata, Y. and Matsumoto, H. 1969. *Proc. Soc. Exp. Biol. Med.* 132:383–385.

Narisawa, T. and Nakano, H. 1973. *Gann* 64:93–95.

Nishida, K. 1959. *Japan J. Chem.* 13:730–737 (in Japanese; English translation available).

Nishida, K., Kobayashi, A. and Nagahama, T. 1955a. *Bull. Agr. Chem. Soc. Japan* 19:77–83.

Nishida, K., Kobayashi, A. and Nagahama, T. 1955b. *Bull. Agr. Chem. Soc. Japan* 19:172–175.

Nishida, K., Kobayashi, A., Nagahama, T., Kojima, K. and Yamane, M. 1956a. *Seikagaku* 28:218–223.

Nishida, K., Kobayashi, A. and Nagahama, T. 1956b. *Bull. Agr. Chem. Soc. Japan* 20:74–76.

O'Gara, R. W., Brown, J. M. and Whiting, M. G. 1964. *Fed. Proc.* 23:1383.

Orgell, W. H. and Laqueur, G. L. 1964. *Fed. Proc.* 23:1378–1380.

Palekar, R. S. and Dastur, D. K. 1965. *Nature* 206:1363–1365.

Polsky, F. I., Nunn, P. B. and Bell, E. A. 1972. *Fed. Proc.* 31:1473–1475.

Porter, E. D. and Teas, H. J. 1971. *Radiation Botany* 11:21–26.

Rabe, A. and Haddad, R. K. 1972. *Fed. Proc.* 31:1536–1539.

Rechcigl, M., Jr. 1964. *Fed. Proc.* 23:1376–1377.
Rechcigl, M., Jr. and Laqueur, G. L. 1968. *Enzym. Biol. Clin.* 9:276–286.
Riggs, N. V. 1954. *Australian J. Chem.* 7:123–124.
Riggs, N. V. 1956. *Chem. Ind. (London)* 1956:926.
Sanger, V. L., Yang, M. and Mickelsen, O. 1972. *Fed. Proc.* 31:1524–1528.
Sargeant, K., Sheridan, A. and O'Kelly, J. 1961. *Nature* 192:1096–1097.
Shank, R. C. and Magee, P. N. 1967. *Biochem. J.* 105:521–527.
Shibuya, C. and Hirono, I. 1973. *Gann* 64:109–110.
Shimada, M. and Langman, J. 1970. *Teratology* 3:119–131.
Smith, D. W. E. 1966. *Science* 152:1273–1274.
Spatz, M. 1964a. *Fed. Proc.* 23:1381–1382.
Spatz, M. 1964b. *Fed. Proc.* 23:1384–1385.
Spatz, M. 1968. *Proc. Soc. Exp. Biol. Med.* 128:1005–1008.
Spatz, M. 1969. *Ann. N.Y. Acad. Sci.* 163:848–859.
Spatz, M. 1970. *Tenth Int. Cancer Congr. Houston* Abstr., pp. 24–25.
Spatz, M. and Laqueur, G. L. 1967. *J. Natl. Cancer Inst.* 38:233–245.
Spatz, M. and Laqueur, G. L. 1968a. *Proc. Soc. Exp. Biol. Med.* 127:281–286.
Spatz, M. and Laqueur, G. L. 1968b. *Proc. Soc. Exp. Biol. Med.* 129:705–710.
Spatz, M., McDaniel, E. G. and Laqueur, G. L. 1966. *Proc. Soc. Exp. Biol. Med.* 121:417–422.
Spatz, M., Smith, D. W. E., McDaniel, E. G. and Laqueur, G. L. 1967a. *Proc. Soc. Exp. Biol. Med.* 124:691–697.
Spatz, M., Daugherty, W. J. and Smith, D. W. E. 1967b. *Proc. Soc. Exp. Biol. Med.* 124:476–478.
Stanton, M. E. 1966. *Fed. Proc.* 25:661.
Steyn, D. C., Van Der Walt, S. J. and Verdoorn, I. C. 1948. *S. Afr. Med. J.* 5:758–760.
Teas, H. J. 1967. *Biochem. Biophys. Res. Commun.* 26:686–690.
Teas, H. J. and Dyson, J. G. 1967. *Proc. Soc. Exp. Biol. Med.* 125:988–990.
Teas, H. J., Sax, H. J. and Sax, K. 1965. *Science* 149:541–542.
Teas, H. J., Dyson, J. G. and Whisenant, B. R. 1966. *J. Georgia Entomol. Soc.* 1:21–22.
Vega, A. and Bell, E. A. 1967. *Phytochemistry* 6:759–762.
Wells, W. W., Yang, M. G., Bolzer, W. and Mickelsen, O. 1968. *Anal. Biochem.* 25:325–329.
Whiting, M. G. 1963. *Econ. Botany* 17:269–302.
Whiting, M. G. 1964. *Fed. Proc.* 23:1343–1345.
Williams, J. N. 1964. *Fed. Proc.* 23:1374–1375.
Williams, J. N. and Laqueur, G. L. 1965. *Proc. Soc. Exp. Biol. Med.* 118:1–4.
Yang, M. G. and Mickelsen, O. 1969. Cycads. In *Toxic constituents of plant foodstuffs*, ed. I. E. Liener, pp. 159–167. New York: Academic Press.
Yang, M. G., Mickelsen, O., Campbell, M. E., Laqueur, G. L. and Keresztesy, J. C. 1966. *J. Nutr.* 90:153–156.
Yang, M. G., Sanger, V. L., Mickelsen, O. and Laqueur, G. L. 1968. *Proc. Soc. Exp. Biol. Med.* 127:1171–1175.
Yang, M. G., Mickelsen, O. and Sanger, V. L. 1969. *Proc. Soc. Exp. Biol. Med.* 131:135–137.
Zedeck, M. S., Sternberg, S. S., Poynter, R. W. and McGowan, J. 1970. *Lab. Invest.* 30:801–812.

Chapter 8

MYCOTOXINS AND OTHER NATURALLY OCCURRING CARCINOGENS

Gerald N. Wogan
Department of Nutrition and Food Science
Massachusetts Institute of Technology
Cambridge, Massachusetts

INTRODUCTION

Several hundreds of chemicals have been shown to have carcinogenic activity in experimental animals, and the carcinogenesis literature is replete with examples of compounds that produce tumors when administered to animals under appropriate conditions. Representatives of many chemical classes are included among these compounds. In a large proportion of such investigations, the carcinogens were used as model compounds in experiments dealing with one or another facet of the carcinogenic process. Useful as information from such experiments may be in contributing to improved understanding of underlying mechanisms, it has not significantly improved elucidation of the etiologic factors involved in causation of cancer in humans, because most of the model compounds involved would probably never be encountered by human populations.

In contrast to the recent elucidation of the relationships between exposure to vinyl chloride and occurrence of angiosarcoma of the liver in men (Bartsch and Montesano, 1975), no definite evidence exists that establishes any single chemical agent as the causative factor for most kinds of cancer in humans. Therefore, in evaluating the possible involvement of carcinogens in this context, it is necessary to place heavy reliance on the adequacy of evidence for carcinogenic activity in animals, and to attempt meaningful extrapolation of that evidence to humans in constructing an evaluation of carcinogenic risk. On the basis of current knowledge, this is a very inexact process, since the frequency and time of appearance of tumors in both animals and humans may be modified by numerous factors, including specific environmental chemicals, nutritional and endocrine status, genetic constitution, and interactions among these and possibly additional modulating influences as yet unidentified.

The number of known synthetic carcinogens is now large and is continuously expanding as additional chemicals are tested for carcinogenic activity. The synthetic chemical carcinogens include the large group of polycyclic aromatic hydrocarbons, aromatic amines, azo dyes, alkylating agents, lactones, N-nitroso compounds, metals, and many other types of compounds. On the basis of all available evidence, there seems to be no strong reason to invoke most of these carcinogens as possible etiologic agents in human cancers, with the possible exceptions of nitrosamines, certain chlorinated hydrocarbons, and a few other compounds that effect humans in various ways, mainly through occupational exposure.

In the recent past, a number of very potent carcinogens of natural origin have been discovered (see Wogan et al., 1974, for review), and the possibility that certain of them may be etiologic factors in human cancers, especially hepatocellular carcinoma, has been extensively investigated and discussed. This group includes aflatoxins and certain other toxic products of fungi, pyrrolizidine alkaloids, bracken fern, and several other plant constituents. Such naturally occurring chemicals can arise from a variety of sources. Most are encountered by humans as a consequence of their presence in either foods or beverages. In some circumstances, carcinogenic agents are present as normal constituents of plants or plant products used as foods, herbal medicines, or teas. Other naturally occurring carcinogens are not usually present, but become contaminants of foods or beverages accidentally, as in the case of compounds produced by spoilage fungi growing on stored food crops.

The purpose of this review is to present a summary of available information on presently known carcinogens of natural origin, especially as this evidence bears on assessment of their significance to humans.

MYCOTOXINS

Aflatoxins

Knowledge about aflatoxins has developed during an era of increasing awareness of the importance of natural as well as anthropogenic chemicals as environmental contaminants. The intensity with which this problem has been investigated is reflected in the large number of publications about it that have appeared since its emergence in 1960. Most of this large literature is beyond the scope of this chapter, which will emphasize recent developments, mainly those having to do with the carcinogenicity of aflatoxins and their mechanisms of action. This field has been the subject of previous specialized reviews (Wogan, 1973; Rodricks, 1969; Wogan, 1968), and the entire subject has been comprehensively surveyed in a monograph (Goldblatt, 1969) and in summary form (Detroy et al., 1971). Those sources give detailed references to the original literature on which the following general summary is based.

The existence of aflatoxins was discovered as a consequence of mass outbreaks of poisoning of poultry, and it is possible that this episode might have been relegated to the miscellaneous problems of agriculture, except for several features of the problem whose importance became increasingly obvious as early developments unfolded.

Important among these was the early recognition that the toxic agents were produced by *Aspergillus flavus*, a common and widely distributed food spoilage fungus. The problem assumed global dimensions when aflatoxins were identified in agricultural products, especially peanut meals, originating in many different parts of the world. Coupled with this information was the eventual discovery that toxin-producing fungal strains could produce aflatoxins whenever conditions permitted their growth on practically any natural substrate, thereby providing for a high probability of appearance of the toxins as contaminants of human foods. Among the most striking features of the problem are the poisonous properties of aflatoxins, and especially their extraordinary potency as hepatocarcinogens in animals. The obvious implications of these various facets of the problem to public health stimulated research into occurrence of the toxins, means for prevention and control of their contamination of human foods, and their toxicology and pharmacology.

In addition to their importance as public health hazards, the aflatoxins have become useful model compounds for investigations in experimental chemical carcinogenesis. In this group of substances, nature has provided compounds of closely related chemical structure but widely differing potency and tissue specificity. Although various members of the series are effective in inducing toxic or other manifestations of biological activity in many different kinds of test systems, there are great variations in carcinogenic response among animal species. The underlying mechanisms responsible for these structure-activity relationships and species differences in responses are unidentified. Their elucidation can reasonably be expected to improve our understanding of some of the mechanisms involved in carcinogenesis and fully warrants continued investigation. This is particularly important in view of increasing evidence that human populations in some parts of the world are being exposed to aflatoxins and that such populations are at higher risk of developing liver cancer than are unexposed groups.

Source and chemical identity. Chemically, the aflatoxins are highly substituted coumarins, and have a fused dihydrofurofuran configuration peculiar to a limited number of compounds of natural origin. The compounds occur in two series, aflatoxin B_1 and derivatives, and aflatoxin G_1 and derivatives. The structure of aflatoxin B_1 is shown in Fig. 1. A total of 13 naturally occurring derivatives have been structurally identified, some of which are also shown in Fig. 1. In the aflatoxin G series, a smaller number of analogs are also known to exist.

The aflatoxins are produced by only a few strains of *Aspergillus flavus* and *A. parasiticus*, fungi whose spores are widely distributed, especially in soil. Organisms that are capable of toxin production generally synthesize only two

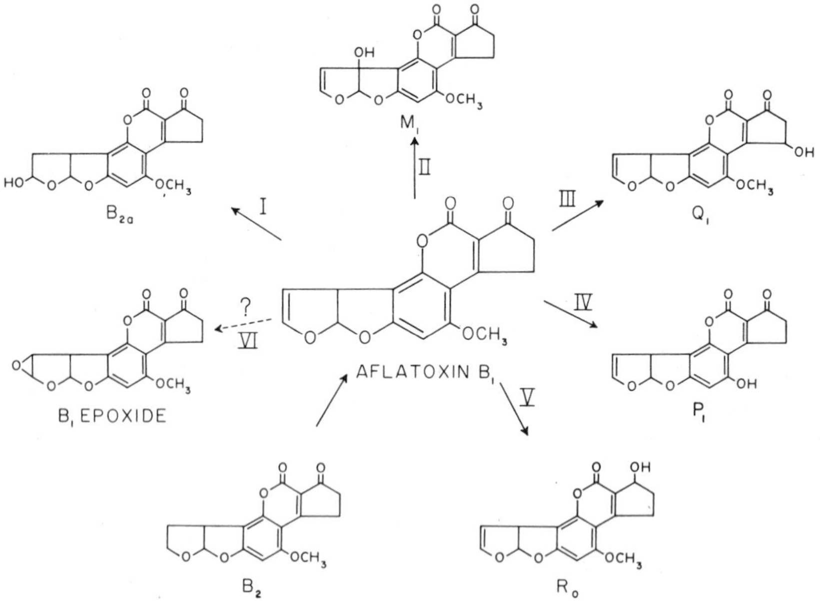

FIGURE 1   Metabolic transformations of aflatoxin B_1.

or three aflatoxins under a given set of conditions. When they occur as food contaminants, aflatoxin B_1 is always present. Although aflatoxins in the G series have sometimes been found in contaminated products, they generally occur less frequently than B_1 and have never been reported in the absence of B_1. This is an important point, since B_1 has the highest potency of the group as a toxin and as a carcinogen.

With respect to substrate, requirements for toxin production are relatively nonspecific, and the mold can produce the compounds on virtually any food (or indeed on simple synthetic media) that will support growth. Thus, any food material can be subject to aflatoxin contamination if it becomes moldy. However, experience has shown that the frequency and levels of aflatoxins found vary greatly among foods collected within a given region and among different regions.

Carcinogenicity in experimental animals and other relevant biological effects. The carcinogenicity, toxicity, and biochemical effects induced in various biological test systems by aflatoxins have been extensively studied, and only a brief summary is possible here to indicate the present status of these facets of the field. Acute or subacute poisoning can be produced in animals by feeding aflatoxin-contaminated diets or by dosing with purified compounds. Although there are wide species differences in responsiveness to acute toxicity, no completely refractory species is known. Symptoms of poisoning are produced in most domestic animals by aflatoxin levels in the feed of 10–100 mg/kg (ppm) or less. As regards lethal potency to experimental animals, the oral or parenteral LD_{50} values are generally in the range of 5-15 mg/kg body weight for aflatoxin B_1. The value for trout, the most sensitive species, is <0.5 mg/kg, and that for the mouse, the least sensitive, is 60 mg/kg. In both acute and subacute poisoning, the liver is the main target organ for aflatoxin B_1. The chief pathologic lesions in liver associated with acute or chronic toxicity are periportal or centrilobular necrosis, bile duct proliferation, and, in some species, cirrhosis.

Many of the biochemical changes induced in various biological systems by aflatoxin B_1 follow a consistent pattern. Administration of the toxin to rats is quickly followed by pronounced inhibition of DNA and RNA polymerases in liver, and similar responses have been observed in human and animal cell cultures. Protein synthesis is also impaired, particularly under conditions where synthesis is strongly influenced by alterations in *de novo* RNA synthesis. Available evidence indicates that polymerase inhibition is an indirect consequence of impaired template activity of chromatin subsequent to toxin-chromatin interaction. Consequently, interaction between aflatoxin or some derivative of it with DNA or another component of chromatin is viewed as the initiating event in the observed series of reactions. Much of the current literature deals with one or another facet of this sequence of biochemical events. Another line of evidence that may be related to the mode of action of the toxins deals with their ability to interact with membranes of the endoplasmic reticulum and thereby alter polysomal binding to those membranes. However, the available evidence is as yet inadequate to explain in detail the biochemical basis of the cytotoxicity and carcinogenic effects of these toxins.

Aflatoxins have been shown to have carcinogenic activity in many species of animals, including rodents, nonhuman primates, birds, and fish. The liver is the organ principally affected, in which the toxins induce hepatocellular carcinomas and other tumor types. However, under some circumstances, significant incidence of tumors at sites other than liver has been recorded, their distribution depending on the specific aflatoxin used, species, strain, and dose level administered.

The majority of published information on aflatoxin carcinogenicity deals with experiments in rats, in which the toxins have a high order of potency. In addition to experiments dealing with dose-response characteristics, influences of such factors as route, dosing regimen, strain, sex, and age have been investigated. Also, effects of various other modifying factors on carcinogenic responses have been evaluated, including diet, hormonal status, liver injury, microsomal enzyme activity, and concurrent exposure to other carcinogenic agents.

Many early experiments involved the feeding of diets containing aflatoxin-contaminated ingredients. Levels of the toxin were determined by chemical assays and manipulated by dilution with uncontaminated material. As a group, these experiments established the fact that aflatoxin levels of 0.1 ppm (mg/kg diet) and higher consistently induced liver carcinomas in rats.

G. N. Wogan

TABLE 1   Dose-Response Characteristics of Aflatoxin B_1
Carcinogenesis in Male Fischer Rats

Dietary aflatoxin level (ppb)	Duration of feeding (wk)	Liver carcinoma incidence	Preneoplastic liver lesions
0	74–109	0/18	0/18
1	78–105	2/22	7/22
5	65–93	1/22	5/22
15	69–96	4/22	13/22
50	71–97	20/25[a]	5/25
100	54–88	28/28[b]	–

[a]Two animals had pulmonary metastases.
[b]Four animals had pulmonary metastases.

This conclusion has been confirmed and extended in later experiments in which purified aflatoxin B_1 was added; the results are summarized in Table 1. It is evident from these observations that the compound has demonstrable carcinogenic properties at a level of 1 ppb (μg/kg diet), and the response is dose-related up to 100 ppb, at which level liver carcinoma developed in all animals surviving for approximately 18 months.

Considerable variation exists among rat strains with respect to sensitivity to carcinogenic effects of low levels of aflatoxins. However, a dietary level of 1.0 ppm consistently induces liver carcinoma at high incidence in several rat strains even when feeding is not continued throughout the entire period of observation, as shown by representative data in Table 2. In contrast, inbred mice showed no evidence of carcinogenic response at this level. In fact, a dietary level of 150 ppm was ineffective in inducing liver tumors in a random-bred mouse strain fed that level for their entire lifespan. On the other hand, infant mice of an F_1 hybrid strain (C57B1 $\times$ C3H) developed a high incidence of hepatocellular carcinomas when given repeated injections of aflatoxin B_1 during the perinatal period.

The primary target organ for aflatoxin B_1 in most rat strains is the liver, in which it induces hepatocellular carcinomas and cholangiocarcinomas, among other lesions. Tumors of other tissues that have been observed in aflatoxin B_1-treated rats include carcinomas of the glandular stomach and mucinous adenocarcinomas of the colon. Both are infrequently observed in rats treated with carcinogens, and although only a relatively small number have been observed in aflatoxin-treated animals, a causative association has been suggested. More recent experiments suggest that the incidence of the colon tumor may be enhanced by vitamin A deficiency.

Published evidence of carcinogenicity of aflatoxin B_1 in nonrodent species is summarized in Table 3. Liver carcinomas have been induced in

TABLE 2 Hepatocarcinogenicity of Aflatoxin B_1 in Rodents

Species	Dosing regimen	Duration of treatment	Period of observation	Liver tumor incidence	Reference
Rat, Fischer	1.0 ppm in diet	33 wk	52 wk	3/6	Svoboda et al., 1966
Rat, Fischer	1.0 ppm in diet	41–64 wk	Same	18/21	Wogan and Newberne, 1967
Rat, Porton	1.0 ppm in diet	20 wk	90 wk	19/30	Butler, 1969
Rat, Wistar	1.0 ppm in diet	21 wk	87 wk	12/14	Epstein et al., 1969
Mouse, Swiss	150 ppm in diet[a]	20 months	Same	0/60	Wogan, 1973
Mouse, C57B1/6NB	1.0 ppm in diet	20 months	Same	0/30	
Mouse, C3HfB/HEN	1.0 ppm in diet	20 months	Same	0/30	
Mouse, hybrid F_1 4 days old	6.0 μg/g b.w.	3 doses ip	80 wk	16/16	Vesselinovich et al., 1972

[a]A mixture of aflatoxins B_1 and G_1 was used in this experiment.

TABLE 3 Hepatocarcinogenicity of Aflatoxin B_1 in Nonrodent Species

Species	Dosing regimen	Duration of treatment	Period of observation	Liver tumor incidence	Reference
Monkey, rhesus (M)	1.655 g total[a]	5.5 yr	8.0 yr	1/1	Gopalan et al., 1972
Monkey, rhesus (F)	1.655 g total	5.5 yr	10.75 yr	1/1	Tilak, 1975
Monkey, rhesus (F)	0.504 g total	6.0 yr	8.0 yr	1/1	Adamson et al., 1973
Marmoset	3.0 mg total	50–55 wk	Same	1/3	Lin et al., 1974
	5.04–5.84 mg total[b]	87–94 wk	Same	2/3	
Tree shrew (M & F)	24–66 mg total	74–172 wk	Same	9/12	Reddy et al., 1976
Ferret	0.3–2.0 ppm in diet	28–37 months	Same	7/9	Butler, 1969
Duck	30 ppb in diet	14 months	Same	8/11	Carnaghan, 1965
Rainbow trout	4 ppb in diet	12 months	Same	15%	Sinnhuber et al., 1968
	8 ppb in diet	12 months	Same	40%	
	20 ppb in diet	12 months	Same	65%	
Rainbow trout embryos	0.5 ppm in water	1 hr	296–321 days	38%	Sinnhuber and Wales, 1974
Salmon	12 ppb in diet[c]	20 months	Same	50%	Wales and Sinnhuber, 1972
Guppy	6 ppm in diet	11 months	Same	7/113	Sato et al., 1973

[a]A mixture of aflatoxins B_1 and G_1 was used in this experiment.
[b]These animals were infected simultaneously with hepatitis virus.
[c]This diet also contained 50 ppm cyclopropenoid fatty acids.

subhuman primates in four separate experiments. Although the total number of positive responses is very small, it seems clear that aflatoxin B_1 is an effective carcinogen for the liver of these species.

Among the remaining animals that have been studied, the rainbow trout and duck appear to be of comparable sensitivity, responding to levels of 4-30 ppb in the diet. Effective levels in the guppy and ferret were in the parts-per-million range, and the salmon responded only when exposed concurrently to aflatoxin B_1 and cyclopropene-containing fatty acids that have a cocarcinogenic property in fish.

Numerous reports have dealt with factors of various kinds that modify the carcinogenic response of rats to aflatoxin B_1, including experimental alteration of nutritional and endocrine status, various types of liver insults, and simultaneous exposure to aflatoxins and other pharmacologically active compounds.

Because of the possibility that exposure to aflatoxins could occur in human populations suffering from malnutrition, the influence of nutritional status on aflatoxin carcinogenesis in rats has received attention by a number of investigators. The effect of dietary protein has been evaluated with somewhat contradictory results. Madhavan and Gopalan (1968) found that rats fed a low (5%) protein diet were sensitized to the toxic effects of aflatoxin, but developed liver tumors at a lower incidence than controls fed a 20% protein ration. On the other hand, Newberne et al. (1966) and Newberne and Wogan (1969) found that diets containing 9% protein resulted in a higher incidence of liver tumors in a shorter period of time than a diet containing 22% protein when both groups of rats were intubated with 375 μg aflatoxin B_1 per animal. The reasons for these disparate results are unclear, and this important problem requires further investigation.

Rogers and Newberne (1969, 1971) have focused attention on the possible importance of simultaneous occurrence of marginal insufficiency of dietary lipotropic agents, such as methionine and vitamin B_{12}, and aflatoxin exposure, and have studied these conditions in rats. Marginal lipotrope deficiency protected rats against doses of aflatoxin B_1 that were lethal to 60-100% of rats on an adequate diet. However, when treated with a carcinogenic regimen, animals with a lipotrope deficiency developed liver tumors much earlier and at a higher frequency than did control animals. The mechanisms responsible for these interactions have not been identified.

Simultaneous administration of aflatoxin B_1 with other pharmacologically active compounds, including other carcinogens, has been investigated. Reddy and Svoboda (1972) studied the effects in rats of lasiocarpine, a pyrrolizidine alkaloid that is carcinogenic and strongly hepatotoxic, on carcinogenesis by feeding aflatoxin B_1 at 2 ppm. They found that the alkaloid did not prevent initiation of liver tumors by aflatoxin, but did alter the pathogenic pattern in which the tumors developed. McLean and Marshall (1971) demonstrated a protective action of phenobarbitone against the carcinogenicity of aflatoxin B_1.

Continuous administration of phenobarbitone in drinking water during a 9 wk period in which aflatoxin B_1 was fed at 5 ppm in the diet resulted in a smaller incidence and delayed appearance of liver tumors than were observed in rats fed aflatoxin alone. These investigators suggested induction by phenobarbitone of liver microsomal enzymes that metabolize the aflatoxin to noncarcinogenic products.

Aflatoxin metabolism. Considerable research has been done on the metabolic fate of aflatoxin B_1, intended mainly to produce data bearing on mechanisms that might explain mode of action and differences in susceptibility to the toxin among various animal species, and possibly in humans. The information generated to date is inadequate to provide complete explanations, but some general outlines of metabolic patterns are beginning to emerge (Wogan, 1973; Patterson, 1973).

Patterns of tissue distribution and excretion of aflatoxin B_1 following oral or parenteral dosing have been studied in several species. Experiments with ^{14}C-labeled toxin indicated that more than 90% of a single dose is excreted within 24 hr by rats. Feces represent the principal excretory route, accounting for up to 75% of the dose, with urine containing an additional 15–20%. Retained radioactivity is present mainly in liver. This pattern of tissue distribution and excretion is generally similar in mice, in rhesus monkeys given a single dose intraperitoneally or orally, and in chickens dosed repeatedly by intubation. In all of these experiments, the identity of the radioactive material retained or excreted is largely unknown, except that unmetabolized aflatoxin B_1 does not account for more than 5% of the total in any instance. In a few cases, major metabolites have been isolated and identified chemically.

All of the metabolic transformations of aflatoxin B_1 known to take place in animals are indicated by the pathways outlined in Fig. 1. The identity of some metabolites has been established from compounds isolated from *in vivo* sources; other have been produced *in vitro*.

Hydroxylated derivatives of aflatoxin B_1 are formed through several routes. Ring hydroxylation at the 4 position (pathway II in Fig. 1), producing M_1, appears to be a common pathway. This derivative has been found in milk, tissues, and urine of animals and people ingesting B_1, and is also produced *in vitro* by liver microsomes of birds, rodents, and primates, including humans (Patterson, 1973). Ring hydroxylation of the carbon atom β to the carbonyl function of the cyclopentenone ring (pathway III) to form aflatoxin Q_1 was recently discovered in monkey liver preparations (Masri et al., 1974) and represents the major *in vitro* conversion by human liver microsomes (Büchi et al., 1974). This pathway seems to be of only minor importance in rodent and bird liver, and free aflatoxin Q_1 has not been found in tissues or excreta of any animal exposed to B_1 *in vivo*.

Aflatoxin P_1, a phenolic derivative, is produced by *O*-demethylation of B_1 (pathway IV). Although this metabolite is a major excretory product in monkeys (Dalezios et al., 1971), the free phenol is only a minor *in vitro* metabolite of liver microsomes of monkeys, mice, and rabbits, and is apparently not formed by other species *in vitro*.

A further pathway leading to a hydroxylated derivative is the hydration of the 2,3 vinyl ether double bond producing the hemiacetal called B_{2a} (pathway I). This transformation is accomplished readily by liver microsomes of the rabbit, guinea pig, mouse, chick, and duck, but much less efficiently by the rat (Patterson, 1973). Nonenzymatic addition of water also occurs readily under strongly acidic conditions.

All of the preceding metabolic transformations have been demonstrated with crude and purified microsomal preparations. An additional conversion leading to a hydroxylated derivative involving an $NADPH_2$-dependent soluble enzyme is the reduction of the cyclopentenone function of aflatoxin B_1 to produce the cyclopentenol called R_0 (or aflatoxicol). This pathway (V) is especially prominent in the livers of rabbits and several avian species, and the reaction is blocked by 17-ketosteroid sex hormones, suggesting that a soluble $NADPH_2$-linked 17-hydroxysteroid dehydrogenase may be involved (Patterson, 1973).

It must be emphasized that current knowledge about aflatoxin metabolism is very incomplete. All of the available information on the relative importance of known pathways is at best semiquantitative in character. This is true because only unconjugated metabolites extractable from excreta or incubation media by organic solvents have thus far been identified. Whenever quantitative experiments using radioactive toxin have been done, permitting accurate monitoring of all substrate and product fractions, it has been found that significant portions, often a majority, of metabolites are not recovered by solvent extraction and thus remain unidentified. These undoubtedly include, among other possible derivatives, conjugates of known metabolites; all such components will remain unidentified until methods are developed for their isolation.

Recent evidence for an additional pathway (VI) seems particularly important to the question of metabolic activation of aflatoxin B_1. Rodent liver microsomes convert the toxin to its reactive 2,3 oxide, which has been trapped as an RNA adduct (Garner, 1973). This system generates a product lethal and mutagenic to bacteria through the production of an electrophilic derivative that reacts with cellular nucleophiles. Although the epoxide itself has not yet been isolated because of its great reactivity, a more stable model compound, aflatoxin B_1 2,3-dichloride has been synthesized (Swenson et al., 1977). This electrophilic analog of the epoxide is more potent than the parent toxin in several biological and chemical assay systems. Thus it seems likely that the epoxidation pathway may represent an important activation step in aflatoxin metabolism. Further indication of the importance of epoxidation of aflatoxin B_1 as an activation reaction is provided by recent experiments which show that aflatoxin B_2, a very much less potent liver carcinogen than B_1, is apparently carcinogenic only after conversion to B_1 as shown in Fig. 1.

Aflatoxins and liver cancer in humans. Aflatoxins are among the few chemically identified and widely disseminated environmental carcinogens for which quantitative estimates of human exposure have been systematically sought. Despite the fact that significant differences in responsiveness are known to exist among animal species, it is reasonable to assume that humans might respond to either acute or chronic effects of the toxins in the event that exposure takes place through contamination of dietary components. It also seems reasonable to assume that the character and intensity of the human response might vary, depending on factors such as age, sex, nutritional status, concurrent exposure to other agents (e.g., herbal medicines), genetic factors, concurrent illness (e.g., viral hepatitis or parasitic infestation), as well as level and duration of exposure to aflatoxins.

As information has accumulated on various aspects of the aflatoxin problem, it has become apparent that the risk of exposure to aflatoxins is much less in technologically developed countries than in developing areas. The lower risk is attributable to the combined effects of several factors contributing to prevention of contamination of foods or food raw materials. The use of such agricultural practices as rapid postharvest drying of crops and controlled storage conditions tends to reduce mold damage in general and thereby also reduce the likelihood of aflatoxin contamination.

In societies not equipped technologically to apply such practices, the risk of aflatoxin exposure is clearly much greater. Since the discovery of aflatoxins, reports have occasionally been made of their identification in many kinds of human foods collected in various parts of the world. Although these findings indicated the widespread geographic nature of the problem, they provided little useful information on human exposure, since samples were randomly collected and it was unknown whether they would actually have been eaten.

Information has recently become available from studies carried out by several groups of investigators in different countries of Africa and Asia. All of these investigations were designed to obtain estimates of aflatoxin intake by populations in which primary carcinoma of the liver occurs at different incidences.

Summary data from four such studies are presented in Table 4, which contains information on aflatoxin ingestion and liver cancer incidence, arranged in order of increasing values for each parameter. It can be seen that aflatoxin ingestion varied over a range of values from 3-5 to 222 ng/kg body weight per day. Estimated liver cancer incidence values extended from a minimum of 2.0 to a maximum of 35.0 cases per 100,000 people per year. There was a positive association between the two parameters, in that high intake values were consistently associated with high incidence rates. The association was most apparent in connection with incidence rates for adult men; larger numbers of cases were involved, so that more precise estimates of disease incidence were obtained.

Taken together, these data provide strong circumstantial evidence of a

TABLE 4 Summary of Current Evidence on Aflatoxin Ingestion
and Liver Cancer Incidence

Population	Dietary aflatoxin intake (ng/kg/day)	Liver cancer[a]					
		In adults (>15 yr)				In total population (both sexes)	
		Men		Women			
		No.[b]	Incidence[c]	No.	Incidence	No.	Incidence
Kenya (high altitude)	3–5	1	3.1	0	0		
Thailand (Songkhla)	5–8	–	–	–	–	2	2.0
Swaziland (highveld)	5–9	9	7.1	2	1.4		
Kenya (medium altitude)	6–8	13	10.8	6	3.3		
Kenya (low altitude)	10–15	16	12.9	9	5.4		
Swaziland (middleveld)	8–15	24	14.8	5	2.2		
Swaziland (Lebombo)	15–20	4	18.7	0	0		
Thailand (Ratburi)	45–77	–	–	–	–	6	6.0
Swaziland (lowveld)	43–54	35	26.7	7	5.6		
Mozambique	222	–	35.0	–	15.7	–	25.4

[a]Periods covered were 1 yr in Thailand, 3 yr in Mozambique, and 4 yr each in Kenya and Swaziland.
[b]Number of cases in study population.
[c]Number of cases per 100,000 population per year.

causal relationship between aflatoxin ingestion and liver cancer incidence in humans. Although this evidence cannot be regarded as proof that aflatoxins are the single cause of liver cell carcinoma in humans, the data are sufficient to indicate that exposure to the carcinogen elevates the incidence of this form of cancer; therefore continued investigations should be made to find effective means for monitoring and control of the occurrence of aflatoxins as food contaminants.

Other Mycotoxins

Sterigmatocystin and derivatives. Sterigmatocystin is a toxic metabolite that has been isolated from cultures of *Aspergillus versicolor, A. Nidulans,* and a *Bipolaris* species (Holzapfel et al., 1966). These organisms were identified in a survey of cereal and legume crops of South Africa for toxin-producing molds. Sterigmatocystin proved to be the principal toxic substance produced by these fungi when toxicity was evaluted by feeding to ducklings. Two derivatives, *O*-demethylsterigmatocystin and aspertoxin, were isolated from aflatoxin-producing cultures of *A. flavus* (Burkhardt and Forgacs, 1968; Rodricks, 1969). These compounds have certain features in common with the aflatoxins, in that the two groups of compounds are among only a small number of naturally occurring oxygen heterocycles that contain the unusual 7,8-dihydrofuro[2,3-6] furan configuration. Aspertoxin carries an OH function on the dihydrofurofuran ring system, and in this respect is similar to aflatoxin M_1.

The toxicity of these compounds has not been extensively studied, but enough information is available to indicate that they could be of significance if they occur as food contaminants. The acute toxicity of sterigmatocystin to rats has been reported (Holzapfel et al., 1966; Purchase and van der Watt, 1968). When sterigmatocystin was given by the oral route, the LD_{50} value was 120-166 mg/kg, while intraperitoneal dosing caused greater toxicity (LD_{50}= 60-65 mg/kg). Liver necrosis was a prominent postmortem finding, with the site of necrotic development differing according to route of administration. Oral dosing resulted in a centrilobular distribution, and intraperitoneal dosing produced periportal necrosis. Severe necrosis of the renal tubules and glomeruli was also observed at high dose levels.

Two lines of evidence demonstrate that sterigmatocystin is carcinogenic to rats. Dickens et al. (1966) found that repeated subcutaneous injection of sterigmatocystin to rats resulted in formation of sarcomas at the injection sites. Subsequently, Purchase and van der Watt (1968 and 1970) showed that oral administration to rats caused hepatocellular carcinomas in a large proportion of survivors. The compound was administered by gavage or by feeding for 52 wk. A high incidence of hepatocellular carcinomas was observed in rats surviving a dose of 1.5-2.25 mg/day, and fibrosis was also present in practically all cases.

No evidence is available on the toxicity of O-methylsterigmatocystin or aspertoxin in mammals, but both compounds are toxic in other bioassay systems (Rodricks, 1969).

Luteoskyrin and cyclochlorotine. Luteoskyrin and cyclochlorotine are hepatotoxic metabolites of *Penicillium islandicum* (Sopp), an organism frequently associated with spoilage of rice. Investigations of this mold and its products were stimulated by experimental findings that cultures of it induce acute and chronic liver damage when fed to animals and by the high incidence of liver diseases, including liver carcinoma, in Asian populations for whom rice is a major dietary component (Uraguchi et al., 1961). Studies of various aspects of the pathology, chemistry, and toxicology of these mycotoxins have been in progress for the past decade (Miyake and Saito, 1965).

Following preliminary observations of hepatotoxicity of rice contaminated with *P. islandicum*, systematic studies were conducted in which rats were fed cultures of the organism (Kobayashi et al., 1959). Continuous feeding for up to 620 days caused fibrosis, bile ductule hyperplasia, and parenchymal cell hyperplasia. Similar observations were made after chronic feeding to mice (Miyake et al., 1960). Definitive association of hepatotoxicity with fungal metabolites was later provided by feeding cultures grown on synthetic medium; mice and rats fed the fungal mats of such cultures developed toxic liver injuries, including acute atrophy, cirrhosis, and hepatoma formation. Integration of chemical techniques and toxicological approaches resulted in the isolation and purification of two major toxic products, luteoskyrin and cyclo-chlorotine. The chronic toxicity and carcinogenicity of the purified myco-toxins was investigated in mice (Uraguchi et al., 1972).

Cyclochlorotine is a cyclic peptide that acts rapidly in causing death of experimental animals; the oral LD_{50} in mice is 6.5 mg/kg. A prominent fea-ture of histopathologic lesions is severe hemorrhagic necrosis of the liver. Chronic administration results in the induction of cirrhosis. The mechanism of action has not been extensively investigated, but removal of the chlorine atoms from the molecule is said to render the compound nontoxic.

More extensive investigations have been conducted into various bio-logical and biochemical properties of luteoskyrin (Enomoto and Ueno, 1974).

This compound is a lipid-soluble pigment that is slow-acting with respect to its induction of liver damage. Its oral LD_{50} in mice is 211 mg/kg. Acute liver injuries of mice and rats surviving a single dose for more than 24 hr include centrilobular necrosis and lipid accumulation. Electron microscopy re-veals mitochondrial damage and cystic dilation of the endoplasmic reticulum. Chronic administration induces periportal fibrosis and a low incidence of nodular hyperplasia. Acute necrotic lesions were induced in the livers of mice fed a semi-synthetic diet deficient in protein and containing 50 ppm luteoskyrin.

Further biochemical investigation has revealed that luteoskyrin impairs mitochondrial structure and function in rat liver. Oxygen uptake and activity of several enzymes involved in oxidative metabolism in rat liver, kidney, and heart homogenates were inhibited by the toxin. Luteoskyrin binds to calf thymus DNA in the presence of Mg^{++}, and also binds with the DNA portion of deoxyribonucleohistone. The DNA-dependent RNA polymerase activity of Ehrlich ascites cells is inhibited by the pigment, presumably as a result of its binding properties. Luteoskyrin is also inhibitory to cell division of the pro-tozoan *Tetrahymena pyriformis.*

These findings indicate that luteoskyrin has a rather wide range of bio-chemical properties, including the ability to interfere with important me-tabolic pathways in liver. The observed changes in function following acute exposure are thought to be associated with the toxicity of this substance to liver cells. As regards its carcinogenic properties, luteoskyrin is carcinogenic in mice, the only species in which adequate investigations have been conducted. Feeding of diets containing the purified compounds at levels such that the daily intake of toxin was 50–500 µg per animal resulted in the induction of liver cell adenomas and carcinomas, as well as hepatic reticuloendotheliomas.

Luteoskyrin and cyclochlorotine are produced in culture by *P. islandicum* (Sopp). Although there are no data based on direct chemical anal-ysis concerning the occurrence of these two mycotoxins in human foods, the toxin-producing fungus has been reported as one of the major isolates from various grains in Japan and Africa, and as a prevalent infection of prepared foods in South Africa. In those areas, exposure to the mycotoxins might therefore occur, but there is no basis on which to estimate levels of intake.

Other fungal metabolites. The search for carcinogenic substances among the metabolic products of fungi has received great impetus from the development of information about aflatoxins, sterigmatocystin, and other mycotoxins of known structure that have been established as carcinogens. One line of endeavor currently being followed involves attempts to identify the toxic agents produced by fungi incriminated in outbreaks of moldy food poisoning of poultry or livestock. One such approach involves studies on *Penicillium viridicatum*, an organism frequently isolated from grain that is toxic to swine and other animals. Various isolates of the organism are known to be capable of producing one or more known mycotoxins, including ochratoxins, citrinin, oxalic acid, and penicillic acid, as well as hepatorenal and photosensitizing toxins of unknown structure (Ciegler et al., 1973). Current research activities include attempts to characterize the toxic responses to culture extracts (McCracken et al., 1974a, 1974b, 1974c), to optimize toxin production (Budiarso et al., 1971), and to identify new mycotoxins (Hutchison et al., 1973; Wilson et al., 1973). One recent report (Zwicker et al., 1973) suggests that some component of culture extracts of *P. viridicatum* may be carcinogenic to mice on prolonged feeding, but the active components have not been identified.

Fungi pathogenic for humans (dermatophytes) have also been examined for possible production of carcinogenic metabolites. Methanolic extracts of *Candida parapsilosis* induced subcutaneous sarcomas in mice following multiple injection. Suggestive evidence of carcinogenicity was also obtained with lipid extracts of species of the genera *Microsporum, Trichophyton, Epidermophyton,* and *Scopulariopsis* (Blank et al., 1968). No attempts have been made to isolate the active materials.

Pyrrolizidine Alkaloids

Pyrrolizidine alkaloids occur in a large number of plants in the genus *Senecio,* and also in species of *Crotolaria, Amsinckia, Heliotropium, Echium,* and *Trichodesma* (Bull et al., 1968). Interest in the compounds was due initially to economic considerations, because of the toxicity of plants containing them to livestock and the consequent losses of animals grazing on pastures in which the toxic plants were present. Not all species of plants in these genera are toxic, and those that are owe their toxicity to the presence of certain pyrrolizidine alkaloids. Despite the fact that these groups of plants are not closely related phylogenetically, their toxic alkaloids all belong to a single chemical group containing the pyrrolizidine nucleus.

Two excellent reviews of the extensive literature on the chemistry and biological properties of these alkaloids have appeared. A monograph by Bull et al. (1968) covers the chemistry, pathogenicity, and other biological properties of the compounds, while a review by McLean (1970) deals with their general toxicology and biochemistry. The interested reader is referred to these publications for comprehensive coverage of the field. The present report considers only aspects pertinent to carcinogenesis together with relevant background information.

With respect to their chemical structures, the pyrrolizidine alkaloids all contain the pyrrolizidine nucleus. Bull et al. (1968) list 102 such compounds for which structural configurations have been established. Not all of these compounds are toxic. All of the toxic alkaloids are ester derivatives of 1-hydroxymethyl-1:2-dehydropyrrolizidine, and structural requirements for toxicity can be summarized as follows: the ring nucleus must be unsaturated in the 1:2 position, the nucleus must be esterified, and one of the ester side chains must contain a branched chain. Although the toxic pyrrolizidine alkaloids are chemically rather stable compounds, they are known to undergo several kinds of metabolic transformation in animal tissues. Important among these are the formation of *N*-oxides; hydrolysis of the ester linkages and conjugation reactions are also known to occur.

A further metabolic change has been proposed as a possible activation mechanism in the formation of a proximate toxin. Current evidence suggests that some or all of the cytotoxic effects of the unsaturated pyrrolizidine alkaloids are caused by pyrrolic metabolites formed by enzymatic dehydrogenation of the alkaloids in liver (Mattocks, 1968). Compared with the parent alkaloids, these metabolites are highly reactive alkylating agents, and react chemically with tissue constituents. Saturated alkaloids that are not hepatotoxic to rats are metabolized to pyrrole-like derivatives that are different from the metabolites of toxic alkaloids. According to the present hypothesis, two requirements must be met for a pyrrolizidine alkaloid to be cytotoxic. First, it must be metabolized *in vivo* to a pyrrole derivative without the loss of its ester groups. Second, the resulting metabolite must possess the structural features required for it to be a chemically reactive alkylating agent. The type of toxic action produced under such circumstances would be determined by the reactivities and number of alkylating centers in the metabolite.

With respect to their various biological properties, the pyrrolizidine alkaloids have been investigated in many different test systems, and some generalizations seem justified for purposes of the present discussion. In field cases of poisoning of domestic animals, a variety of syndromes have been observed. Under various circumstances the prominent features of these have included acute and chronic liver damage, lung damage, neurological symptoms, and a hemolytic syndrome. The kind of syndrome that develops depends on the species of animal, type of plant consumed, total amount of alkaloid consumed, and pattern of consumption.

In experimental studies, the pattern of toxicity depends mainly on the dose of alkaloid employed. Single high doses cause acute liver necrosis, while smaller doses give rise to a chronic liver lesion characterized by megalocytosis, which progresses long after dosing has been discontinued; smaller doses also cause progressive lung damage. Young animals are more susceptible than adults to the chronic liver effects.

Until recently, there has been disagreement about the carcinogenic activity of pyrrolizidine alkaloids. McLean (1970) tabulated published reports of liver tumors following administration of several alkaloid preparations to rats and chickens. The following points emerge from a consideration of those data. Positive findings (i.e., induction of hepatomas) were reported in animals dosed with retrorsine, isatidine (retrorsine N-oxide), monocrotaline, seneciphylline, and mixed alkaloids of *Senecio jacobea*. Retrorsine and isatidine appeared to be carcinogenic in those experiments. In a total of 201 animals surviving various dosing regimens, hepatomas were reported in 53 (25%). Only two of these were reported to be metastasizing liver tumors. A total of 11 animals (5%) had "other tumors."

McLean (1970) summarized evidence suggesting that pyrrolizidine alkaloids are *not* carcinogenic in three categories. First, in extensive studies on rats, Bull et al. (1968) found no evidence of carcinogenic activity of alkaloids from *Heliotropium* or *Crotalaria*. Second, in the numerous reports of poisoning by pyrrolizidine in domestic animals, there has been no indication of tumor induction. Similarly, despite evidence of acute poisoning of humans (e.g., in Jamaica), elevated liver cancer incidence has not been observed in the affected populations. A third consideration is lack of agreement among pathologists in distinguishing regenerative liver nodules from hepatomas and the resulting uncertainty with respect to the nodular lesions seen in chronic alkaloid poisoning.

Two recent studies have produced more definitive information on the carcinogenicity of compounds in this class. Svoboda and Reddy (1972) found that repeated intraperitoneal injection of lasiocarpine into rats resulted in the induction of malignant tumors in several tissues, including the liver. The liver tumors were successfully transplanted through five generations of rats. In experiments on monocrotaline, Newberne and Rogers (1973) found that liver cell carcinomas were produced in rats by multiple administration of the alkaloid by stomach tube. The carcinogenicity of the compound was enhanced by feeding a diet marginally deficient in lipotropic agents.

Thus, to date, four pure alkaloids (retrorsine, isatidine, lasiocarpine, and monocrotaline) have been found carcinogenic in rats, but adequate tests are not available for other members of this class. Some plant materials known to contain pyrrolizidine alkaloids, the identities of which are unknown or only partially established, have also been shown to be carcinogenic in experimental animals. On the present evidence, therefore, it seems justified to undertake further tests on untested alkaloids to which humans may possibly be exposed.

Bracken Fern

Bracken fern, *Pteridium aquilinium*, is distributed throughout the world. It has been known for a long time that it is poisonous to livestock, particularly to cattle (Kingsbury, 1964). Two quite different toxicity syndromes can result from ingestion of fresh or dried bracken. One is clearly attributable to the presence of a thiaminase in the plant, and it can effectively be reversed or prevented by adequate replacement of the vitamin. The second, occurring mainly in cattle and sheep grazing on bracken, comprises a syndrome whose main symptoms resemble those caused by ionizing radiation or by radiomimetic chemicals. The characteristics of the latter syndrome and attempts to identify the active agents have recently been reviewed (Evans, 1968, 1970). Indications that bracken fern also contains carcinogenic substances have been provided through chronic feeding studies, which are discussed below.

The components of bracken responsible for its radiomimetic and carcinogenic properties have not yet been chemically identified. It has not been rigorously proved that the same substances are responsible for these two properties, but attempts at isolation of active materials have strengthened the assumption that this is true. The present state of knowledge concerning the chemistry of the active material was summarized as follows by Leach et al. (1971).

Isolation of the radiomimetic component has been hampered by lack of a convenient bioassay system and by instability of the substance. A material that is mutagenic, carcinogenic, and acutely lethal to mice was extractable with hot ethanol. Subsequent purification procedures yielded a chromatographically homogeneous substance that is carcinogenic and toxic. Mass spectrometric data indicate a molecular weight of 156 and an empirical formula of $C_7H_8O_4$. The substance is nonaromatic and highly unstable with respect to its biological activity, and its chemical reactivity suggests the possible presence of a lactone in the molecular structure.

Published information on the carcinogenic properties of bracken fern has mainly derived from studies on fresh or dried plants or plant extracts, and little work has been done with highly purified material. Consequently, it is impossible to estimate accurately the potency of the active component.

Several general observations are warranted by the limited data available. Tumors induced in rats (Evans and Mason, 1965; Hirono et al., 1970; Pamukcu and Price, 1969; Pamukcu et al., 1970b; Schacham et al., 1970) and in Japanese quail (Evans, 1968) by chronic administration of the plant or ethanol extracts consist primarily of intestinal adenocarcinomas, mainly of the ileum, with relatively fewer papillomatous lesions or carcinomas of the urinary bladder. The induction of intestinal tumors is noteworthy in view of the rarity with which they occur spontaneously in rodents and the small number of chemical carcinogens that induce them experimentally. On the other hand, Swiss mice (Evans, 1968) respond to similar exposure by the development of lung adenomas, indicating a significant species difference in response.

The studies of Hirono et al. (1970) indicate that bracken prepared according to Japanese tradition—immersion in hot water—retains its carcinogenic properties for rats, although at an apparently reduced potency. The water used for processing was not carcinogenic under the conditions of the experiment.

Pamukcu et al. (1970b) reported that the incidence of urinary bladder tumors in rats fed bracken is increased by simultaneous administration of thiamine. Intestinal tumors appeared at a high incidence in bracken-treated rats whether or not thiamine was administered.

Published data also provide evidence relevant to the etiology of urinary bladder tumors in cattle. This disease, frequently observed in various parts of the world, has been associated epidemiologically with chronic bovine hematuria and also with the geographic distribution of bracken fern (Pamukcu, 1963). The fact that bracken contains a carcinogen for the urinary bladder of cattle is demonstrated by experiments in which a high incidence of bladder carcinomas and papillomatous lesions was induced after feeding for periods of 9 months to more than 4 yr (Pamukcu et al., 1967; Price and Pamukcu, 1968). Occurrence of tumors was invariably preceded by hematuria. The guinea pig responds to bracken feeding in the same way as cattle, developing both hematuria and bladder tumors (Evans, 1968). The relatively brief exposure and short latent period required for tumor production indicate a high sensitivity to the carcinogenic stimulus in these animals.

Pamukcu et al. (1966), in attempting to substantiate the association between consumption of bracken fern and the field syndrome in cattle, studied fractions of urine from cows fed the plant. They found evidence for the presence in urine of one or more substances that were carcinogenic when implanted as cholesterol pellets into the urinary bladders of mice. It was not established whether the active material was originally present in bracken or whether it was a metabolite produced in the animals. Using a similar assay technique, the same investigators later showed that active materials were also present in methanolic extracts of the plant (Pamukcu et al., 1970a).

The existence of carcinogenic substances in bracken fern, which is established by these experiments, has several public health implications. Human exposure to the substances could take place through several routes. Direct consumption of bracken by humans is known to occur in Japan (Hirono et al., 1970) as well as in other parts of the world. The implications of this fact are obvious, and the suggestion has been made that this practice might be associated with the relatively high incidence of stomach cancer in Japan and North Wales (Evans et al., 1971).

Indirect consumption might also occur. It has been established that the carcinogenic agent in bracken is readily transferred from mother to offspring in mice through placenta and milk (Evans et al., 1972). Passage of the toxic substance into milk of cattle fed the fern has also been demonstrated (Evans et al., 1972). These observations have important implications for humans, since they suggest the possibility of exposure through consumption of milk or possibly meat of animals grazing on bracken pastures. This kind of exposure could affect larger populations over longer periods than direct consumption, which is restricted to a brief period during which the tender fronds ("fiddle-heads") are available. The possibility that milk may become contaminated also has obvious importance with respect to early exposure of infants and children, for whom milk may represent a major portion of the diet.

Betel

Betel chewing is a long-established practice in Oriental countries. The chewing quids are composed mainly of betel nut and lime, with or without tobacco and spices. A possible link between betel chewing and cancer of the mouth has been suggested (Muir and Kirk, 1960). Although it is generally considered that betel and tobacco together are required for cancer induction, there is some evidence that tobacco alone may be sufficient to induce oral cancer (Friedell and Rosenthal, 1941).

Several experimental approaches have been employed in attempts to establish the carcinogenic properties of betel and to identify the active principles. One line of experimentation has been based on the hypothesis that alkaloids in the betel may be carcinogenic. The metabolism of two of these, arecoline and arecaidine, has been studied in the rat (Boyland and Nery, 1969). Both compounds were found to be converted into mercapturic acid derivatives and may therefore be considered to be biological alkylating agents.

Several attempts have been made to produce evidence of betel carcinogenicity in animal assays. In one such study, DMSO extracts of betel nuts induced tumors of the mucosa of the hamster cheek pouch when painted thrice weekly for 21 wk (Suri et al., 1971). A weak carcinogenic response was found in experiments in which betel quids containing tobacco were placed into surgically prepared cheek pouches in baboons at thrice weekly intervals for periods up to 42 months (Hamner, 1972). On the other hand, implantation of beeswax pellets containing various components of betel quids into hamster cheek pouches failed to induce tumors in another experiment (Dunham and Herrold, 1962).

Thus, the putative role of betel in the induction of oral cancer in humans suggested by epidemiologic evidence remains to be established experimentally.

Other Plant Carcinogens

Safrole and related compounds. Safrole (4-allyl-1,2-methylenedioxybenzene) is a component of many essential oils such as star anise oil, camphor oil, and sassafras oil. It also occurs in oil of mace, ginger, California bay laurel, and cinnamon leaf oil. Until recently, it was used as a flavoring agent in soft drinks and other food products. Its use for these purposes was discontinued after it was discovered that the compound has hepatocarcinogenic activity in rodents.

Toxicity and carcinogenesis evaluations have been conducted on safrole, and also on two structurally related compounds, isosafrole and dihydrosafrole. The three compounds have LD_{50} values in rats of 1950, 1340, and 2260 mg/kg, respectively. Chronic liver damage, including induction of liver adenomas, was observed in rats fed 0.1 or 1.0% safrole in diets deficient in riboflavin, tocopherol, and protein (Homburger et al., 1961). It was subsequently found that riboflavin deficiency intensified the hepatotoxicity of diets containing 1% safrole (Homburger et al., 1962). Carcinogenic properties of safrole were established by the induction of tumors in rats fed high levels of the compound for 2 yr. Animals fed 0.5% safrole developed malignant liver tumors at high incidence (14 of 50 animals), whereas lower levels (0.1%) induced benign tumors at lower incidence (Hagan et al., 1965; Long et al., 1963).

An interesting structure-activity pattern emerges from similar studies on dihydrosafrole and isosafrole. Isosafrole fed at 0.5% of the diet induced hepatocellular carcinomas in 3 of 50 rats, and is therefore a weaker hepatocarcinogen for the rat than safrole (Homburger and Boger, 1968). On the other hand, dihydrosafrole fed at 1.0% of the diet induced no liver tumors in rats, but did produce papillary epidermoid carcinomas of the esophagus at a 75% incidence; 50% of the tumors were judged to be malignant. The response was dose-related, since the compound at 0.5% induced esophageal tumors at 74% incidence (35% malignant), and 0.25% at 20% (5% malignant) (Long and Jenner, 1963).

Thus, in rats safrole and isosafrole appear to be hepatocarcinogens, but dihydrosafrole is carcinogenic for esophagus. The same pattern does not appear to hold for the mouse. In two inbred mouse strains, all three compounds induced hepatomas, and no esophageal tumors were reported (Innes et al., 1969). The three compounds were not of equal potency, however. When administered by stomach tube (464 mg/kg daily) for 4 wk, then in the diet (1,112 ppm) for 78 wk, safrole and dihydrosafrole induced hepatomas in 27 of 33 mice and 10 of 34 mice, respectively. Isosafrole administered at a lower dose (215 mg/kg, then 517 ppm) induced hepatomas in 6 of 34 mice.

It has been shown recently that subcutaneous injection of safrole into infant mice (on 1, 7, 14, and 21 days of age) induced hepatomas (58%) and pulmonary adenocarcinomas in survivors killed at 1 yr of age (Epstein et al., 1969).

Studies of the metabolism of safrole, isosafrole, and dihydrosafrole in the rat revealed that metabolites were excreted in bile and urine with a slow and prolonged excretion pattern. The compounds with unsaturated side chains were more readily modified chemically than dihydrosafrole. Although the active carcinogenic form of safrole has not been identified, 1'-hydroxysafrole has been identified as a new urinary metabolite in rats, and 1'-acetoxysafrole as a reactive derivative of the compound (Borchert et al., 1971).

Compounds active by parenteral routes. Many natural products have been reported to have carcinogenic properties on the basis of local tumor induction resulting from parenteral, usually subcutaneous, injection. Although most such evidence falls outside the purview of this review, some substances in this class deserve brief consideration.

Tannic acid is a powerful hepatotoxic agent when administered topically or by injection. In one set of experiments, about 56% of rats surviving tannic acid injection for longer than 100 days developed liver tumors. Moreover, simultaneous dosing with tannic acid and 2-acetylaminofluorene induced more liver tumors and a greater degree of malignancy than did the synthetic carcinogen alone (Mosonyi and Korpassy, 1953). Because commercial preparations of tannic acid, such as those used in these experiments, are poorly characterized mixtures of substances, it is not possible to identify the active components in such studies.

Other plant toxins. Petasites japonicus, a form of coltsfoot said to be used as an herbal remedy or food in Japan, was found to induce hemangioendothelial sarcomas of the liver and liver cell carcinomas when dried flower stalks of the plant were fed to rats for periods of 220 days (Hirono et al., 1973).

Fusel oil from potatoes, administered orally or subcutaneously to Wistar rats, resulted in extensive liver damage and papillomas and carcinomas of the esophagus and forestomach (Gibel et al., 1968).

SUMMARY

The geographical pathology of human cancers suggests the involvement of environmental carcinogenic factors. The number of possible carcinogens that might constitute the total carcinogenic burden is potentially quite large, and in many instances either the compounds themselves or precursors capable of forming them are widely distributed in the environment. Both factors create a large potential for exposure, which is probably long-term and low-level in character, which makes it particularly difficult to establish cause-and-effect relationships. Field epidemiology based on exposed populations is inherently limited in sensitivity because of the long latency period and low frequency of the disease in the general population. For these reasons, in making assessments of public health risks represented by carcinogens, heavy reliance must be placed on evidence of carcinogenicity in experimental animals coupled with estimates of the extent to which human populations are exposed to specific carcinogens.

On this basis, of the various chemical carcinogens known to induce cancer in experimental animals, the strongest evidence of involvement exists for the aflatoxins in the induction of liver cancer. Others possibly involved include sterigmatocystin and possibly other mycotoxins; certain pyrrolizidine alkaloids; cycasin and related glycosides; and carcinogenic nitrosamines or nitrosamides formed through the interaction of nitrite and nitrosatable substances in the environment. It is impossible to assess the importance of other known carcinogens, such as the chlorinated hydrocarbons, even though some of them are widely distributed in the environment. Although many other natural and synthetic liver carcinogens are known, there seems no reason to implicate them as etiologic agents in the absence of further evidence.

REFERENCES

Adamson, R. H., Correa, P. and Dalgard, D. W. 1973. *J. Natl. Cancer Inst.* 50:549–553.
Alpert, M. E., Hutt, M. S. R., Wogan, G. N. and Davidson, C. S. 1971. *Cancer* 28:253–260.
Bartsch, H. and Montesano, R. 1975. *Mutat. Res.* 32:93–113.
Bills, D. D., Hildrum, K. I., Scanlan, R. A. and Libbey, L. M. 1973. *J. Agric. Food Chem.* 21:876–877.
Blank, F., Chin, O., Just, G., Meranze, D. R., Shimkin, M. B. and Wieder, R. 1968. *Cancer Res.* 28:2276.
Borchert, P., Miller, E. C. and Miller, J. A. 1971. *Proc. Am. Assoc. Cancer Res.* 12:34.
Boyland, E. and Nery, R. 1969. *Biochem. J.* 113:123.
Büchi, G. H., Muller, P. M., Roebuck, B. D. and Wogan, G. N. 1974. *Res. Commun. Chem. Pathol. Pharmacol.* 8:585–592.
Budiarso, I. T., Carlton, W. W. and Tuite, J. 1971. *Toxicol. Appl. Pharmacol.* 20:194.
Bull, L. B., Culvenor, C. C. J. and Dick, A. T. 1968. In *Frontiers of biology*, eds. A. Neuberger and E. L. Tatum. New York: Wiley.
Burkhardt, H. J. and Forgacs, J. 1968. *Tetrahedron* 24:717–720.
Butler, W. H. 1969. In *Aflatoxin: Scientific background, control and implications*, ed. L. A. Goldblatt, pp. 223–236. New York: Academic Press.
Carnaghan, R. B. A. 1965. *Nature (Lond.)* 208:308.
Ciegler, A., Fennell, D. I., Sansing, G. A., Detroy, R. W. and Bennett, G. A. 1973. *Appl. Microbiol.* 26:271.
Dalezios, J. I., Wogan, G. N. and Weinrab, S. 1971. *Science* 171:584–585.
Detroy, R. W., Lillehoj, E. B. and Ciegler, A. 1971. In *Microbial Toxins*, eds. A. Ciegler, S. Kadis, and S. J. Ajl, vol. 6, pp. 4–178. New York: Academic Press.
Dickens, F., Jones, H. E. H. and Wayneforth, H. B. 1966. *Br. J. Cancer* 20:134–144.
Dunham, L. J. and Herrold, K. M. 1962. *J. Natl. Cancer Inst.* 29:1047.
Durham, W. F. and Williams, C. H. 1972. *Annu. Rev. Entomol.* 17:123–148.
Edwards, C. A. 1970. In *Persistent pesticides in the environment*. Cleveland, Ohio: CRC Press.
Enomoto, M. and Ueno, I. 1974. In *Mycotoxins*, ed. I. F. H. Purchase, pp. 302–326. Amsterdam: Elsevier.
Epstein, S. M., Bartus, B. and Farber, E. 1969. *Cancer Res.* 29:1045–1050.
Epstein, S. S., Fujii, K., Andrea, J. and Mantel, N. 1970. *Toxicol. Appl. Pharmacol.* 16:321–334.
Evans, I. A. 1968. *Cancer Res.* 28:2252.
Evans, I. A. 1970. Bracken fern toxin. *10th Int. Cancer Congr.*, Houston, Texas.
Evans, I. A. and Mason, J. 1965. *Nature (Lond.)* 208:913.
Evans, I. A., Widdop, B., Jones, R. S., Barber, G. D., Leach, H., Jones, D. L. and Mainwaring-Burton, R. 1971. *Biochem. J.* 124:28P.
Evans, I. A., Jones, R. S. and Mainwaring-Burton, R. 1972. *Nature (Lond.)* 237:107.
Fiddler, W., Piotrowski, E. G., Pensabene, J. W., Doerr, R. C. and Wasserman, A. E. 1972a. *J. Food. Sci.* 37:668–670.
Fiddler, W., Pensabene, J. W., Doerr, R. C. and Wasserman, A. E. 1972b. *Nature (Lond.)* 236:307.

Fishbein, L. 1974. *Annu. Rev. Pharmacol.* 14:139–156.
Friedell, H. L. and Rosenthal, L. M. 1941. *J. Am. Med. Assoc.* 116:2130.
Garner, R. C. 1973. *Chem. Biol. Interact.* 6:125–129.
Gibel, W. von, Wildner, G. P. and Lohs, K. 1968. *Arch. Geschwulstforsch.* 32:115.
Goldblatt, L. A. 1969. In *Aflatoxin: Scientific background, control and implications*, ed. L. A. Goldblatt. New York: Academic Press.
Gopalan, C., Tulpule, P. G. and Krishnamurthi, D. 1972. *Food Cosmet. Toxicol.* 10:519–521.
Hagan, E. C., Jenner, P. M., Jones, W. I., Fitzhugh, O., Long, E. L., Brouwer, J. G. and Webb, W. K. 1965. *Toxicol. Appl. Pharmacol.* 7:18–24.
Hamner, J. E. 1972. *Cancer* 30:1001.
Hawksworth, G. and Hill, M. J. 1971. *Br. J. Cancer* 25:520.
Heisler, E. C., Siciliano, J., Krulick, S., Porter, W. L. and White, J., Jr. 1973. *J. Agric. Food Chem.* 21:970–973.
Hirono, I., Shibuya, C., Fushimi, K. and Haga, M. 1970. *J. Natl. Cancer Inst.* 45:179.
Hirono, I., Shimizu, M., Fushimi, K., Mori, H. and Kato, K. 1973. *Gann* 64:527.
Holzapfel, C. W., Purchase, I. F. H., Steyn, P. S. and Gouws, L. 1966. *S. Afr. Med. J.* 40:1100–1101.
Homburger, F. and Boger, E. 1968. *Cancer Res.* 28:2372–2374.
Homburger, F., Kelley, T., Friedler, G. and Russfield, A. B. 1961. *Med. Exp.* 4:1–11.
Homburger, F., Kelley, T., Baker, T. R. and Russfield, A. B. 1962. *Arch. Pathol.* 73:118–125.
Hutchison, R. D., Steyn, P. S. and van Rensburg, S. J. 1973. *Toxicol. Appl. Pharmacol.* 24:507.
IARC Monographs on the Evaluation of Carcinogenic Risk of Chemicals to Man, vol. 1. 1972. Lyon, France: International Agency for Research on Cancer.
IARC Monographs on the Evaluation of Carcinogenic Risk of Chemicals to Man, vol. 5. 1974. Lyon, France: International Agency for Research on Cancer.
Innes, J. R. M., Ulland, B. M., Valerio, M. G., Petrucelli, L., Fishbein, L., Hart, E. R., Pallotta, A. J., Bates, R. R., Falk, H. L., Gart, J. J., Klein, M., Mitchell, I. and Peters, J. 1969. *J. Natl. Cancer. Inst.* 42:1101–1114.
Keen, P. and Martin, P. 1971. *Trop. Geogr. Med.* 23:44–53.
Kingsbury, J. M. 1964. In *Poisonous plants of the United States.* Englewood Cliffs, N.J.: Prentice-Hall.
Kobayashi, A. and Matsumoto, H. 1965. *Arch. Biochem. Biophys.* 110:373–380.
Kobayashi, Y., Uraguchi, K., Sakai, R., Tatsuno, T., Tsukioka, M., Noguchi, Y., Tsunoda, H., Miyake, M., Saito, M., Enomoto, M., Shikata, T. and Ishibo, T. 1959. *Proc. Jap. Acad.* 35:501–506.
Laqueur, G. L. and Spatz, M. 1968. *Cancer Res.* 28:2262–2267.
Laqueur, G. L., Michelsen, O., Whiting, M. G. and Kurland, L. T. 1963. *J. Natl. Cancer Inst.* 31:919–951.
Leach, H., Barber, G. D., Evans, I. A. and Evans, W. C. 1971. *Biochem. J.* 124:13P.
Lijinsky, W. and Epstein, S. S. 1968. *Nature (Lond.)* 225:21–23.
Lijinsky, W., Keefer, L., Conrad, E. and Van de Bogart, R. 1972b. *J. Natl. Cancer Inst.* 49:1239–1249.
Lin, J. J., Liu, C. and Svoboda, D. J. 1974. *Lab. Invest.* 30:267–278.

Long, E. L. and Jenner, P. M. 1963. *Fed. Proc.* 22:275.

Long, E. L., Nelson, A. A., Fitzhugh, O. G. and Hansen, W. H. 1963. *Arch. Pathol.* 75:595–604.

Madhavan, T. V. and Gopalan, C. 1968. *Arch. Pathol.* 85:133–137.

Magee, P. N. 1968. *Food Cosmet. Toxicol.* 9:491–503.

Magee, P. N. and Barnes, J. M. 1967. *Adv. Cancer Res.* 10:163–246.

Masri, M. S., Haddon, W. F., Lundin, R. E. and Hsieh, D. P. H. 1974. *Agric. Food Chem.* 22:512–515.

Matsumoto, H. and Strong, F. M. 1963. *Arch. Biochem. Biophys.* 101:299–310.

Mattocks, A. R. 1968. *Nature (Lond.)* 217:723–728.

McCracken, M. D., Carlton, W. W. and Tuite, J. 1974a. *Food Cosmet. Toxicol.* 12:79.

McCracken, M. D., Carlton, W. W. and Tuite, J. 1974b. *Food Cosmet. Toxicol.* 12:89.

McCracken, M. D., Carlton, W. W. and Tuite, J. 1974c. *Food Cosmet. Toxicol.* 12:99.

McLean, A. E. M. and Marshall, A. 1971. *Br. J. Exp. Pathol.* 52:322–329.

McLean, E. K. 1970. *Pharmacol. Rev.* 22:429–483.

Miyake, M. and Saito, M. 1965. In *Mycotoxins in foodstuffs*, ed. G. N. Wogan, pp. 133–146. Cambridge, Mass.: MIT Press.

Miyake, M., Saito, M., Enomoto, M., Shikata, T., Ishiko, T., Uraguchi, K., Sakai, F., Tatsuno, T., Tsukioka, M. and Sakai, Y. 1960. *Acta Pathol. Jap.* 10:75–123.

Mosonyi, M. and Korpassy, B. 1953. *Nature (Lond.)* 171:791.

Muir, C. S. and Kirk, R. 1960. *Br. J. Cancer* 14:44.

Newberne, P. M. and Rogers, A. E. 1973. In *Plant foods for man*, ed. P. M. Newberne, pp. 23–31.

Newberne, P. M. and Wogan, G. N. 1969. *Toxicol. Appl. Pharmacol.* 11:51A.

Newberne, P. M., Harrington, D. H. and Wogan, G. N. 1966. *Lab. Invest.* 15:962–969.

Oser, B. L. and Oser, M. 1962. *Toxicol. Appl. Pharmacol.* 4:70–77.

Pamukcu, A. M. 1963. *Ann. N.Y. Acad. Sci.* 108:938.

Pamukcu, A. M. and Price, J. M. 1969. *J. Natl. Cancer Inst.* 43:275.

Pamukcu, A. M., Olson, C. and Price, J. M. 1966. *Cancer Res.* 26:1745.

Pamukcu, A. M., Göksoy, S. K. and Price, J. M. 1967. *Cancer Res.* 27:917.

Pamukcu, A. M., Price, J. M. and Bryan, G. T. 1970a. *Cancer Res.* 30:902.

Pamukcu, A. M., Yalciner, S., Price, J. M. and Bryan, G. T. 1970b. *Cancer Res.* 30:2671.

Patterson, D. S. P. 1973. *Food Cosmet. Toxicol.* 11:287–294.

Payne, W. J. 1973. *Bacteriol. Rev.* 37:409–452.

Peers, F. G. and Linsell, C. A. 1973. *Br. J. Cancer* 27:473–484.

Peers, F. G., Gilman, G. A. and Linsell, C. A. 1976. *Int. J. Cancer* 17:167–176.

Phillips, W. E. 1968. *J. Agric. Food Chem.* 16:88–91.

Price, J. M. and Pamukcu, A. M. 1968. *Cancer Res.* 28:2247.

Purchase, I. F. H. and van der Watt, J. J. 1968. *Food Cosmet. Toxicol.* 6:555–556.

Purchase, I. F. H. and van der Watt, J. J. 1969. *Food Cosmet. Toxicol.* 7:135–139.

Purchase, I. F. H. and van der Watt, J. J. 1970. *Food Cosmet. Toxicol.* 8:289–295.

Reddy, J. K. and Svoboda, D. 1972. *Arch. Pathol.* 93:55–60.
Reddy, J. K., Svoboda, D. J. and Rao, M. S. 1976. *Cancer Res.* 36:151–160.
Rodricks, J. V. 1969. *J. Agric. Food Chem.* 17:457–461.
Rogers, A. E. and Newberne, P. M. 1969. *Cancer Res.* 29:1965–1972.
Rogers, A. E. and Newberne, P. M. 1971. *Nature (Lond.)* 229:62–63.
Sander, J. 1971. *Arzneim. Forsch.* 21:1572–1580; 1707–1713; 2034–2039.
Sato, S., Matsushima, T., Tanaka, N., Sagimura, T. and Takashima, F. 1973. *J. Natl. Cancer Inst.* 50:765–778.
Scanlan, R. A., Lohsen, S. M., Bills, D. D. and Libbey, L. M. 1974. *J. Agric. Food Chem.* 22:149–150.
Schacham, P., Philp, R. B. and Gowdey, C. N. 1970. *Am. J. Vet. Res.* 31:191.
Schmal, D. and Osswald, H. 1967. *Experientia* 23:497–513.
Schweinsberg, F. and Sander, J. 1972. *Hoppe Seylers Z. Physiol. Chem.* 353:1671–1676.
Sebranek, J. G., Cassens, R. G., Hoekstra, W. G., Winder, W. C., Podebradsky, E. V. and Kielsmeier, E. W. 1973. *J. Food Sci.* 38:1220–1223.
Sen, N. P., Smith, D. C. and Schwinghamer, L. 1969. *Food Cosmet. Toxicol.* 7:301–307.
Shank, R. C., Bhamarapravati, N., Gordon, J. E. and Wogan, G. N. 1972a. *Food Cosmet. Toxicol.* 10:171–179.
Shank, R. C., Gordon, J. E., Wogan, G. N., Nondasuta, A. and Subhamani, B. 1972b. *Food Cosmet. Toxicol.* 10:71–84.
Shank, R. C., Wogan, G. N., Gibson, J. B. and Nondasuta, A. 1972c. *Food Cosmet. Toxicol.* 10:61–69.
Shuval, H. I. and Gruener, N. 1972. *Am. J. Public Health* 62:1045–1051.
Sinnhuber, R. O. and Wales, J. H. 1974. *Fed. Proc.* 33:247.
Sinnhuber, R. O., Wales, J. H., Ayres, J. L., Engebrecht, R. H. and Amend, D. L. 1968. *J. Natl. Cancer Inst.* 41:711–718.
Spatz, M. 1964. *Fed. Proc.* 23:1384–1385.
Spatz, M. 1969. *Ann. N.Y. Acad. Sci.* 163:848–859.
Sternberg, S. S., Popper, H., Oser, B. L. and Oser, M. 1960. *Cancer* 13:780–786.
Suri, K., Goldman, H. M. and Wells, H. 1971. *Nature (Lond.)* 230:383.
Svoboda, D. J. and Reddy, J. K. 1972. *Cancer Res.* 32:908–912.
Svoboda, D., Grady, H. and Higginson, J. 1966. *Am. J. Pathol.* 49:1023–1051.
Swenson, D. H., Lin, J. K., Miller, E. C. and Miller, J. A. 1977. *Cancer Res.* 37:172–181.
Tannenbaum, S. R., Sinskey, A. J., Weisman, M. and Bishop, W. 1974. *J. Natl. Cancer Inst.* 53:79–84.
Tilak, T. B. G. 1975. *Food Cosmet. Toxicol.* 13:247–249.
Tomatis, L., Partensky, C. and Montesano, R. 1973. *Int. J. Cancer* 12:1–20.
Uraguchi, K., Sakai, F., Tsukioka, M., Noguchi, T., Tatsuno, T., Saito, M., Enomoto, M., Ishiko, T., Shikata, T. and Miyake, M. 1961. *Jap. J. Exp. Med.* 31:435–461.
Uraguchi, K., Saito, M., Noguchi, Y., Takahasi, K., Enomoto, M. and Tatsumo, T. 1972. *Food Cosmet. Toxicol.* 10:193–207.
van Rensburg, S. J., van der Watt, J. J., Purchase, I. F. H., Pereira Cautinho, L. and Markham, R. 1974. *S. Afr. Med. J.* 48:2508a–d.
Vesselinovich, S. D., Mihailovich, N., Wogan, G. N., Lombard, L. S. and Rao, K. V. N. 1972. *Cancer Res.* 32:2289–2291.
Wales, J. H. and Sinnhuber, R. O. 1972. *J. Natl. Cancer Inst.* 48:1529–1530.
Wilson, B. J., Yang, D. T. C. and Harris, T. M. 1973. *Appl. Microbiol.* 26:633.

Wogan, G. N. 1968. *Cancer Res.* 28:2282–2287.
Wogan, G. N. 1973. In *Methods in cancer research*, vol. 7, ed. H. Busch, pp. 309–344. New York: Academic Press.
Wogan, G. N. and Newberne, P. M. 1967. *Cancer Res.* 27:2370–2376.
Wogan, G. N., Paglialunga, S. and Newberne, P. M. 1974. *Food Cosmet. Toxicol.* 12:681–685.
Zwicker, G. M., Carlton, W. W. and Tuite, J. 1973. *Food Cosmet. Toxicol.* 11:989.

Chapter 9

EPIDEMIOLOGY OF AFLATOXIN CARCINOGENESIS

Ronald C. Shank

Department of Community and Environmental Medicine
Department of Medical Pharmacology and Therapeutics
College of Medicine
University of California, Irvine
Irvine, California

INTRODUCTION

The first species in which a chemical was shown to be carcinogenic was the human (Pott, 1775), and it was 140 yr later that chemical carcinogenesis was first demonstrated in experimental animals (Yamagiwa and Ichikawa, 1918). In most of the human cases, detection of the carcinogenicity of a compound was associated with occupational exposure where the population at risk was readily recognizable (chimney sweeps, dye workers, radium dial painters, asbestos mine workers, etc.). It was not until the association was made between cigarette smoking and lung cancer that a general population was recognized as being at risk. Another major event in the study of cancer has been the association of tumors in humans with exposure to a compound already known to be carcinogenic in experimental animals. In 1968 diethylstilbestrol was shown to induce testicular tumors in mice (Canter and Shimkin, 1968); in 1971 Greenwald et al. and in 1972 Herbst et al. associated treatment of pregnant women with diethylstilbestrol with the development of vaginal adenocarcinoma in their daughters when they reached the ages of 15-19 yr. In this case, the carcinogenicity of diethylstilbestrol in humans became evident after review of the medical histories of the cancer patients and their mothers.

As is shown in this chapter, there is strong epidemiological evidence to support the suggestion that the mold-derived toxins, aflatoxins, have a causal role in the development of liver cancer in human beings. What makes the studies discussed below unique is that they are the first apparently successful attempt to deliberately seek out a human response to a compound first proven to be highly carcinogenic to experimental animals. The aflatoxin story is important not only as an example of a quantitative study in cancer epidemiology but also as a possible turning point in cancer epidemiology, where investigators begin to anticipate cancer problems in human beings before they occur. Our knowledge of the carcinogenicity of a wide variety of chemicals can serve as an armamentarium to be used to prevent exposing humans to compounds suspected, on the basis of structure and animal testing, of being carcinogenic. Indeed, following the aflatoxin studies, one now sees efforts to determine whether N-nitroso compounds, well-established animal carcinogens, are responsible for human tumors (Sander, 1967; Lijinsky and Epstein, 1970; Migasena and Changbumrung, 1974; Weisburger and Raineri, 1975).

HISTORICAL BACKGROUND

Occurrence of Aflatoxins in the Environment

The aflatoxins were discovered in Brazilian peanut meal used as a protein supplement in poultry diets and associated with the deaths of more than 100,000 young turkeys in England in 1960 (Blount, 1961). At the same time, peanut meals from Uganda and Tanganyika were shown responsible for the acute deaths of ducklings in eastern Africa (Asplin and Carnaghan, 1961), and cottonseed meals were associated with trout hepatoma problems in California hatcheries (Wolf and Jackson, 1963). The large number of animals and the variety of species involved in these instances of oilseed toxicity served as a focus for research by highly competent investigators, many in England. No doubt the aflatoxin problem had been encountered several times long before 1960 (see Allcroft, 1969; Halver, 1969), but with the initiation of studies at the Central Veterinary Laboratory at Weybridge and the Tropical Products Institute in London in 1960, rapid progress was made, and within a year a mixture of the aflatoxins was isolated as toxic metabolites of a ubiquitous mold, *Aspergillus flavus* (Sargeant et al., 1961). LeBreton et al. (1962) and Salmon and Newberne (1963) reported the induction of liver cancer in rats fed diets containing peanut meal, and Barnes and Butler (1964) clearly demonstrated the carcinogenicity of purified aflatoxins. With the realization that the aflatoxins were possibly widespread contaminants of human food supply and the suggestion that they may be involved in human liver cancer (LeBreton et al., 1962; Oettlé, 1965), a worldwide study of aflatoxins and mycotoxins in general was begun.

Depending on harvesting practices and processing techniques, the aflatoxins can be sporadic, frequent, or almost constant contaminants of oilseeds (especially peanuts and cottonseed) and grains (especially corn). Sorghum and cassava are less frequent sources of the aflatoxins. Less obvious sources have been garlic, dried chili peppers, dried fish (Shank et al., 1972b), and cows' milk (Allcroft and Roberts, 1968; Jacobsen et al., 1971).

Geographic Distribution of Human Liver Cancer

For most of the world, primary liver cancer is an uncommon disease with an incidence of approximately two cases per year for a general population (male and female, all ages) of 100,000 (Doll et al., 1966; Segi and Kurihara, 1972). Among certain populations in Africa (Higginson and Oettlé, 1960; Oettlé, 1964; Prates and Torres, 1965), southern India and Japan (Berman, 1951; Stewart, 1965), and Southeast Asia (Yeh and Cowdry, 1954; Shanmugaratnam, 1956; Marsden, 1958; Bhamarapravati and Virranuvatti, 1966), the rate for liver cancer is unusually high. In most high-incidence areas agricultural practices in harvesting and storage of crops and climate are such as to favor mold growth and aflatoxin production (Geneva is an exception; Tuyns and Obradovic, 1975), and in 1965 Oettlé proposed a mycotoxin hypothesis to explain the etiology of primary cancer of the liver in Africa. Similar agricultural practices and climate occur in portions of South America, yet reports of high liver cancer rates have not been forthcoming; this apparent anomaly has not yet been explained.

In most of the world the sex ratio for primary liver cancer is between 1.0 and 1.5 to 1 (M:F) (Segi and Kurihara, 1972). In Uganda (Alpert et al, 1968) and Kenya (Peers and Linsell, 1973), the sex ratio is 3:1; in other areas where tumor incidence is high, the sex ratios are even greater: Singapore—3.5:1 (Simons et al., 1971); Swaziland—5:1 (Keen and Martin, 1971); Mozambique—5.4:1 (Prates and Torres, 1965); and Thailand—between 5 and 6 to 1 (Viranuvatti and Satapanakul, 1962; Shank et al., 1972d).

Not only is the sex ratio different in the high-incidence areas, but so is the age at which the tumors occur. Liver cancer rates peak between the ages of 35–45 yr in Uganda (Alpert et al., 1968) and Mozambique (Prates and Torres, 1965), 40–59 in Thailand (Viranuvatti and Satapanakul, 1962; Shank et al., 1972e), and 50–59 in Singapore (Simons et al., 1971). In countries where the incidence is low, age distributions show that cases in the young are rare and that the rate increases after the age of 45 yr and does not peak as it does in the high-incidence areas.

The above-cited studies in Africa and Asia have also demonstrated that the increase in liver tumor incidence in these areas represents an increase primarily in the hepatocellular carcinoma rate, although cholangiocarcinomas and mixed-cell tumors are also seen.

There has been much discussion on the role of cirrhosis in human liver cancer (see Higginson, 1963; Mori, 1967; Davies, 1973). It is often stated that 40, 60, or even 90% of all liver cancer in humans arises in cirrhotic livers, implying a causal relationship. In fact, considering all cases of cirrhosis, liver cancer is unusual. Hepatocarcinoma occurs in about 0.3% of the cirrhotic livers in Mexico (Lopez-Corella et al., 1968) and in about 2% of the cases in the United States (see Davies, 1973). In areas where liver cancer, but not necessarily cirrhosis, is more frequent, a higher proportion of cirrhotic livers develop carcinomas; thus about 20% of the cirrhosis cases in Uganda develop tumors (Alpert et al., 1969), 23% in Thailand (Bhamarapravati and Virranu-vatti, 1966), and 51% of the female and 62% of the male cirrhotics in Mozambique (Prates and Torres, 1965). These are associations with the post-necrotic, macronodular, multilobular type of cirrhosis and not with Laënnec's cirrhosis of the micronodular monolobular type. Cirrhosis seems to occur concomitantly with liver cancer and not necessarily as a precursor or causative factor in the etiology of human hepatoma.

Investigators have been searching for an environmental agent that could integrate the findings on cirrhosis and liver cancer. It was noted that liver cancer occurs with higher frequency where kwashiorkor (severe protein mal-nutrition) is prevalent (see Higginson, 1963). Uncomplicated kwashiorkor, however, does not lead to cirrhosis, even though cirrhosis is widespread in areas where kwashiorkor and liver cancer correlate well. Also, kwashiorkor occurs frequently in parts of Central America, but liver cancer apparently is rare.

Nutrition does have a significant effect on carcinogenesis, as discussed in the chapter by Mehlman in this volume. Especially pertinent are the studies of Newberne and Rogers, who have demonstrated that rats fed a diet marginally deficient in lipotropes and treated with aflatoxin B_1 develop hyperplastic nodules 1-2 days after toxin exposure and hepatocarcinomas in 6 months; animals fed a nutritionally adequate diet and treated with aflatoxin develop the nodules several weeks after exposure and tumors only after a year (Rogers and Newberne, 1971). The dietary deficiency results in fatty livers but not cirrhosis. A greater deficiency will result in cirrhosis but does not seem to potentiate aflatoxin carcinogenesis (Rogers and Newberne, 1969).

Parasitic diseases can lead to cirrhosis; schistosomiasis (bilharziasis) occurs at a high rate in Lorenzo Marques (Prates and Torres, 1965), and opisthorciasis is endemic in northeastern Thailand (Viranuvatti and Satapana-kul, 1962); in both these areas, hepatomas occur at increased rates. In Egypt, however, schistosomiasis is common but liver cancer is not; in western Africa (Mauritania and Senegal), liver cancer is not unusual but schistosomiasis is (Oettlé, 1964).

Viral hepatitis, especially after repeated attacks, can lead to liver cir-rhosis, and viral hepatitis is common in most liver cancer areas; thus, it is tempting to ascribe to viral hepatitis a causative role in liver cancer. The correlation does not withstand scrutiny, however, for areas high in viral hepatitis can be low in liver cancer and in some areas of mixed races where all are susceptible to the infection, only one race will demonstrate an increased liver cancer risk (see Higginson, 1963). Several reports demonstrate an in-creased frequency in the appearance of hepatitis-associated antigen in hepa-toma patients (Prince et al., 1970; Bagshawe et al., 1971; Tong et al., 1971; Vogel et al., 1972), but others do not (Smith and Blumberg, 1969; Wright et al., 1969; Simons et al., 1971; Welsh et al., 1972). It is unfortunate that apparently few have asked what proportion of a population with a history of viral hepatitis develops liver cancer and/or cirrhosis and compared the rate with that for a population free of viral hepatitis.

Plant toxins such as the pyrrolizidine alkaloids have been suggested (Schoental, 1968) as probable environmental agents responsible for human liver cancer, for these compounds are common in areas where liver cancer is shown to be carcinogenic (Svoboda and Reddy, 1972; Newberne and Rogers, 1973a); however, no one has yet been able to provide epidemiological evidence to support the hypothesis.

Reddy and Svoboda (1972) obtained liver tumors with concomitant postnecrotic cirrhosis with aflatoxin B_1 in rats treated with lasiocarpine, a pyrrolizidine alkaloid, which at the dose used did not by itself cause cirrhosis. However, the simultaneous development of cirrhosis did not affect the induction time or incidence of hepatomas caused by aflatoxin.

Sun et al. (1971) in a study of the effect of cirrhosis on aflatoxin carcinogenesis demonstrated that rats with antecedent CCl_4-induced postnecrotic cirrhosis developed more hepatomas in a shorter time than did rats with ethanol-induced fatty livers or normal rats, when treated with aflatoxin B_1; aflatoxin alone does not induce cirrhosis. They interpreted their results as suggesting that the regenerative liver cells in the cirrhotic nodules are more susceptible to the carcinogenic effects of the aflatoxin. The effect of cirrhosis may be more complex than stimulation of regeneration, as Rogers et al. (1971) have shown that partial hepatectomy is without effect on aflatoxin B_1 carcinogenesis in two strains of rat. Evidence continues to accumulate that indicates aflatoxin B_1 must be metabolized to the active carcinogenic form, probably an epoxide (Garner, 1973); it would be interesting to look at the effect cirrhosis has on hepatic activation of aflatoxin.

There is no reason why several of these factors, such as hepatitis, cirrhosis, and a toxin, cannot be required in concerted action to produce hepatocellular carcinomas. It could well be that a liver, stressed by an attack of viral hepatitis and a chronically poor diet, or by cirrhosis, or parasites, develops tumors in response to a toxic insult from an environmental agent such as aflatoxin, whereas without the precedent stress, exposure to the toxin may not be sufficient to cause tumors. The remainder of this chapter concentrates on evidence specifically concerning the possible role aflatoxins may have in human liver cancer.

FIELD ASSOCIATIONS FOR AFLATOXINS AND HUMAN LIVER CANCER

The epidemiological evidence pertaining to the association between aflatoxins and human liver cancer has recently been reviewed (Campbell and Stoloff, 1974; Shank, 1975a,b). All of the work has been done in Africa (Uganda, Swaziland, Kenya, and Mozambique) and Southeast Asia (the

Philippines and Thailand). These studies are discussed chronologically, with emphasis on the comparability of results from the various studies.

Uganda

The first major epidemiological study of the association between aflatoxins and human liver cancer took place in Uganda in 1966–1967 (Alpert et al., 1971). Climate is temperate in the mountains of the southwest, subtropical in the plains and marshes of the south, and arid in the northern semideserts; such variation provides a suitable field for study of the effects that differences in mold growth could have on human health.

From September 1966 to June 1967, samples of food from home granaries or local village markets were collected throughout Uganda by medical students on vacation leave and by staff on visits to district hospitals and dispensaries. The foods sampled were typical of those kept in storage or sold for human consumption. Samples were sealed and refrigerated until air freighted to the United States where they were analyzed by extraction and thin-layer chromatography for aflatoxins B_1, B_2, G_1, and G_2 (Eppley, 1966); identity of aflatoxins B_1 and G_1 were confirmed by derivatives formation according to Andrellos and Reid (1964).

Of the 480 food samples analyzed for aflatoxins, 142 (30%) were positive. The types of foods sampled and the aflatoxin concentrations reported are summarized in Table 1. Approximately 30% of the samples contained aflatoxins, most (61% of the contaminated samples) contained less than 100 μg total aflatoxins/kg sample. Peanuts accounted for 32% of the samples collected; 18% of the peanut samples were contaminated, and 8 of 27 (30%) contaminated peanut samples contained more than 1 mg total aflatoxins/kg. Of four contaminated samples of cassava, two contained more than 1 mg aflatoxins/kg. Beans (72%) were the most frequently contaminated commodity.

TABLE 1   Concentrations of Aflatoxins in Ugandan Foodstuffs[a]

| | | | Percent contaminated | | | |
| | | | Total aflatoxin concentration (μg/kg sample) | | | |
Foodstuff	No. assayed	No. contaminated	1–100	100–1000	> 1000	All
Beans, peas	83	49	67	22	10	59
Maize, peanuts	201	49	49	35	16	24
Cereal grains	162	40	75	15	15	25
Cassava	34	4	0	50	50	12
Total	480	142	61	25	15	30

[a]From Alpert et al. (1971).

Analysis of the geographic distribution of aflatoxin contamination in Uganda revealed that three districts had particularly high frequencies of contamination: Toro district (23 of 29 samples, or 79% contaminated); Masaka district (26 of 43 samples, 61%); and Karamoja (46 of 105 samples, 44%). In other districts the small number of samples examined prevented comparison.

The geographical distribution of liver cancer in Uganda was determined using the records of the Kampala Cancer Registry, Makerere University College Medical School biopsy service, and district hospitals over the period from 1964 to 1966. Of the total 403 cases collected, 310 were biopsy-proved cases of primary hepatic carcinoma and 93 were clinically diagnosed; other studies have shown that clinical diagnosis of hepatoma in Uganda is approximately 85% accurate (Davies and Owor, 1960; Alpert et al., 1969). These represent the total number of hepatoma cases diagnosed in all of Uganda (approximately 6 million tribal people) during the 3-yr survey; 48 of the patients were not Ugandan Africans.

For most of the tribes, the hepatoma incidence was between 1.0 and 2.7 cases/100,000 population (all ages, both sexes) per yr; the frequency of aflatoxin contamination varied between 10 and 23% (Table 2). The Hutu and Tutsi immigrants to Buganda Province had an incidence of 3.0 compared to 2.0 cases/100,000 per yr for a comparable indigenous population. Aflatoxin contamination of foodstuffs collected from this area of Uganda was at a frequency of about 29% (43 of 149 samples). In Karamoja District, where aflatoxins were found in 44% of 105 samples assayed for the Pokot (Suk) and Karamojang tribes, the incidence was 6.8 cases/100,000 per yr (a combination of 10.7/100,000 for the Pokot and 3.5/100,000 for the Karamojang; M. E. Alpert, personal communication, 1975). Most of the food samples from the Toro district came from the Bwamba tribespeople, who apparently prefer to let their food spoil before consumption. Aflatoxin contamination was high in these samples, but unfortunately most of these people lived outside Uganda in neighboring Congo. At the time of the study it was not possible to obtain liver cancer incidence figures from the Congo for the Bwamba people (Alpert et al., 1971; M. E. Alpert, personal communication, 1975). As summarized in Table 2, the results do support an association between aflatoxin contamination of foodstuffs and the distribution of human liver cancer.

Philippines

In 1967 Campbell and co-workers (Campbell and Salamat, 1971) began assaying Philippine food products for aflatoxins and found that the two largest sources of the toxin in the human dietary were peanut butter and maize. Almost all of 149 samples of peanut butter contained aflatoxins, one sample as much as 8600 μg/kg; the average contamination was 213 μg aflatoxin B_1/kg. Whole peanuts were slightly less contaminated; 80 of 100 samples contained aflatoxin B_1, with an average concentration of 98 μg/kg. Of

TABLE 2 Hepatoma Incidence and Aflatoxin Contamination in Uganda[a]

Area	Tribe	Hepatoma incidence	No. assayed	Percent contaminated	Total aflatoxin concentration (μg/kg sample)		
					1–100	100–1000	>1000
Toro	Bwamba	—	29	79	10	31	38
Karamoja	Pokot (Suk) and Karamojang	6.8[b]	105	44	24	15	5
Buganda	Buganda	2.0	149	29	23	4	1
	Immigrants	3.0					
West Nile	West Nile tribes	2.7	26	23	19	4	0
Acholi	Acholi	2.7	26	15	15	0	0
Busoga	Soga	2.4	39	10	5	5	0
Ankole	Ankole	1.4	37	11	11	0	0

[a]From Alpert et al. (1968, 1971).
[b]M. E. Alpert, personal communication, 1975.

98 maize samples 95 contained an average of 110 μg aflatoxin B_1/kg (Campbell and Stoloff, 1974).

The two largest sources of aflatoxin in the Philippine diet appear to be eaten by well-defined elements of the population (Campbell and Salamat, 1971). Peanut butter is consumed principally by children, and maize is limited chiefly to the people of the south central island of Cebu; rice, the staple of most of the Philippines, sampled in the raw state contained insignificant amounts of aflatoxins. These results suggest that the general population in the Philippines probably is not exposed to as much aflatoxin in the long-term daily diet as are the people of Uganda; if the association between aflatoxin and human liver cancer is real, then the hepatoma rates in the Philippines should be low. Unfortunately, liver cancer incidence has not been measured directly, but the rates reported by Campbell and Salawat (1971) are indeed low (range 0.15–1.17; whole country, 0.80).

Swaziland

Keen and Martin (1971) examined the possible association between aflatoxins and human liver cancer in Swaziland. A cancer registry was established in 1964 and the records from 1964 to 1968 listed 90 cases of primary liver cancer, 75 male and 15 female. This gave a crude annual rate of 8.6/100,000 males (all ages) and 1.6/100,000 females (all ages). It was also evident that Shangaan immigrants living in Swaziland were at a higher risk for hepatoma than were the Swazis. A geographical distribution for hepatoma incidence was also apparent.

Chemical analysis of peanuts revealed a geographical distribution for aflatoxins that correlated with hepatoma incidence (Table 3). Residents of the lowveld of Swaziland had a relative risk for primary cancer of the liver more than four times greater than for residents in the highveld. Geographical distribution for liver cancer within individual areas also agreed with frequency of aflatoxin contamination of peanuts. Tribal groups were interviewed regarding eating habits for peanuts. The Shangaans indicated that they ate more peanuts for longer periods and in a stored powder form more often than did the Swazis; the Shangaans have a higher liver cancer incidence. Swazis who

TABLE 3   Hepatoma Risk and Aflatoxin Contamination of Peanuts
in Swaziland[a]

Geographic area	No. liver cancer cases	Crude rate of hepatoma	Aflatoxin contamination of peanuts (%)
Lowveld	44	9.7	60
Middleveld	34	4.0	57
Highveld	11	2.2	20

[a]From Keen and Martin (1971).

develop liver cancer tend to live in areas with Shangaans, who apparently influence the eating habits of the Swazis; these Swazis eat peanuts more often than do Swazis living elsewhere.

Kenya

The Murang'a district of the central province of Kenya was the site of an extensive study of the geographical distributions of human hepatoma and aflatoxin consumption, not just aflatoxin contamination of foodstuffs (Peers and Linsell, 1973). The study was conducted as a check on feasibility, methodology, and general design; an unusually high incidence of liver cancer was not anticipated, and although peanuts are not a component of the diet, toxin contamination of the local foodstuffs was expected. The area offered three distinct terrains with a high-altitude area at 12,000 ft, a middle area of about 6000 ft, and a low area down to 3500 ft. Climates and crops varied with altitude, providing different diets for the three areas. The total population in the district was 344,854, with approximately 40,000 in the high-altitude area, 160,000 in the middle area, and 145,000 in the low area.

A dietary survey was conducted over a period of 21 months. The samples collected for aflatoxin analysis were of the main meal of the day; eight samples were collected from each of 16 locations ("cluster centers") in each of the three altitude areas, four times a year. In addition to the food sample, one sample of local beer from each cluster per survey was assayed for aflatoxins.

Of 808 diet samples from the high-altitude area assayed, almost 5% were contaminated with aflatoxin B_1; the mean concentration for all samples assayed was 0.121 μg aflatoxin B_1/kg wet diet. For the middle and low areas approximately 7 and 10% of the diet samples assayed were contaminated, with mean aflatoxin B_1 concentrations of 0.205 and 0.351 μg/kg, respectively. The frequency of aflatoxin contamination of local beers was approximately the same as observed for the diets in each of the three altitude areas, with mean aflatoxin B_1 concentrations of 0.050, 0.069, and 0.167 μg/l for the high, middle, and low areas, respectively.

These data were used to calculate the mean aflatoxin B_1 ingestion for the residents of the three areas, assuming the daily intake was 2 kg food/70 kg adult and, for the men only, an additional 2 liters of beer. These figures are given in Table 4 and indicate an aflatoxin consumption ratio of 1.0, 1.6, and 3.0 for men and 1.0, 1.7, and 2.9 for women in the high, middle, and low altitude areas.

Liver cancer incidences were calculated from cases occurring from 1967 to 1970 and obtained through the cancer registry. Criteria used to include cases were (1) histological confirmation, (2) positive α-fetoprotein test, or (3) clinical diagnosis followed by death within 6 months. The incidence rate for primary liver cancer in the three altitude areas is given in Table 4 and correlates well with aflatoxin ingestion.

TABLE 4   Aflatoxin Consumption and Hepatoma Incidence in Kenya[a]

| Altitude area | Average daily aflatoxin B_1 intake (ng/kg body weight) | | Hepatoma incidence | | | |
| | | | Cases/adult population[b] (1967-1970) | | Cases/100,000 adults/yr | |
	Male	Female	Male	Female	Male	Female
Low	14.81	10.03	16/30,949	9/41,375	12.92	5.44
Middle	7.84	5.86	13/30,105	6/45,693	10.80	3.28
High	4.88	3.46	1/8,027	0/10,885	3.11	(< 1/10,000/4 yr)

[a]From Peers and Linsell (1973).
[b]16 yr of age and older.

Peers and Linsell (1973) calculated a regression line for aflatoxin ingestion correlated with hepatoma incidence, combining the data for males and females; $y = 19.06 \log x - 10.16$, where y is the hepatoma incidence/100,000 adults per yr and x is the mean daily aflatoxin B_1 ingestion in ng/kg body weight. If these data are treated separately for males and females, which seems justified from (1) the high aflatoxin intake for males, (2) the apparent difference in slopes of the two regression lines, and (3) the apparent sex difference in primary liver cancer incidence in Africa and Asia, then the regression lines are $y = 20.83 \log x - 9.88$ for males and $y = 12.97 \log x - 7.73$ for females. The importance of these regression lines, if they represent a causal relationship, is that they show that human males respond to a given dose with a greater incidence of liver cancer than do females.

Thailand

A project was begun in the latter part of 1967 to examine the extent to which mycotoxins might be associated with human liver disease in Southeast Asia. Interest focused on Thailand because of reports of high frequencies of primary hepatomas among autopsies (Bhamarapravati and Virranuvatti, 1966) and because climate and agricultural practices appeared to permit extensive fungal invasion of foodstuffs.

The overall study was designed to be executed in three phases. The first phase was a market survey to determine (1) which molds frequently invade human foods and foodstuffs, (2) which mycotoxins are elaborated by these molds in the foodstuffs, (3) which food commodities are the major sources of the various mycotoxins, and (4) what the seasonal and geographical distributions of these mycotoxin contaminations are. This phase was conducted over a 23-month period, principally in Thailand and to a lesser extent in Hong Kong and Malaysia, with the collaboration of Dr. James B. Gibson of the University of Hong Kong and Dr. Y. H. Chong of the Institute for Medical Research in Kuala Lumpur. The climates and agricultural practices in Hong Kong and

Malaysia were similar to those in Thailand and these areas were included in the market survey, thus providing a larger base upon which an epidemiological survey could be established. The study in Malaysia was not extended beyond the initial exploratory phase as it was anticipated that there would be serious difficulty in obtaining histopathologic evidence of liver disease among the Muslim people. The market survey in Hong Kong was completed (Shank et al., 1972a, b).

Table 5 summarizes the results of the market survey for Thailand. As was seen in Uganda and many places elsewhere, peanuts and maize were the most frequently and most highly contaminated foodstuffs. Cereal grains, especially rice, however, were not seriously contaminated; this probably reflects better agricultural practices used for these commodities. Rice was stored in the husk and often showed signs of surface contamination by molds; the rice was milled shortly before use, however, and the polished grain seldom contained aflatoxins.

The second phase of the project was designed as a pilot study of the epidemiology of aflatoxin consumption and the incidence of human liver cancer. Based on the results of the market survey and a preliminary investigation of hospital records regarding cancer cases, it was decided to conduct the second phase wholly in Thailand. At the completion of the pilot study, it was decided that the third phase, a formal epidemiological study of the association between dietary aflatoxins and human liver cancer was not necessary, as reasonable evidence for an association had already been obtained in the pilot study; the considerable expense of a large-scale epidemiological study could not be justified.

The dietary survey (Shank et al., 1972c) in nine villages in central, western, and southern Thailand indicated that considerable amounts of aflatoxin were being consumed. Chemical analyses were done on plate samples collected from all meals for three 2-day periods over a period of 1 yr to cover all three seasons. Toxin intakes were calculated by multiplying the concentration of aflatoxins in the foods by the amounts of the foods eaten by the combined body weights of the household members who ate the contaminated

TABLE 5 Concentrations of Aflatoxins in Thai Foodstuffs[a]

Foodstuff	No. assayed	No. contaminated	Total aflatoxin concentration (μg/kg sample)	
			Mean (all samples)	Maximum
Peanuts, maize	278	46	614	12,256
Beans, peas	462	4	4	1,620
Cereal grains	408	3	< 1	248
Sago	65	3	5	294

[a]From Shank et al. (1972b).

TABLE 6   Aflatoxin Consumption and Hepatoma Incidence in Thailand[a]

Area	Average daily aflatoxin intake (ng/kg body weight)		Highest single-day intake (ng/kg body weight)	Liver cancer incidence (cases/100,000/yr)[b]
	B_1	Total	Total aflatoxins	
Singburi	51–55	73–81	13,082	–
Ratburi	31–48	45–77	3,224	6.0
Songkhla	(5–6)[c]	(5–8)[c]	(1,072)[c]	2.0

[a]From Shank et al. (1972c, d).
[b]General population, all ages.
[c]One woman consumed 1,072 ng aflatoxins/kg body weight in 1 day and 380 ng/kg the following day, greatly in excess of what any other members of the surveyed households in the entire Songkhla area consumed; exclusion of these particular intakes reduces the area average to nil.

foods, and average consumption was expressed as ng/kg body weight/day. As these intakes are calculated on a family basis, some individual intakes would be higher.

The average daily aflatoxin consumptions for the people of the three survey areas are given in Table 6. Variation within families over the three seasons and between families within any one season was great. The highest concentrations of aflatoxins in plate samples were found in Singburi in cabbage fried with pork and garlic (B_1, 748 μg/kg sample; total, 1299 μg/kg) and sun-dried fish (B_1, 679 μg/kg; total, 795 μg/kg food). Rice, the staple food of Thailand, was lightly contaminated (frequency of 1-3%) in Singburi and Songkhla but in Ratburi, 10% of the plate samples of rice contained aflatoxins. Maximum concentrations of total aflatoxin were 600 μg/kg sample in Singburi, 180 μg/kg in Ratburi, and 71 μg/kg in Songkhla. Clearly, rice served at meals is a greater source of aflatoxins than could be predicted on the basis of the market survey. Dried chili peppers and garlic often are contaminated with aflatoxins and are common ingredients in Thai cookery. Peanuts, frequently contaminated, were consumed sporadically as snacks, usually by children, and were often hand-sorted by the consumer immediately before ingestion, making estimation of aflatoxin intake from peanuts most difficult. Peanut consumption in Thailand probably produces a variation in aflatoxin intake on a baseline established by daily sources of the toxin.

While the dietary survey was in progress, the incidence of hepatoma in two of the same areas was measured directly. Physicians stationed in provincial hospitals in rural towns near the dietary survey villages obtained liver viscerotomy specimens from 21-33% of the persons aged 15 yr or more who lived and died in the defined populations (Shank et al., 1972d). Of the 97,867 residents (all ages) of the Songkhla study area, two residents (males aged 32 and 58 years) died with primary liver cancer within the 12-month study period. In the Ratburi study area, population 99,537 residents (all ages), six residents (5 males ages 41-88 yr and one female aged 68 yr) died with primary hepatomas in the same period.

The hepatoma incidence data are related to the aflatoxin consumption data in Table 6. Based on examination of hospital records for many years and interviews with local physicians, it was expected that the incidence of primary liver cancer in the Singburi area (where aflatoxin consumption was highest) would be one of the highest in the country. At the time the hepatoma survey was to begin in Songkhla, Ratburi, and Singburi, an epidemic of cholera broke out on the eastern border of Thailand, and the director of the major hospital in Singburi, an expert on cholera, was called upon by the government to go to the cholera area to aid in controlling the epidemic. This removed a key figure in the hepatoma survey of the Singburi area, and therefore the incidence of liver cancer in that area had to be measured indirectly, as the dividend of prevalence over duration. The prevalence study on almost 60,000 people in the Singburi area failed to detect any cases of primary liver cancer (Shank et al., 1972e), and it was regarded as necessary to have a study population some ten times greater to conduct a point prevalence study, a requirement that was logistically impractical to meet.

The conclusion of the overall study in Thailand was that presumptive epidemiological evidence was obtained supporting the hypothesis that aflatoxins played a role in the cause of liver cancer in the Thai population.

Mozambique

Mozambique has been reported to have the highest incidence of primary liver cancer in the world (Prates and Torres, 1965), and the obvious question is whether aflatoxin consumption in this area is also high. Van Rensburg et al. (1974) measured the extent of aflatoxin contamination of prepared food in the district of Inhambane, on the Channel coast between Lorenzo Marques and Beira. Chemical analyses of 880 meals indicated a mean total aflatoxin contamination of 7.8 μg/kg (wet weight) for all prepared food; from this a mean daily per capita consumption of 222.4 ng total aflatoxins/kg body weight was estimated.

The liver cancer incidence rate was determined from data obtained through health records from South African gold mines for workers originating from the Inhambane district. The hospital rate, based on 460 histologically confirmed cases but judged to be an underestimate, was 16 cases/100,000 per yr for the adult population. Adding the data from the miners' health records from 1969 to 1971, the incidence rate was calculated to be 25.4/100,000 per yr, with a sex ratio of 2.2 (M:F).

Only a few years ago Mozambique was regarded as somewhat of an anomaly in the aflatoxin hypothesis of human hepatocarcinogenesis. Early reports from Mozambique estimated the age-specific incidence rate of cancer of the liver and biliary passages in males to be almost 110/100,000 per yr and for females, 29/100,000 per yr (Prates and Torres, 1965). Such high rates would require unreasonably high levels of dietary contamination, making it difficult to see how aflatoxin consumption could have a causative role. For example, using the regression line of Peers and Linsell (1973), in order to observe an incidence rate of 110/100,000 men per yr, the aflatoxin intake would be expected to approach 2 mg/kg body weight per day, five orders of magnitude greater than was seen in Kenya and Thailand. The results of Van Rensburg et al. (1974) seem to dispel the anomaly and, in fact, are in good agreement with those from Kenya and Thailand.

Indeed, if the data correlating aflatoxin consumption with the geographical distribution of liver cancer incidence in Kenya, Mozambique, and Thailand are pooled, regression lines with high correlation coefficients can be determined separately for males and females, as shown in Fig. 1. Incidence of primary liver cancer for the three countries has been expressed as the number of cases observed per 100,000 individuals of all ages per year. The data from Kenya express aflatoxin consumption in terms of aflatoxin B_1, whereas the Mozambique data are in terms of total aflatoxins without indication of the proportions at which individual aflatoxins occured; Thailand data have been reported in terms of both aflatoxin B_1 and total aflatoxins. For Fig. 1

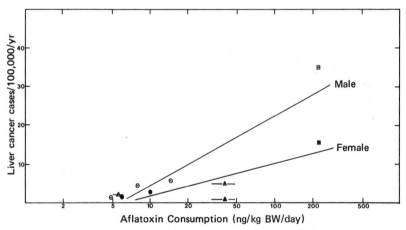

FIGURE 1 Correlation between incidence rate of primary liver cancer in Kenya, Mozambique, and Thailand and the consumption of aflatoxin. Regression lines were determined by the method of least squares from pooled data reported for Kenya (circles; Peers and Linsell, 1973), Mozambique (squares; Van Rensburg et al., 1974), and Thailand (triangles; Shank et al., 1972c, d), separately for males (open symbols) and females (closed symbols). Liver cancer incidence is expressed as the annual rate of cases per 100,000 males or females, all ages. Aflatoxin consumption is expressed as aflatoxin B_1 ingestion, except for Mozambique where "total aflatoxin" ingestion is used. The regression line for males is $y = 18.08 \log x - 13.51$, $r = 0.90$, $0.02 > p > 0.01$, and for females, $y = 8.61 \log x - 6.73$, $r = 0.87$, $0.05 > p > 0.02$.

aflatoxin consumptions have been expressed in terms of aflatoxin B_1 for Kenya and Thailand, but as total aflatoxins for Mozambique. As the B_1 form constitutes the major portion of total aflatoxins in most food samples, this probably introduces little error. In Kenya and Thailand no liver cancer cases were seen in three female subpopulations; these instances were not used as determinants in the regression analysis, as no cases seen in 100,000 persons in 1 yr is not 0/100,000 but rather, less than 1/100,000. The regression line for males, for the pooled data, is $y = 18.08 \log x - 13.51$, with a correlation coefficient of 0.90 for four degrees of freedom ($0.02 > p > 0.01$); for females the regression line is $y = 8.61 \log x - 6.73$, with a correlation coefficient of 0.87 for two degrees of freedom ($0.05 > p > 0.02$). It must be remembered, however, that the lines are only approximations and are valid only for the data used to derive them; one should be cautioned against extrapolating to the intercept of the abscissa to determine the amount of aflatoxin that could be consumed without producing tumors. There is no guarantee that the line remains linear for lower (or higher) exposures, and one must always distinguish between a zero incidence and an incidence that is less than 1 per population size.

SPECIAL PROBLEMS

Field Laboratory Assay for Aflatoxins

The importance of a well-equipped and well-staffed laboratory near the site of sample collection cannot be overemphasized. Such a laboratory is vital to the support of the epidemiological aspects of programs investigating environmental toxicants and human disease.

Many assay methods have been proposed for the aflatoxins. If the method is to be used continually for large numbers of samples in or near the field, then it must be simple, portable, and readily understandable to technicians. One such method is that proposed by Eppley (1966). It requires little equipment and it can be used with little modification on a wide variety of samples. The Eppley method was used in Thailand for the analysis of oilseeds, grains, sauces, fermented meats, dried fruits, cooked vegetables, soups, curry dishes, dried fish, cakes, oils, alcoholic beverages, and autopsy specimens (Shank et al., 1971a, 1972b,c). The equipment could be packed into a four-wheel drive vehicle and transported to remote clinics and dispensaries and the assays done literally at the site.

With most of the aflatoxin assay methods, it is often desirable, if not necessary, to confirm the identities of the compounds. Several chemical derivative methods are available for this (Andrellos and Reid, 1964; Pohland et al., 1970; Stack et al., 1972). Artifacts confounding the aflatoxin fluorescence-based assays abound in plant and animal products. Some artifacts occur naturally as a component of the product, such as the fluorescent artifacts in oats (Shotwell et al., 1968), sweet potatoes (Peers and Linsell, 1973), and human liver, urine, and feces (Shank et al., 1971a). Other metabolites of fungi, such as food-borne *Macrophomina phasioli* (Maubl) Ashby, falsely appear as aflatoxins in peanuts, maize, sunflower seed meal, cocoa, and cassava (Crowther, 1968). It was the experience of the team in Thailand that in over 10,000 aflatoxin assays, virtually all the artifacts could be detected as separate from true aflatoxins by performing thin-layer chromatography with three different solvent systems: 4–8% acetone in chloroform, 3% methanol in chloroform, and benzene-ethanol-water (46:35:19 v/v) (Shank et al., 1972b).

Interactions Affecting Aflatoxin Carcinogenesis

No one has yet reported data on what effect nutrition, infection, or cointoxication may have on the association between dietary aflatoxin and human liver cancer. In the section Geographic Distribution of Human Liver Cancer, various environmental agents other than the aflatoxins are discussed as possible factors in the etiology of liver cancer. While there may not be much support that these agents directly cause liver cancer, they may have profound effects on aflatoxin carcinogenesis. Rogers and Newberne (1971) halved hepatoma induction time by feeding aflatoxin-treated rats a diet marginally deficient in lipotropes. The same effect of diet has been shown on monocrotaline (a pyrrolizidine alkaloid) carcinogenesis (Newberne and Rogers, 1973a). Rats treated with aflatoxin B_1 and maintained on diets marginal in vitamin A content develop colon carcinomas as well as hepatocellular carcinomas (Newberne and Rogers, 1973b). These findings raise important questions. Are the diets in Uganda, Swaziland, Kenya, Mozambique, and Thailand nutritionally deficient in such ways as to potentiate the carcinogenicity of the aflatoxin in the food supplies? If people in Central and South America are exposed to high levels of aflatoxins but do not develop liver tumors (which has not been proven), could the explanation be found in nutritional differences in diets?

National vital statistics in Thailand indicated that the greatest frequency of liver cancer in that country occurred in the northeast. This was also the area where liver fluke infestation was endemic. Cholangiocellular carcinomas as well as hepatocellular carcinomas were often seen there where the majority of the adult population develops opisthorciasis. Studies on the effect of *Opisthorcis viverrini* on aflatoxin B_1 carcinogenesis in laboratory animals have recently begun in Thailand (T. Glinsukon, personal communication, 1975). Studies should also be carried out on the effect of viral hepatitis infections on laboratory animals given carcinogenic doses of aflatoxins.

Cointoxication is another area that needs investigation. It is reasonable that where conditions permit contamination of the human food supply by aflatoxin, other mycotoxins may also be present. Study of a sample of leftover cooked rice associated with the death of a young Thai boy (Bourgeois et al., 1971a) demonstrated that the rice was heavily contaminated with aflatoxins and three toxigenic molds in addition to *A. flavus*. One of these molds, *A. clavatus* (Glinsukon et al., 1974), was shown to produce the highly toxic mycotoxin, cytochalasin E (Büchi et al., 1973; Glinsukon et al., 1975a, b), and two quinazolone tremorgens (Clardy et al., 1975). How these myco-toxins affect the toxicity of aflatoxin B_1 is not known. Plant toxins, such as the pyrrolizidine alkaloids, may also be in the diet or used as herbal medi-cines. Recently, it was appreciated that various naturally occurring secondary and tertiary amines can undergo intragastric *N*-nitrosation in the presence of nitrite to form carcinogenic nitroso compounds (Sander, 1967); if this occurs where dietary aflatoxin concentrations are high, there may be a synergistic effect on tumor production. We tend to evaluate the risk of each environ-mental carcinogen individually when we, in our environment, undoubtedly encounter the compounds in multiple ways. All these problems need thorough examination.

Measuring Toxin Consumption

Market surveys are useful for establishing geographical and seasonal distributions for aflatoxin contamination of foodstuffs, but they should not be the sole basis for calculating the amounts of toxin consumed by people. The Thailand study provides a good example because both a market survey and a dietary (plate) survey were carried out. The market survey indicated that peanuts and maize were the most contaminated foodstuffs, and thus one might conclude that these products were the chief sources of the toxin in the diet; raw rice was virtually toxin-free. Maize is not a popular food item in Thailand and is thus only a minor source of aflatoxins in the diet. Peanuts are consumed as snacks and estimation of aflatoxin intake from peanuts is most difficult. Rice is often cooked in quantity and stored unrefrigerated until eaten and thus is a significant source of aflatoxin in the Thai diet, even though the market samples of rice were seldom contaminated with the toxin.

Dietary surveys are only second-best, however, for it is nearly impossible in a free population to measure all sources of the toxin at all times. It would be more desirable to measure the toxin or one of its metabolites in blood, urine, or feces. Campbell and co-workers (1970) were able to measure the urinary excretion of aflatoxin M_1, a B_1-hydroxylated derivative, in Philippine children unintentionally consuming contaminated peanut butter; their data suggest that aflatoxin M_1 could be detected in a 24-hr urine sample when children consumed 10–15 μg of aflatoxin B_1 in 24 hr. This is two orders of magnitude greater than the mean aflatoxin consumption levels measured in populations in Kenya and Thailand that demonstrated elevated hepatoma rates. Nevertheless, if methods with greater sensitivity for aflatoxin M_1, or perhaps methods for other metabolites, such as aflatoxin Q_1, produced by human liver (Büchi et al., 1974), can be achieved, this approach to measuring aflatoxin consumption may become practical.

The epidemiological studies discussed in this chapter were attempts to associate current rates of aflatoxin consumption with a chronic disease probably induced many years before becoming clinically detectable. Toxin consumption was measured in populations in which patients bearing hepatomas most likely experienced induction of the tumors well before consumption of aflatoxin was measured. Many of the hepatoma patients studied in the late 1960s (in Uganda, Kenya, and Thailand) were aged 45–50 yr; if the tumor induction period was 25–30 yr, the patients would have been in the early part of their third decade (aged 20–25 yr) when tumor induction began. This would have been in the early 1940s, the time of World War II. No answer has been found to the question of whether aflatoxin consumption today can be related to a like exposure 25–30 yr earlier, and it seems unlikely that anyone would chose to do a 40-yr prospective study on aflatoxin consumption and liver cancer.

Measuring Hepatoma Incidence

A disease incidence expressed as a rate is defined as the number of cases of the disease that occur in a specified population in a specified period of time. In most situations one cannot determine the true number of liver cancer cases that come into being in a human population, and the incidence rate of this disease is therefore measured indirectly, as seen in the above studies. Liver cancer is not always simple to diagnose clinically, and it is necessary to know how often clinical diagnoses are accurate for the study population before cases so recognized can be included in the determination of incidence rates; confirmation can be done reliably only by histopathological examination.

Even in areas where liver cancer incidence is high, one is looking for 10–20 cases in a general population of 100,000 people over a period of 12 months. Detection of so few cases in such a large population requires a great number of man-hours. If the survey population is smaller than 100,000 and the incidence rate is between 10 and 20, then the survey will have to be conducted for several years in order to detect a sufficient number of cases to provide statistical reliability to the data. Finding liver cancer cases in such large general populations is simplified by surveying only that portion of the population older than 15 yr of age, as liver cancer rarely occurs in the younger population; in many countries the younger age group can be 40% or more of the general population and their exclusion from the survey represents a significant savings in time and resources.

Not only is it difficult to determine accurately the true number of cases of primary liver cancer occurring in a given period, but it can also be difficult to know the exact population from which the cases have been drawn. Patients within and without the prescribed survey population may be attracted to or repelled from the clinical center for detection due to the reputation of the staff. Patients may not always disclose the true location of their residence. The composition of the survey population may be complicated by migrations.

It is important that the survey population be exactly defined before the survey begins to eliminate bias and that all liver cancer cases of bona fide residents only be used to calculate the incidence rate of the disease.

Incidence rate can be calculated as the dividend of the point prevalence rate (the number of cases existing in a specified population at one specific time) divided by the duration of the disease from onset to termination. For diseases of low incidence rate and short duration, such as primary liver cancer, this method is usually not feasible. The Thailand study (Shank et al., 1972e) may provide an example; in the Songkhla area the incidence rate was measured directly in a survey population of 97,867 (all ages) as 2.0 new cases of primary liver cancer/100,000 people per yr. A second population, 101,718 people, all ages, in the same area was selected for the determination of the point prevalence of the disease, and no cases were found. Duration was also measured and found to be 1.3 months from time of diagnosis until time of death; thus, a survey population of approximately 500,000 people in the Songkhla area would be required to provide just one case of primary liver cancer in a prevalence field study. Survey of such large populations was not feasible.

ACUTE AFLATOXICOSIS IN HUMANS

If an environmental contaminant like aflatoxin can be present in the diet long enough and at concentrations sufficient to induce liver cancer, it is reasonable to expect instances of short exposure to high levels inducing an acute response. Three reports of possible acute aflatoxicoses in areas where liver cancer is prevalent may offer a different approach to relating an environmental toxin to liver cancer in man.

Taiwan Report

Ling and co-workers (1967) studied an outbreak of apparent intoxications of 26 persons in two Taiwan farming villages. The symptoms included edema of the lower extremities, abdominal pain, vomiting, and palpable liver; fever was not reported in any of the cases. The victims were limited to members of households that had consumed moldy rice for periods up to 3 wk. Chemical assays were performed on one or two rice samples from the affected households; aflatoxin B_1, 200 μg/kg sample, was found in two of the samples. Three of the victims, children 4–8 yr old, died but autopsies were not done. The evidence to incriminate aflatoxins in this episode is not strong.

Uganda Report

Serck-Hanssen (1970) reported a suspected case of aflatoxin poisoning in Uganda. A 15-yr-old African boy with symptoms closely resembling the Taiwan cases died 6 days after onset of illness. In this case, an autopsy was performed and revealed pulmonary edema, a flabby heart, and diffuse hepatic necrosis. Histopathologic examination indicated pulmonary edema and congestion, interstitial edema of the heart, and centrilobular necrosis and a mild fatty liver. A younger brother and sister became ill at the same time but recovered. The main components of the diets of these children were cassava, beans, fish, and meat. Samples of cassava taken from the home contained 1.7 mg aflatoxins/kg sample, and thus the cassava, if eaten for a few weeks, may have provided a lethal dose to the boy if he was as sensitive to the toxin as is the African monkey (Alpert and Serck-Hanssen, 1970).

Reye's Syndrome in Thailand

While the association study of aflatoxin consumption and human liver cancer was in progress in Thailand, a disease in northeastern Thailand, previously thought to be an encephalitis, was determined as Reye's syndrome and called locally Udorn encephalopathy or EFDV, encephalopathy and fatty degeneration of the viscera (Bourgeois et al., 1969). It is a disease confined to children up to adolescence but particularly prevalent in the age range 1-8 yr. Reye's syndrome (Reye et al., 1963) is characterized by a short prodrome of several hours, vomiting, convulsions, and coma usually ending in death 24-48 hr after onset. Histopathologic examination reveals a severe fatty liver, fat accumulation in the proximal tubules of the kidney and in the myocardium, and severe cerebral edema.

The consumption of leftover cooked rice, heavily contaminated with aflatoxin, was associated with the death of a 3-yr-old Thai boy who suffered from Reye's syndrome (Bourgeois et al., 1971a). The boy had eaten the rice and apparently only that rice for 2 days prior to the onset of illness. After a brief prodromal period the boy developed fever, vomiting, coma, and convulsions; 12 hr later he was admitted to the hospital with severe hypoglycemia (24 mg glucose/100 ml) and died 6 hr later. Autopsy and histopathology confirmed the diagnosis of Reye's syndrome.

This case prompted a reexamination of acute aflatoxin poisoning in the monkey. The median lethal dose for crystalline aflatoxin B_1 in the macaque was determined using 24 young female monkeys (Shank et al., 1971b), and the investigators noted a marked similarity between acute aflatoxicosis in this species and Reye's syndrome in children (Bourgeois et al., 1971a). The monkey tissues were chemically assayed for aflatoxin B_1, which was readily recoverable from animals that died as long as 6 days after a single oral administration (Shank et al., 1971b).

If aflatoxin B_1 was as persistent in tissues of children supposedly poisoned by the toxin as it was in the tissues of poisoned macaques, then the toxin should be recoverable from the human tissues at the time of death. Autopsy specimens from 22 of 23 cases of Reye's syndrome contained detectable levels of aflatoxin B_1; the highest levels were 93 μg/kg in a liver specimen, 123 μg/kg in stool, 127 μg/kg in stomach and intestinal contents, and 8 μg/ml in bile (Shank et al., 1971a). Trace amounts of aflatoxin B_2 were also detected. The concentrations of aflatoxin B_1 in the livers of two of the Reye's syndrome cases were of the same magnitude as the levels in livers of monkeys that received about twice the LD_{50}. The LD_{50} for aflatoxin B_1 in the young macaque is 7.8 mg/kg body weight for a test period of 6 days (Shank et al., 1971b). Material similar to aflatoxin M_1 was found in trace amounts in 2 of 51 urine specimens from Reye's syndrome cases. Eight of the urine specimens contained a blue fluorescent material with an R_f value identical to that of aflatoxin B_1. Aflatoxins could be detected in only trace amounts in specimens from 10 of 13 children aged 1-7 yr who died from causes other than Reye's syndrome and in 1 of 2 youths, aged 17 and 20 yr, who died in road accidents. It was suggested that the trace amounts of the toxin in these control cases probably reflect the chronic low-level ingestion of aflatoxin in this area of Thailand as predicted from a survey of mycotoxin contamination of market foods (Shank et al., 1972b).

Aflatoxins have also been found in autopsy specimens by Becroft and Webster (1972) in two cases of Reye's syndrome in New Zealand and by I. Dvorackova (personal communication, 1974) in six cases in Czechoslovakia. Aflatoxins have not been reported to occur in Reye's syndrome cases in the United States. Collins (1974) has found intranuclear inclusions in pancreatic acinar cells in four cases occurring in New York and Massachusetts and draws attention to the similarity between these inclusions and those seen in the macaques acutely poisoned with aflatoxin B_1 (Bourgeois et al., 1971a).

In the United States, where the disease is rare, it has been suggested that Reye's syndrome may be a viral disease, probably associated with outbreaks of chicken pox or influenza B (Glick et al., 1970). Such an etiology could explain the seasonal variation of the disease and the prodromal symptoms, including occasional fever and upper respiratory tract infections; but a viral etiology does not explain the lack of family involvement, the lack of patho- logical findings characteristic of known viral diseases, or the inability to associate a virus with the disease in other areas, especially Thailand, where Reye's syndrome occurs with high incidence (Olson et al., 1971).

In spite of the evidence associating aflatoxins with Reye's syndrome in Thailand, New Zealand, and Czechoslovakia, some aspects of the disease are difficult to explain solely on the basis of intoxication. In particular, they include (1) lack of sibling involvement, (2) rarity of reports of "sublethal" doses, and (3) in spite of the ubiquity of toxigenic strains of *Aspergillus flavus* (producers of the aflatoxins), the improbability that children in such diverse places were exposed to and could ingest lethal quantities of the poison.

Epidemiologic information on Reye's syndrome is sparse, but what is available suggests a variation in causality in different world areas. The disease may represent a final common response to a variety of insults both toxic (e.g., mushroom, ackee, aflatoxin poisoning) and infectious. The question raised by Bradford and Latham (1967) as to whether Reye's syndrome represents a single disease entity warrants more attention; if it is a single entity, its etiology most likely depends on more than a single specific agent.

Analysis of the data from northeastern Thailand, where the prevalence of the disease is the highest ever reported, indicates that in addition to exposure to viruses and mycotoxins, chronic mild dietary protein deficiency and infections are common, especially infections by liver fluke (*Opisthorchis viverrini*) and intestinal parasites (Sadun, 1955a,b; U.S. Department of Defense, 1962). The higher incidence of Reye's syndrome in Thailand may reflect interactions between these environmental factors. While the primary factor may be intoxication in all Reye's syndrome cases, it may be that a secondary factor in U.S. cases is a viral infection and in Thai cases a diet marginally deficient in protein and/or lipotropic factors. If such synergisms occur and if the specific elements of the synergism differ from one geographic area to another, then a diversity of causative patterns conceivably would emerge in support of Bradford and Latham's (1967) contention that Reye's syndrome is not a single disease entity. Also, this would help explain epidemiologic findings on seasonal variations, involvement of a specific age group, lack of family involvement, and lack of clustering of patients within the epidemic areas.

Bourgeois et al. (1971a) suggested that the pathogenesis of Reye's syndrome is initiated by a toxic, nutritional, or infectious insult resulting in a subclinical liver injury, which may be manifested by fatty metamorphosis. A second injury to the liver, possibly acute aflatoxicosis, results in hypoglycemia, accumulation of metabolites such as ammonia and free fatty acids resulting in further injury and fatty degeneration of the liver, kidney, and heart. The hypoglycemia, elevated blood ammonia, and electrolytic imbalances could produce the central nervous system changes and be responsible for the convulsions, coma, and death.

The reason for discussing Reye's syndrome here is that there may be an association between the disease and liver cancer in Thailand. Reye's syndrome occurs with greatest frequency in the northeastern portion of Thailand, and it is this same area that appears to have a high liver cancer rate. The incidence of liver cancer has not been measured directly in that area, but a review of hospital records covering all provinces of Thailand for several years indicated that the northeast had the greatest number of reported cases of liver cancer per capita; however, in many instances histopathology was not done and diagnosis therefore was not confirmed. In Thailand it may be that Reye's syndrome, as a manifestation of acute aflatoxicosis, identifies a population at increased risk for liver cancer; moreover, survivors of the acute disease may have an especially high risk for liver cancer. If there is an association between acute aflatoxicosis and liver cancer, then areas with high liver cancer rates should also produce at least a few cases of acute poisoning. Evidence available today can only provide two additional reports to support this suggestion: the death of the African boy associated with aflatoxin-contaminated cassava in Uganda where the rate of liver cancer is increased (reviewed above) and the outbreak of disease in Taiwan associated with moldy rice (also reviewed above); Yeh and Cowdry (1954) have reported an elevated incidence rate of liver cancer in Taiwan.

CONCLUSIONS

One argument that is often directed at suggestions relating an environmental contaminant and a human cancer is that humans are not exposed to the levels of the carcinogen needed to produce tumors in experimental animals, and therefore, there is little risk to humans from such compounds. This may seem to be true of the aflatoxins, as it is difficult to appreciate how nanogram per kilogram body weight quantities could induce carcinoma in humans. It is important here to emphasize the incredible potency of aflatoxin B_1 to induce liver tumors. Wogan et al. (1974) have obtained liver carcinomas in 10% of the rats fed diet containing only 1 μg aflatoxin B_1/kg diet; one-tenth this dietary level will produce liver tumors in trout (Halver, 1969). More specifically, young adult rats (250 g) eating 15 g food/day containing 1 μg aflatoxin B_1/kg diet consume aflatoxin at a rate of 60 ng/kg body weight per day; the expected tumor incidence in such a group of animals would be 10,000/100,000 over their life span. The human consumption of aflatoxin B_1 in Kenya and Thailand was up to approximately 50 ng/kg body weight per day, and the corresponding tumor incidence was 6 cases/100,000 people per yr, not per life span. (The human studies measured average intakes, when in fact individual intakes may well have exceeded these levels.) Aflatoxin intakes in Thailand and Kenya, then, are comparable to carcinogenic levels for the rat and trout.

All of the investigations of the relation between aflatoxin ingestion and human liver cancer have been successful in correlating the two, and these studies have been done in Uganda, Swaziland, Kenya, Mozambique, and Thailand. In each case, a dose-response relationship is apparent. One can conclude, then, that there is strong presumptive evidence that aflatoxin is a human carcinogen and appears to be responsible, at least in part, for some of the primary liver cancers that develop in populations in Africa and Southeast Asia. The evidence, however, is only circumstantial, a causal relation has not been proven, and it is unlikely that it could be proven due to the objections of conducting a prospective study in which aflatoxin consumption is monitored for decades in large populations in which hepatocellular carcinoma rates are measured. Nevertheless, it seems clear that sufficient evidence is now available that indicates a high probability that aflatoxins are a human health hazard, and great effort should be made to minimize human exposure to these compounds.

SUMMARY

The evidence relating aflatoxin consumption and human liver cancer consists of the following observations:

1. Aflatoxin B_1 is the most potent hepatocarcinogen for experimental animals yet recognized.
2. All animal species tested in studies on the carcinogenicity of aflatoxin B_1 have developed liver carcinoma, although interspecies sensitivities vary greatly.
3. Human liver contains enzymes capable of metabolizing aflatoxin B_1, although the proximate carcinogen for aflatoxin B_1 has not yet been established.
4. Geographical areas of Uganda and Swaziland with extensive contamination of foodstuffs by aflatoxins are also the areas where the incidence of human liver cancer is increased.
5. Dose-response relationships for aflatoxin ingestion and human primary liver cancer have been observed in Kenya, Mozambique, and Thailand, and the relationships are in quantitative agreement in the three independent studies.
6. In Thailand, the geographical distribution of Reye's syndrome, a children's disease circumstantially associated with aflatoxin consumption, parallels the geographical distribution of primary liver cancer.

Circumstances that favor human consumption of aflatoxin are also likely to favor consumption of other mycotoxins and food-borne toxicants, and only a few such contaminants have been the subject of epidemiologic investigations in relation to human liver cancer; such compounds (e.g., sterigmatocystin, pyrrolizidine alkaloids), however, do not even remotely approach the carcinogenic potency of aflatoxin B_1 (as demonstrated in the rat and the trout). Also, little attention has been given to the effects of interactions of genetic predisposition, nutritional variations, or infectious diseases on aflatoxin carcinogenicity in human populations. It is concluded that the available evidence strongly supports the suggestion that aflatoxins play a role in the etiology of primary liver cancer in human populations of Africa and Southeast Asia where mold damage in the food supply is frequent.

REFERENCES

Allcroft, R. 1969. In *Aflatoxin. Scientific background, control, and implications*, ed. L. A. Goldblatt, p. 239. New York: Academic Press.
Allcroft, R. and Roberts, B. A. 1968. *Vet. Rec.* 82:116–118.
Alpert, E. and Serck-Hanssen, A. 1970. *Arch. Environ. Health* 20:723–728.
Alpert, M. E., Hutt, M. S. R. and Davidson, C. 1968. *Lancet* 1:1265–1267.

Alpert, M. E., Hutt, M. S. R. and Davidson, C. 1969. *Amer. J. Med.* 46:794–802.

Alpert, M. E., Hutt, M. S. R., Wogan, G. N. and Davidson, C. S. 1971. *Cancer* 28:253–260.

Andrellos, P. J. and Reid, G. R. 1964. *J. Assoc. Offic. Anal. Chem.* 47:801–803.

Asplin, F. D. and Carnaghan, R. B. A. 1961. *Vet. Rec.* 73:1215–1219.

Bagshawe, A. F., Parker, A. M. and Jindani, A. 1971. *Brit. Med. J.* 1:88–89.

Barnes, J. M. and Butler, W. H. 1964. *Nature* 202:1016.

Becroft, D. M. O. and Webster, D. R. 1972. *Brit. Med. J.* 4:117.

Berman, C. 1951. *Primary carcinoma of the liver.* London: Lewis.

Bhamarapravati, N. and Virranuvatti, V. 1966. *Amer. J. Gastroent.* 45:267–275.

Blount, W. P. 1961. *Turkeys* 9:52.

Bourgeois, C., Keschamras, N., Comer, D. S., Harikul, S., Evans, H., Olson, L., Smith, T. and Beck, M. R. 1969. *J. Med. Assoc. Thailand* 52:553–565.

Bourgeois, C., Olson, L., Comer, D., Evans, H., Keschamras, N., Cotton, R., Grossman, R. and Smith, T. 1971a. *Amer. J. Clin. Pathol.* 56:558–571.

Bourgeois, C. H., Shank, R. C., Grossman, R. A., Johnsen, D. O., Wooding, W. L. and Chandavimol, P. 1971b. *Lab. Invest.* 24:206–216.

Bradford, W. D. and Latham, W. C. 1967. *Amer. J. Dis. Child.* 114:152–156.

Büchi, G., Kitaura, Y., Yuan, S. S., Wright, H. E., Clardy, J., Demain, A. L., Glinsukon, T., Hunt, N. and Wogan, G. N. 1973. *J. Amer. Chem. Soc.* 95:5423–5425.

Büchi, G. H., Miller, P. M., Roebuck, B. D. and Wogan, G. N. 1974. *Res. Comm. Chem. Pathol. Pharmacol.* 8:585–592.

Campbell, T. C. and Salamat, L. 1971. In *Symposium on mycotoxins in human health*, ed. I. F. H. Purchase, pp. 271–280. London: Macmillan.

Campbell, T. C. and Stoloff, L. 1974. *J. Agr. Food Chem.* 22:1006–1015.

Campbell, T. C., Caedo, J. P., Jr., Bulatao-Jayme, J., Salamat, L. and Engel, R. W. 1970. *Nature* 227:403.

Canter, H. Y. and Shimkin, M. B. 1968. *Cancer Res.* 28:386–387.

Clardy, J., Springer, J. P., Büchi, G., Matsuo, K. and Wightman, R. 1975. *J. Amer. Chem. Soc.* 97:663–665.

Collins, D. N. 1974. *Lab. Invest.* 30:333–340.

Crowther, P. C. 1968. *Analyst* 93:623–624.

Davies, J. N. P. 1973. In *The liver*, ed. E. A. Gall and F. K. Mostofi, p. 361. Baltimore: Williams and Wilkins.

Davies, J. N. P. and Owor, R. 1960. *E. Afr. Med. J.* 37:249–254.

Doll, R., Muir, C. and Waterhouse, J., eds. 1966. *Cancer incidence in five continents*, vol. 1. Geneva: International Union Against Cancer.

Eppley, R. M. 1966. *J. Assoc. Offic. Anal. Chem.* 49:1218–1223.

Garner, R. C. 1973. *FEBS Letters* 36:261–264.

Glick, T. H., Likosky, W. H., Levitt, L. P., Mellin, H. and Reynolds, D. W. 1970. *Pediatrics* 46:371–377.

Glinsukon, T., Yuan, S. S., Wightman, R., Kitaura, Y., Büchi, G., Shank, R. C., Wogan, G. N. and Christensen, C. M. 1974. *Plant Foods for Man* 1:113–119.

Glinsukon, T., Shank, R. C., Wogan, G. N. and Newberne, P. N. 1975a. *Toxicol. Appl. Pharmacol.* 32:135–146.

Glinsukon, T., Shank, R. C. and Wogan, G. N. 1975b. *Toxicol. Appl. Pharmacol.* 32:158–167.

Greenwald, P., Barlow, J. J., Nasca, P. C. and Burnett, W. S. 1971. *N. Engl. J. Med.* 285:390–392.

Halver, J. E. 1969. In *Aflatoxin. Scientific background, control, and implications*, ed. L. A. Goldblatt, pp. 265–266. New York: Academic Press.

Herbst, A. L., Kurman, R. J., Scully, R. E. and Poskanzer, D. C. 1972. *N. Engl. J. Med.* 287:1259–1264.

Higginson, J. 1963. *Cancer Res.* 23:1624–1633.

Higginson, J. and Oettlé, A. G. 1960. *J. Natl. Cancer Inst.* 24:584–671.

Jacobson, W. C., Harmeyer, W. C. and Wiseman, H. G. 1971. *J. Dairy Sci.* 54:21–24.

Keen, P. and Martin, P. 1971. *Trop. Geogr. Med.* 23:44–53.

LeBreton, E., Frayssinet, C. and Boy, J. 1962. *Compt. Rend. Acad. Sci.* 255:784–786.

Lijinsky, W. and Epstein, S. S. 1970. *Nature* 225:21–23.

Ling, K.-H., Wang, J.-J., Wu, R., Tung, T.-C., Lin, C.-K., Lin, S.-S. and Lin, T.-M. 1967. *J. Formosan Med. Assoc.* 66:517–525.

Lopez-Corella, E., Ridaura-Sanz, C. and Albores-Saavedra, J. 1968. *Cancer* 22:678–685.

Marsden, A. 1958. *Brit. J. Cancer* 12:161–176.

Migasena, P. and Changbumrung, S. 1974. *J. Med. Assoc. Thailand* 57:175–178.

Mori, W. 1967. *Cancer* 20:627–631.

Newberne, P. M. and Rogers, A. E. 1973a. *Plant Foods for Man* 1:23–31.

Newberne, P. M. and Rogers, A. E. 1973b. *J. Natl. Cancer Inst.* 50:439–448.

Oettlé, A. G. 1964. *J. Natl. Cancer Inst.* 33:383–439.

Oettlé, A. G. 1965. *S. African Med. J.* 39:817–825.

Olson, L. C., Bourgeois, C. H., Cotton, R. B., Harikul, S., Grossman, R. A. and Smith, T. J. 1971. *Pediatrics* 47:707–716.

Peers, F. G. and Linsell, C. A. 1973. *Brit. J. Cancer* 27:473–484.

Pohland, A. E., Yin. L. and Dantzman, J. G. 1970. *J. Assoc. Offic. Anal. Chem.* 53:101–102.

Pott, P. 1775. *Chirurgical observations relative to the cataract, the polypus of the nose, the cancer of the scrotum, the different kind of ruptures and the mortification of the toes and feet.* London.

Prates, M. D. and Torres, F. O. 1965. *J. Natl. Cancer Inst.* 35:729–757.

Prince, A. M., Leblanc, L., Krohn, K., Masseyeff, R. and Alpert, M. E. 1970. *Lancet* 2:717–718.

Reddy, J. K. and Svoboda, D. 1972. *Arch Pathol.* 93:55–60.

Reye, R. D. K., Morgan, G. and Baral, J. 1963. *Lancet* 2:749–752.

Rogers, A. E. and Newberne, P. M. 1969. *Cancer Res.* 29:1965–1972.

Rogers, A. E. and Newberne, P. M. 1971. *Nature* 229:62–63.

Rogers, A. E., Kula, N. S. and Newberne, P. M. 1971. *Cancer Res.* 31:491–495.

Sadun, E. H. 1955a. *Amer. J. Hygiene* 62:81–115.

Sadun, E. H. 1955b. *Amer. J. Hygiene* 62:116–155.

Salmon, W. D. and Newberne, P. M. 1963. *Cancer Res.* 23:571–575.

Sander, J. 1967. *Arch. Hyg. Bakt.* 151:22–28.

Sargeant, K., Sheridan, A., O'Kelly, J. and Carnaghan, R. B. A. 1961. *Nature* 192:1096–1097.

Schoental, R. 1968. *Cancer Res.* 28:2237–2246.

Segi, M. and Kurihara, M. 1972. *Cancer mortality for selected sites in 24 countries*, no. 6 (1966–1967), p. 104. Tokyo: Japan Cancer Society.

Serck-Hanssen, A. 1970. *Arch. Environ. Health* 20:729–731.

Shank, R. C. 1975a. In *Handbook on mycotoxins and mycotoxicoses*, ed. T. D. Wyllie and L. G. Morehouse, in press. New York: Academic Press.

Shank, R. C. 1975b. In *Advances in chemistry series: Symposium on mycotoxins and toxic phytoalexins*, ed. R. F. Gould, in press. Washington, D.C.: American Chemical Society.

Shank, R. C., Bourgeois, C. H., Keschamras, N. and Chandavimol, P. 1971a. *Fd. Cosmet. Toxicol.* 9:501–507.

Shank, R. C., Johnsen, D. O., Tanticharoenyos, P., Wooding, W. L. and Bourgeois, C. H. 1971b. *Toxicol. Appl. Pharmacol.* 20:227–231.

Shank, R. C., Wogan, G. N. and Gibson, J. B. 1972a. *Fd. Cosmet. Toxicol.* 10:51–60.

Shank, R. C., Wogan, G. N., Gibson, J. B. and Nondasuta, A. 1972b. *Fd. Cosmet. Toxicol.* 10:61–69.

Shank, R. C., Gordon, J. E., Wogan, G. N., Nondasuta, N. and Subhamani, B. 1972c. *Fd. Cosmet. Toxicol.* 10:71–84.

Shank, R. C., Bhamarapravati, N., Gordon, J. E. and Wogan, G. N. 1972d. *Fd. Cosmet. Toxicol.* 10:171–179.

Shank, R. C., Siddhichai, P., Subhamani, B., Bhamarapravati, N., Gordon, J. E. and Wogan, G. N. 1972e. *Fd. Cosmet. Toxicol.* 10:181–191.

Shanmugaratnam, K. 1956. *Brit. J. Cancer* 10:232–246.

Shotwell, O. L., Shannon, G. M., Goulden, M. L., Milburn, M. S. and Hall, H. H. 1968. *Cereal Chem.* 45:236–241.

Simons, M. J., Yap, E. H., Yu, M., Seah, C. S., Chew, B. K., Fung, W. P., Tan, A. Y. O and Shanmugaratnam, K. 1971. *Lancet* 1:1149–1151.

Smith, J. B. and Blumberg, B. S. 1969. *Lancet* 2:953.

Stack, M. E., Pohland, A. E., Dantzman, J. G. and Nesheim, S. 1972. *J. Assoc. Offic. Anal. Chem.* 55:313–314.

Stewart, H. L. 1965. In *Primary hepatoma*, ed. W. S. Burdette, pp. 31–36. Salt Lake City: University of Utah Press.

Sun, S.-C., Wei, R.-D. and Schaeffer, B. T. 1971. *Lab. Invest.* 24:368–372.

Svoboda, D. S. and Reddy, J. K. 1972. *Cancer Res.* 32:908–913.

Tong, M. J., Sun, S.-C., Schaeffer, B. T., Chang, N.-K., Lo, K.-J. and Peters, R. L. 1971. *Ann. Intern. Med.* 75:687–691.

Tuyns, A. J. and Obradovic, M. 1975. *J. Natl. Cancer Inst.* 54:61–64.

U.S. Department of Defense. 1962. *Nutrition survey in the Kingdom of Thailand, October–December 1960.* Interdepartmental Committee on Nutrition for National Defense.

Van Rensburg, S. J., Van der Watt, J. J., Purchase, I. F. H., Coutinho, L. P. and Markham, R. 1974. *S. African Med. J.* 48:2508a–2508d.

Viranuvatti, V. and Satapanakul, C. 1962. *Proc. 9th Pacific Sci. Congress, 1957* 17:416–429.

Vogel, C. L., Anthony, P. P., Sadikali, F., Barker, L. F. and Peterson, M. R. 1972. *J. Natl. Cancer Inst.* 48:1583–1588.

Weisburger, J. H. and Raineri, R. 1975. *Toxicol. Appl. Pharmacol.* 31:369–374.

Welsh, J. D., Brown, J. D., Arnold, K., Chandler, A. M., Mau, H. M. and Thuc, T. K. 1972. *Lancet* 1:592.

Wogan, G. N., Paglialunga, S. and Newberne, P. M. 1974. *Fd. Cosmet. Toxicol.* 12:681–685.

Wolf, H. and Jackson, E. W. 1963. *Science* 142:676–678.

Wright, R., McCollum, R. W. and Klatskin, G. 1969. *Lancet* 2:117–121.

Yamagiwa, K. and Ichikawa, K. 1918. *Cancer Res.* 3:1–29.

Yeh, S. and Cowdry, E. V. 1954. *Cancer* 7:425–436.

Chapter 10

ORGANOHALOGEN CARCINOGENS

H. P. Burchfield and Eleanor E. Storrs
Gulf South Research Institute
New Iberia, Louisiana

INTRODUCTION

Nitrosamines and polynuclear arenes are carcinogens that, unknown to us until recently, have polluted our environment since the early days of civilization, since they are produced by such age-old processes as the curing and frying of bacon and burning of wood and fossil fuels. Natural products that are carcinogens are probably older than humans themselves. Cycasin, a potent hepatocarcinogen, is produced by palmlike plants of the order Cycadales, which are known to have existed in the Mesozoic Era about 65–225 million years ago.

Thus some environmental carcinogens are formed incidentally as by-products of food preparation or heating of homes and factories, while others have nothing whatever to do with the direct activities of humans. Cancerlike changes have been found in million-year-old dinosaur bones, and in humans the disease has been recognized since earliest times, and occurs in all human populations. It is now estimated that 60–90% of cancers may be caused by chemicals, and the rate has increased to where cancer is now the second leading cause of death in the United States.

To our knowledge, no one produces carcinogenic polynuclear arenes in bulk quantities, and nitrosamines are not used to a major extent by the chemical industry. However, organohalogen compounds, aromatic amines, and some other industrial chemicals are manufactured in bulk, and this development took place only during the past century. It is known that some members of these groups cause cancer. Of these, organohalogen compounds are probably the most ubiquitous in occurrence. Not only are they used extensively as intermediates in the manufacture of other chemicals, but many of their end-use products contain halogen, and some of these—because of their use as pesticides and their high chemical stabilities—have become distributed throughout the biosphere. This is not to say that all organohalogen compounds are carcinogens: a few are, some have borderline activity, and others are inactive by presently known biologic test methods.

However, because of their recent introduction into chemical technology, high production volume, and ubiquitous presence in the biosphere, their potentials for good and harm should be scrutinized more closely than is done for any other group of ehcmicals. This conclusion is dramatized by a recent disaster in Hopewell, Virginia, where a plant manufacturing Kepone (chlordecone) caused illness among factory workers, contaminated the community, and led to widespread pollution of surrounding waterways. In experiments recently concluded under the sponsorship of the National Cancer Institute, Kepone was shown to be carcinogenic to rodents.

NATURAL ABUNDANCE OF HALOGENS IN THE BIOSPHERE

At the beginning of the Cambrian Period, about 570 million years ago, marine organisms dominated the world; there are no fossil records of land or freshwater creatures that lived on our planet at that time. For this reason, and because of a rough similarity between the salt contents of seawater and blood, it is believed that life developed from prebiotic organic compounds in oceans or pools that did not differ greatly in salinity from the oceans of today. The amounts of carbon compounds in seawater when life began are unknown. However, in our time inorganic chloride is about 700 times more abundant in the seas than carbon (Table 1), which is the core element of all organic compounds. Although bromine is rare in the earth's crust, it is enriched in seawater, which is its principal industrial source. Iodine is sparingly present in seawater as iodide, which is concentrated selectively by seaweeds; these were formerly processed commercially for recovery of this element. Fluorine is primarily a terrestrial element, most often found in the mineral fluorite; yet it is twice as abundant in the seas as nitrogen, without which the genetic codes inscribed in DNA and the enzymes that execute their orders would not exist.

Thus life began in a nurturing fluid abundant in inorganic halides. While

TABLE 1   Abundance of Elements in the Environment (ppm)
Compared to Amounts of Covalently Bonded Elements in
the Human Body (Excluding Hydrogen and Oxygen)

Element	Earth's crust	Seawater	Human body
Carbon	250	28	180,000
Nitrogen	20	0.7	30,000
Sulfur	260	904	2,500
Chlorine	130	19,400	0
Bromine	2.5	67	0
Fluorine	650	1.3	0
Iodine	0.05	0.06	0.5

these are essential to many metabolic activities, they were not incorporated extensively into organic molecules by higher plants and mammals during biochemical evolution. However, even though organohalogen compounds are rare in nature, a few are synthesized by living organisms. Thus their exclusion from the biosphere by natural selection was not absolute.

The only organohalogen compounds known to be essential to mammalian life are iodinated amino acids—thyroxine and related compounds—which play key roles in the function of the thyroid gland. Although only 1 mg of iodine per week is needed by humans to ensure normal levels of thyroxine secretion, its absence, although rare, leads to endemic goiter and myxedema.

Organochlorine compounds are synthesized by some bacteria and fungi that inhabit the soil. A few of these are beneficial to humans, including the antibiotics chloramphenicol and chlortetracycline, which have been widely used in the treatment of infectious diseases. Less beneficial, but of some practical use, is fluoroacetate, or gifblaar poison, which is synthesized by a South African plant (*Dichapetalum cymosum*). This compound is highly toxic to humans, and its sodium salt has been used as a water-soluble rodenticide.

The first organobromine compound found in nature was 3,5-dibromo-tyrosine, which is a constituent of a coral skeleton. However, the seaweed *Asparagopsis taxiformis* has been found to contain at least 42 organohalogen compounds in its essential oil (Burreson et al., 1976), 36 of which contain bromine.

This plant, which is highly prized for its odor and flavor, is the favorite edible seaweed in Hawaii, but there has never been a single case of illness attributed to its use. The principal constituent of the oil is bromoform, which has been used as a sedative (Table 2). Since chloroform was recently shown to be carcinogenic, this bromine analog should also be tested. Many other compounds found in this oil could be carcinogenic, and some, such as 1,3,3-tribromo-1,2-epoxypropane, are almost certain to be mutagenic to *Salmonella* and other bacterial tester strains.

Nevertheless, organohalogens are virtually excluded from biosynthesis among higher plants and animals. This could be caused by a number of things, including the limited capacity of enzymes to form and break C—X bonds, their monovalency, the unsuitability of halocarbons for storing metabolic energy, and the capacity of some of them to react spontaneously with DNA to produce lethal mutations.

The first of these, enzyme incapacity, is certainly not a primary barrier since in specific instances halocarbons are synthesized by some bacteria, algae, higher plants, and animals, sometimes in good yields. Most halocarbons can be metabolized, some rapidly and others very slowly, and living organisms have elaborated dechlorinases and dehydrochlorinases for this purpose. Also, continued feeding of chlorinated hydrocarbons to experimental animals activates microsomal enzymes that accelerate the catabolism of these and other xenobiotics.

TABLE 2   Abundance of Most Prevalent of
42 Organohalogen Compounds in Essential
Oil of *Asparagopsis taxiformis*

Compound	% in oil
$CH-Br_3$	80
$CH-Br_2I$	5
$CH-Br-I_2$	2
$I-CH_2-CH_2-OH$	1
$CH_3-CO-CH-Br_2$	2
$CH_3-CO-C-Br_3$	1
$Br_2-C=CH-CH-Br_2$	2
$Br_2-C=CH-CO-CH-Br_2$	2

The monovalency of halogens in organic compounds is a major barrier to their metabolic use since they cannot take part in forming the long-chain backbones and cross-links of the biopolymers that are essential to all life forms. These functions can be performed only by di- and polyvalent elements and groups such as carbon, nitrogen, oxygen, sulfur, and inorganic phosphate. The only general metabolic role for halogens is substitution for hydrogen, and here the results may be more often bad than good.

Long-chain polyhalogenated hydrocarbons could not compete with lipids and carbohydrates for storage and retrieval of metabolic energy. Even though they are soluble in lipids and in some cases have similar physicochemical properties, they are thermodynamically inefficient, and the end products of oxidation (X^-, X_2, or even X_2O) would be far less convenient to dispose of than water.

It is well known that alkylating agents can cause mutations and in some cases cancer, and many organohalogen compounds are alkylating agents. Hence compounds causing lethal mutations would be rejected automatically from the genetic code. These and related topics will be the principal subjects discussed in this article.

USES, PRODUCTION, AND RISKS

The virtual exclusion of organohalogens from the biosphere by natural selection over a period of 3 billion years was precipitously ended by humans a century and a half ago, with most of the major developments taking place in the last 25-50 yr. The technologic results have been spectacularly beneficial, but some side effects harmful to public health and the environment have been observed which could cause serious problems in the future if they are not brought under control.

Chloroform, first synthesized in 1831, was used as a general anesthetic in 1847, and it and other organic compounds provided the sedation and relief from pain needed for the development of modern surgery. Before that time, patients usually died of shock if an operation lasted more than 20 min. Chloroform has now been replaced by its safer and more effective halogen relatives halothane and methoxyflurane.

Within the past 50 yr, organohalogen compounds have become established in medicine as antiseptics, antitussive agents, diuretics, antihistamines, analgesics, sedatives, and tranquilizers. Chlorambucil is used for the treatment of leukemias and some solid tissue tumors; chloroquine was developed as a substitute for quinine for treatment of malaria during World War II; chlorpromazine and chlorpheniramine are major psychotropic drugs—and these are only a sampling of many well-known names. The resources of the physician for the relief of pain, control of physiologic imbalances, palliation of mental disease, and treatment of infections and malignant diseases would be cruelly reduced without synthetic organohalogen compounds.

Most of us are potential patients whose lives and comfort may now or someday depend on the judicious use of organohalogen drugs. Few of us would condemn them if we were fully aware of the consequences.

The impact of organohalogen compounds on agriculture has also been great. The discovery of synthetic pesticides containing chlorine during and shortly after World War II resulted in dramatic improvements in the protection of crops from destruction by insects and fungus diseases. While natural products and inorganic compounds such as rotenone and lead arsenate had been used as insecticides since the 19th century, they were far less effective than DDT, lindane, and the chlorocyclopentadienes. For the first time, the concept of pest-free crops became feasible, and control of insects that carry human diseases became, in a few cases, almost a reality. In our haste to condemn DDT for its adverse side effects, we should not forget that the scientist who discovered its insecticidal properties was awarded a Nobel Prize in recognition of the great value of this compound to humanity for control of disease vectors and protection of crops.

Although less heralded, synthetic organic fungicides rapidly replaced bordeaux mixture and other inorganics during the same decades in which organohalogen insecticides were introduced. Examples of early organochlorine fungicides include chloranil, which was used for the protection of seed, and dichlone, which was used for the protection of fruit and foliage against a variety of fungus diseases. These have since been replaced by compounds such as quintozene, dyrene, captan, chlorothalonil, and dichloran, which are more effective fungicides but which also contain chlorine.

Research on plant hormones in the 1930s led to the discovery of the selective herbicidal properties of 2,4-dichlorophenoxyacetic acid, which marked the birth of chemical weed control. It was soon found that related chlorophenoxy acids were valuable plant growth regulators, and within a few decades a host of new haloorganic herbicides was developed. The names of some of these reveal their halogen content: fluometuron, chloropropham, bromoxynil, and ioxynil.

The industrial and commercial applications of organohalogen compounds are almost innumerable. They are used as solvents for the extraction of natural products, dry cleaning fluids, degreasing agents, fuel additives, fumigants, and intermediates for the synthesis of a multitude of other organic compounds. Polychlorobiphenyls (PCBs) are used as dielectric fluids in the construction of transformers, and chlorofluorocarbons are used as refrigerants and also as aerosol propellants for the dispersal of a multitude of household products.

Some polymers containing halogen are valued because they are fireproof, while others, like neoprene, are highly resistant to solvents, oils, and weathering. Polyvinyl chloride (PVC) leads all other plastics in volume produced and is almost ubiquitous in the packaging industry. In fact, both chlorine and vinyl chloride are classified as bulk chemicals, which means that they are produced in quantities of at least one-half million tons annually.

Although the halogen industry is huge, it is not growing in all sectors. In 1970 the production of chlorine in the United States reached 9.8 million tons, but by 1975 it had fallen to 9.3 million tons, substantially less than in 1974. About 70% of the chlorine produced is used for the manufacture of organic chemicals, 12% for water treatment, and the rest for miscellaneous uses.

The decrease in chlorine production coincided with a decline in production of most basic chemicals in 1971. However, forces are at work which may cause it to lag behind other chemicals in a resurgent economy.

It has been known for many years now that DDT and other hard pesticides are persistent in the environment, become concentrated as they move up in the food chain, and are stored in the tissues of almost all of the world's population. There is no direct evidence at this time that storage of low levels of these compounds in tissues is harmful to human health; however, ordinary prudence suggests that this is an unnatural condition, which should be eliminated when acceptable alternatives for pest control can be found. Finding acceptable alternatives has not been achieved in all cases, judging from the experience of cotton growers in Louisiana, where the use of DDT was banned in 1972 and tobacco bud worm infestation of the crop became a serious problem several years later. It is well known that use of DDT had to be reinstated in California to combat the tussock moth.

Concern about the persistence of organohalogens in the environment was exacerbated when it was found that another group of organohalogen compounds, the PCBs, are as widely distributed in the environment as DDT, are concentrated in the food chain, and are difficultly biodegradable. It was not reassuring to the public to learn that some closely related compounds—polybromobiphenyls—had been accidentally mixed with cattle feed in the Midwest, or that the community of Hopewell, Virginia, was contaminated with Kepone by a carelessly operated manufacturing plant.

However, it is not only the problems of persistent residues, hazards to wildlife, and occasional accidents that have caused grave doubts about the safety of organohalogen compounds, since some of them are carcinogenic to humans and experimental animals. Good evidence exists that vinyl chloride, the most important monomer in the plastics industry, has caused angio-sarcomas in factory workers. It is not reassuring to know that this compound has been used as a propellant for household aerosol sprays. Based on long-term, carefully controlled laboratory tests, it has been shown that DDT and many other chlorinated hydrocarbon insecticides are carcinogenic to some rodents, although it is not yet clear how these data can be extrapolated to humans.

The specter has arisen that organohalogen compounds formed inadvertently in the environment could be carcinogenic or otherwise toxic. About 1.1 million tons of chlorine are used annually for water purification. Water, of course, contains many organic impurities, some of natural origin and others anthropogenic. Inevitably some of these are chlorinated during treatment, which leads to the introduction into drinking water of a vast miscellany of organohalogen compounds, the toxicities of which are still unknown.

Some scientists now claim that use of billions of aerosol spray cans powered by chlorofluorocarbons will lead to accumulation of these compounds in the upper atmosphere in concentrations high enough to attenuate the earth's ozone layer. They reason that photochemical decomposition of these compounds releases chlorine atoms, which then destroy ozone. Depletion of ozone would lead to an increased incidence of skin cancer, since this layer shields the earth's surface from shortwave ultraviolet light, which is known to cause cancer. The basic premise is sound since most biologists believe that life did not emerge from the seas and become established on land until sufficient ozone had formed from photosynthetic oxygen to screen out lethal radiation. However, the ozone attenuation theory has been challenged on the ground that chlorine atoms in the stratosphere can combine with nitrogen oxides to form chlorine nitrate. Nevertheless, another seed of doubt has been sown concerning the risk/benefit ratio of organohalogen compounds to humanity.

Despite the tenuous nature of some of the evidence linking organohalogen compounds to cancer, the risk is real and should cause objective concern. Cancer is the second leading cause of death in the United States today, and eventually afflicts one out of four persons. Epidemiologic maps show that the incidence of cancer tends to be highest in industrial areas. Experts in the field variously estimate that 60–90% of cancers are caused by environmental chemicals. In addition, it is well established that biological alkylating agents usually cause mutations and sometimes cause cancer. Many organohalogen compounds are biological alkylating agents. Finally, vinyl chloride and chloromethyl methyl ether cause cancer in humans, and chlorinated hydrocarbon insecticides cause cancer in experimental animals.

Thus the evidence for linking cancer to halogen compounds is strong. Nevertheless, these compounds should not be condemned as a group. A world without drugs, pesticides, water purification plants, sealed plastic containers, and other products of civilization would soon revert to a condition where infectious diseases and malnutrition would replace cancer as leading causes of death.

One of the wonders of halogen chemistry is the great range of physical and chemical properties that can be achieved by manipulation of a comparatively small number of variables. Therefore, by skillful molecular engineering it should be possible to retain the benefits of organohalogen compounds at minimal risk.

In the following sections, several groups of halogen compounds are discussed which have the potential of causing cancer. Their uses and physicochemical properties vary enormously. If, by continued research, it becomes possible to identify accurately the physicochemical properties of molecules that contribute to carcinogenesis, it should be possible to avoid these features in the design of molecules intended for beneficial uses.

ALKYLATING AGENTS, MUTAGENICITY, AND CARCINOGENICITY

Interrelations

Many organic compounds are mutagenic and at least potentially carcinogenic because they cause base pair subsitutions in DNA as a result of replication errors. Some of these compounds are halogen analogs of nucleic acid bases, such as bromodeoxyuridine, while others are alkylating agents, some of which are also halogen derivatives. Another class of compounds also cause base pair substitution reactions, but these arise as errors in DNA repair rather than replication. Still other compounds can lead to insertions or deletions of base pairs; members of all three groups are potentially carcinogenic.

Polyfunctional alkylating agents (those in which one molecule contains two or more chemically reactive groups) can damage genetic material by forming cross-links between strands of DNA or between DNA and chromosomal proteins. Since interstrand cross-links prevent the DNA duplex from undergoing the complete strand separation necessary for proper gene replication, bi- and polyfunctional agents often produce lethal mutations. However, in addition to cross-linking DNA, polyfunctional agents can react with one strand of DNA only, and in special cases could react with two nucleic acid bases on the same strand. Many polyfunctional alkylating agents are used in cancer chemotherapy, and some of these can also cause cancer (Harris, 1976).

The most common, although not necessarily the most damaging, site of attack for most alkylating agents is the N-7 position of guanine in nucleic acids, nucleotides, or nucleosides. Three-dimensional models of DNA show that the N-7 position of guanine is sterically vulnerable since it is situated in the wide groove of the DNA double helix. Under nonphysiologic conditions, other positions of nucleic acid bases, including guanine, adenine, and cytosine, can also be alkylated; but it is not known whether these reactions are important in the *in vivo* alteration of genetic material. Thus it appears certain that steric as well as electronic effects play key roles in the reactions of biological alkylating agents with genetic materials, just as they do with fungi (Burchfield and Storrs, 1976).

It would be very convenient in the laboratory and very inexpensive for the government if it were possible to correlate directly *in vitro* rates of alkylation of DNA by various chemicals with mutagenicity, and mutagenicity with carcinogenicity. In a very general way, such a relationship appears to exist. However, there are some extremely important exceptions to this, particularly among organohalogen compounds, so that a variety of experimental approaches are required. Factors that mitigate against quantitative correlation include differences in volatility, capacities of compounds for differentially permeating cell membranes, hydrolysis rates, detoxication by notarget metabolites in body fluids and cytoplasm, and residence times of carcinogens in tissues caused by a combination of these factors. For example, DDT has a very long residence time in mammalian tissues because of its low volatility and high solubility in lipids; however, vinyl chloride, a gas above −13.9°C, undoubtedly has a short residence time, but continuous exposure of factory workers to it over prolonged periods of time ultimately can result in the induction of liver cancer.

An important factor invalidating the use of the *in vitro* reaction kinetics of alkylating agents with DNA as an index of carcinogenicity is the fact that some organohalogen compounds do not combine with genetic materials directly, but must first be converted enzymatically to ultimate carcinogens by reactions such as hydrolysis, dehalogenation, or epoxidation.

A more direct correlation can be obtained by measuring the capacities of candidate carcinogens for causing various types of mutations in living organisms. The most widely known system has been *Salmonella typhimurium*, used in combination with microsomes to convert premutagens to ultimate mutagens (Ames, 1971, 1972; Ames et al., 1975; Franz and Malling, 1975; McCann et al., 1975; McCann and Ames, 1976). *Escherichia coli* has also been used extensively (Bridges, 1972; Kondo, 1973; Mohn et al., 1974; Green and Muriel, 1976).

The *in vitro* malignant transformation of human and animal cells in tissue culture by chemicals has been used to detect carcinogenicity, and is generally considered to be a more direct index of activity than tests made with microorganisms (Heidelberger, 1973; Bridges, 1974; Altanerova, 1975). Williams (1976) has shown that DNA damage in rat liver cell cultures by carcinogens was evidenced by the induction of DNA repair, measured as unscheduled DNA synthesis.

Other techniques used for the detection of mutagens include examination of yeast cells for mutations following their injection into rats treated with carcinogens (Fahrig, 1976); analysis of sister chromatid exchange formation *in vivo* in mouse spermatogonia (Allen and Latt, 1976); and measurement of excision repair in human peripheral blood lymphocytes (Slor, 1973). Mutagenesis studies with more complex organisms include studies with higher plants (Ehrenberg, 1971); *Drosophila melanogaster* (Abrahamson and Lewis, 1971); and the wasp *Habrobracon* (Smith and Von Borstel, 1971); and a study of dominent lethal mutations in mice (Bateman and Epstein, 1971). Methods used for direct measurement of carcinogenicity in rodents will be described in a later section of this review.

None of these tests in their present state of development give a completely satisfactory direct correlation between mutagenicity and carcinogenicity. As one worker put it, "To use this kind of test (mutagenicity) as a test for carcinogenicity is a bit like looking under the lamppost for a coin lost a block away because of the availability of light" (Rubin, 1976). However, tests for mutagenicity are short and simple, while those for carcinogenicity are long and expensive. To solve this dilemma, Bridges (1974) has suggested that these tests be carried out in three tiers, using microbial assays to detect mutagens, mammalian and human tissue cultures to measure neoplastic cellular transformations, and long-term experiments with living animals to detect cancer. In this system, the cost per test will range from a few hundred dollars per compound for preliminary screening to several hundred thousand dollars per compound for definitive carcinogenesis bioassay studies on living animals.

However, even this system will not satisfy everyone, since there are some who question the validity of extrapolating lifetime carcinogenicity tests on rodents to humans. Is the formation of fatty hepatomas in some strains of hybrid mice during lifetime feeding studies with high doses of chemical a true index of the hazards of these compounds to humans?

The only organohalogen compounds that are known by direct evidence to be a threat to humans are those, such as vinyl chloride, chloromethyl ethers, and possibly benzoyl chloride, which have been shown statistically to cause cancer in factory workers; yet we cannot morally wait until we find cancer in humans to justify banning or restricting the use of potentially hazardous compounds. Therefore, despite the tenuous and incomplete relationships between alkylating power, mutagenicity, and carcinogenicity among organohalogen compounds, it is essential to examine the existing evidence in detail to delineate areas of ignorance in order to define more precisely where additional experimental and theoretical work must be done.

Haloalkanes

The simplest and best known of biological alkylating agents are haloalkanes and derivatives. Iodoacetate, for example, was used by biochemists as a selective inhibitor for thiol-dependent enzymes long before methyl iodide was found to be carcinogenic (Druckrey et al., 1970). All of these compounds react with nucleophilic substrates, but the rates at which these reactions take place are highly dependent on the nature of the halogen and the presence of other substituent groups in the molecule.

The halogens are differentiated from one another by the number of electron shells and therefore by the total number of electrons they contain. The so-called valence electrons become more distant from the nucleus as the number of shells increases. Consequently, the valence electrons are most firmly held by the fluorine nucleus and least firmly held by the iodine nucleus, as indicated by bond lengths and C–X bond energies (Table 3). All of these elements are more electronegative than hydrogen on the Pauling scale, and the energies of C–X bonds are less than those of C–H bonds, except for fluorine. Consequently, alkyl iodides are much more reactive with nucleophilic substrates than are alkyl fluorides, and many of these compounds can replace hydrogen substituted on group VA and VIA elements in S_N1 and S_N2 reactions. The nature of the halogen atoms also governs volatility (Table 3), which could be a factor in determining whether exposure to them is likely to be by dermal contact, inhalation, or other routes.

To determine whether alkyl halides are carcinogenic, Poirier et al. (1975) injected male and female mice of the A/Heston (A/He) strain intraperitoneally with three doses of alkyl halides three times weekly for a total of 24 doses. Fewer injections of some of the compounds were made because of toxicity. At the end of 24 wk, the animals were killed and the lungs examined for adenomas. Of 15 alkyl halides evaluated, nine were found to cause lung tumors at a confidence level of $p < 0.05$ and one at a level of $p < 0.01$ (Table 4).

The four most active carcinogens were alkyl iodides, which would be expected because of the high reactivities of these compounds with electron-rich centers. Surprisingly, however, ethyl iodide was not carcinogenic, and *sec*-butyl iodide ranked seventh in activity. Of the remaining active compounds, three were alkyl bromides and two chlorides. The authors concluded that chemicals with primary structures are less active than those with secondary or tertiary structures, although they pointed out that there were

TABLE 3 Physical Constants of Hydrogen and Halides

Element	Relative negativity	C–X Bond energy (kcal/mol)	Bond length (Å) CH_3X	Boiling point (°C) CH_3X
H	2.1	102	1.09	−164
I	2.5	53	2.14	+42.5
Br	2.8	67	1.94	+3.5
Cl	3.0	81	1.73	−23.8
F	4.0	108	1.39	−78.4

TABLE 4   Alkyl Halides Causing Pulmonary
Adenomas in Mice with Confidence
Level of <0.05[a]

Rank	Compound	Lowest effective dose (mmol/kg)
1	Methyl iodide	0.31
2	n-Butyl iodide	2.6
3	Isopropyl iodide	7.0
4	n-Propyl iodide	17.6
5[+]	sec-Butyl bromide	21.8[b]
5	Isobutyl bromide	21.8
5	tert-Butyl bromide	21.8
6	tert-Butyl chloride	32.4
7	sec-Butyl iodide	32.6
8	sec-Butyl chloride	35.0

[a]Poirier et al., 1975.
[b]Significant at $p < 0.01$.

exceptions to this, such as methyl iodide, which was most active, and
tert-butyl iodide, which was negative. This does not agree with the relative
reactivities of straight-chain and branched alkyl chlorides in reactions in which
Cl is replaced with I (Table 5). In these reactions, chain branching results in
greatly reduced chemical reactivity compared with that of n-butyl chloride.
However, it may be premature to draw too many conclusions from these
studies. Only 20 mice were used at each dose level of chemical, and with one
exception the level of confidence that the experimental groups had more
tumors than the control groups was only $p < 0.05$. Thus the evidence is good
that many alkyl halides cause tumors, with methyl iodide probably being the
most active, but it may not be precise enough to allow for direct correlation
between chemical structure and biological activity. On the other hand,
chemical kinetics is a precise science, but only one factor is measured out of
many that could contribute to oncogenic activity.

TABLE 5   Relative Reactivities of
Alkyl Chlorine in Reactions in
Which Cl is Replaced with I

Compound	Relative rate
n-Propyl chloride	1.00
Isopropyl chloride	0.013
sec-Butyl chloride	0.020
sec-Amyl chloride	0.044
tert-Butyl chloride	0.010

Since alkyl halides are, in theory and in fact, carcinogens, it is of interest that they are also mutagens because of the great current efforts to relate mutagenicity to carcinogenicity.

Simmon and Poirier (1976) evaluated the direct mutagenicity of 12 alkyl halides to histidine-independent revertants of *E. coli* WP2 (hcr⁻) by 8 hr exposures to the chemicals. All ethyl, propyl, and butyl halides studied were mutagenic to one or more strains. The most active compounds were ethyl bromide, ethyl iodide, and isopropyl iodide. Chain branching generally increased mutagenic activity, these compounds being 5 to 20 times more active than the corresponding *n*-isomers. As in the carcinogenicity tests, this does not correlate well with *in vitro* kinetic measurements, which show that *n*-propyl chloride is about 65 times more reactive than isopropyl chloride with nucleophilic substrates whereas isopropyl iodide is among the most powerful mutagens.

In general, increasing the chain lengths of the alkyl halides diminished their mutagenic activities. This also does not correlate well with the *in vitro* reactivities of these compounds with nucleophilic substrates, as increased chain length has only minor effects on reactivity for compounds containing two or more carbon atoms. The alkyl chlorides were generally less mutagenic than the bromides and iodides, which correlates well with the bond energies of these compounds. At this time there is only a general correlation between alkylating power, mutagenicity, and carcinogenicity among alkyl halides. The fact that ethyl iodide was a potent mutagen to bacteria but did not cause a significant increase in lung adenomas in mice is of special concern. Perhaps the reason lies more in the inadequacies of available test methods than in the basic theory. The need to resolve this and other discrepancies will provide a fertile field for future work.

Compounds containing halogen atoms on adjacent carbon atoms (vicinal substitution) are generally more reactive than those containing a single halogen, and this could enhance affinity for DNA. 1,2-Dibromoethane, a widely used industrial chemical and gasoline additive, is mutagenic to *S. typhimurium* (Ames, 1971) and was later found to be carcinogenic (Powers et al., 1975). The closely related compound 1,2-dibromo-3-chloropropane has also been reported to be carcinogenic (Olson et al., 1973).

However, this general relationship between mutagenicity and carcinogenicity breaks down badly when compounds containing two or more halogens on the same carbon atom (geminal substitution) are considered. In general, these compounds are much less reactive chemically than monohalogen compounds or vicinal dihalides because of steric hindrance, and they do not yield precipitates of AgX on treatment with $AgNO_3$, which is a widely used and simple test for reactive halogens.

Yet chloroform was found to be highly carcinogenic to Osborne-Mendel rats and B6C3F1 mice in a screening program supported by the National Cancer Institute (Anon., 1976b). "The most significant observation

($p < 0.0016$) was kidney epithelial tumors in male rats, with incidences of 0% in controls, 8% in the low-dose groups, and 24% in the high-dose groups. Although an increase in thyroid tumors was also observed in treated female rats, this finding was not considered biologically significant. Mice were started on test at 35 days and sacrificed between 92–93 wk. Initial dose levels were 100 and 200 mg/kg for males and 200 and 400 mg/kg for females. These levels were increased after 18 wk to 150 and 300 mg/kg for males and 250 and 500 mg/kg for females, so that the average levels were 138 and 277 mg/kg and 238 and 477 mg/kg, respectively. Survival rates and weight were comparable for all groups except high-dose females, which had a decreased survival. Highly significant increases ($p < 0.001$) in hepatocellular carcinoma were observed in both sexes of mice, with incidences of 98 and 95% for males and females at the high dose and 36 and 80% for males and females at the low dose, compared with 6% in both matched and colony control males, 0% in matched control females, and 1% in colony control females. Nodular hyperplasia of the liver was observed in many low-dose male mice that had not developed hepatocellular carcinoma.

However, these results are entirely at variance with those obtained by Uehleke et al. (1976) on the mutagenicity of chloroform. They investigated the activity of this compound, using *S. typhimurium* TA 1535 and *E. coli* K-12 to detect base pair substitution mutations and *S. typhimurium* TA 1538 to detect frame-shift mutations. The chloroform was activated with rabbit liver microsomes. Although the positive controls (dimethylnitrosamine and benzo[a]pyrene) were active under these conditions, chloroform and/or its metabolites were not mutagenic.

A similar discrepancy also exists for carbon tetrachloride. Reuber and Glover (1967a, 1967b, 1968, 1970) found that subcutaneous injection of this compound into Japanese, Wistar, Black Rat, and Sprague-Dawley rats caused liver damage, including formation of hepatocellular carcinomas as well as hyperplastic nodules and cirrhosis. Tumors of the liver were observed in rats after repeated inhalation of CCl_4 (Costa et al., 1963). This and other evidence in the literature indicates that CCl_4 is carcinogenic to many strains of rats when administered subcutaneously or by inhalation.

This is inconsistent with the results of McCann and Ames (1976), who found that CCl_4 is not mutagenic in their *Salmonella*/microsome test system. However, they are attempting to modify the *in vitro* metabolic activation system for its detection. The nonmutagenicity of CCl_4 was also reported by Uehleke et al. (1976), using both *S. typhimurium* and *E. coli* as test organisms. Significantly, it was found that ^{14}C-labeled CCl_4 was bound preferentially to liver endoplasmic protein and lipid following ip injection. The authors concluded that the primary metabolic intermediates of the halocarbons tested are short-lived radicals, carbonium ions, or carbanions, which would not easily reach targets distant from the endoplasmic reticulum—in other words, they could not reach and thus react with DNA. Yet, even though mutations did not take place, CCl_4 is carcinogenic to rats. Thus there are still unresolved discrepancies between alkylating power, carcinogenicity, and mutagenicity even among simple alkyl halides.

Haloalkenes

Haloalkenes may be either more or less reactive than haloalkanes, depending on the position of the double bond. Allyl halides are very much more susceptible to nucleophilic substitution of the halogen atom than are alkyl halides because of the following resonance structures.

The first of these promotes S_N1 reactions and the second S_N2 reactions. Hence, under all conditions these compounds are highly reactive, and they would be expected to be at least mutagenic if not carcinogenic.

In many vinyl halides, the C–X bond is stronger than it is in ordinary alkyl halides because of the interaction of the electrons of the halogen with those of the double bond.

Moreover, the carbon atom to which the halogen is attached does not carry a partial positive charge, as does the corresponding carbon atom in typical alkyl halides, and as a result, nucleophilic substitution of the halogen in many vinyl halides does not occur. Thus most of them are not alkylating agents. Therefore, it may have been surprising to some to learn that vinyl chloride is carcinogenic to experimental animals (Van Duuren et al., 1968).

Vinyl chloride (1) boils at $-13.8°C$ so that most exposure to it is probably respiratory. Inhalation studies by Viola et al. (1971), Maltoni and Lefemine (1975), and Keplinger et al. (1975) showed that vinyl chloride causes hepatic angiosarcomas, adenomas, and adenocarcinomas of the lung, neuroblastoma of the brain, lymphomas, and other tumors in a variety of animal species. The toxicity of vinyl chloride-polyvinyl chloride has been reviewed in a monograph published by the New York Academy of Sciences (Selikoff and Hammond, 1972).

In an epidemiologic study of people exposed to vinyl chloride, Waxweiler et al. (1976) found an excessive number of deaths due to cancer of the same four sites: the liver, lung, lymphatic system, and central nervous system. The epidemiologic and pathologic findings indicated that vinyl chloride was the causative agent.

Vinyl chloride by itself is a slow-acting mutagen. Exposure of *S.*

typhimurium TA 1530 in a soft agar layer to 20% vinyl chloride in air in the absence of microsomes caused a linear increase in mutagenicity as a function of incubation time, the mutation rate reaching 20 times the spontaneous rate at 24 hr (Bartsch and Montesano, 1975). It seems unlikely that this could be due to the direct action of vinyl chloride; it is more probable that it was caused by the formation of spontaneous breakdown products, or the action of bacterial enzyme systems.

It has been found that the mutagenic effects of vinyl chloride to this same bacterial tester strain are enhanced by mouse or rat liver extracts. This leads to the possibility that vinyl chloride is activated by enzymatic conversion to chloroethylene oxide (2) or chloroacetaldehyde (3) (Goethe et al., 1974).

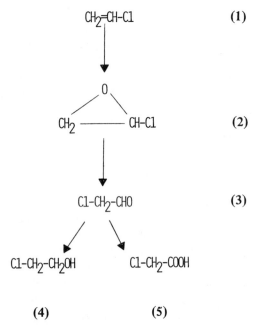

$$CH_2=CH-Cl \qquad\qquad (1)$$

$$
\begin{array}{c}
\text{O} \\
CH_2 \!-\!\!-\!\!-\!\!-\!\!-\! CH-Cl \qquad\qquad (2)
\end{array}
$$

$$Cl-CH_2-CHO \qquad\qquad (3)$$

$$Cl-CH_2-CH_2OH \qquad\qquad Cl-CH_2-COOH$$

$$(4) \qquad\qquad\qquad (5)$$

This is not unexpected since almost all chloroethenes undergo metabolic transformations in living organisms, the first step usually being epoxidation. Symmetrically substituted epoxides are rather stable. However, in the case of vinyl chloride epoxide (2), its polarity decreases stability and leads to an intermolecular rearrangement (Greim et al., 1975) that results in rapid conversion of chloroethylene oxide (2) to chloroacetaldehyde (3). Rannug et al. (1976), comparing the capacities of four possible metabolites of vinyl chloride to cause direct base pair mutations in *S. typhimurium* TA 1535, found that chloroethylene oxide was about 450 times more active than chloroacetaldehyde when the comparison was based on exposure doses defined as the time-independent concentrations of the compounds in the treatment solutions, integrated between the times of beginning and terminating the experiment. The third metabolite, 2-chloroethanol (4), caused a small increase in mutation frequency, twice the control value, only at the highest concentration tested. A fourth substance, chloroacetic acid (5), a urinary excretion product of vinyl chloride, was not mutagenic. Thus, of the four metabolites, chloroethylene oxide is the most powerful mutagen, but it is probably less persistent in tissues than chloroacetaldehyde, which is also mutagenic. The evidence suggests that one or both of these forms may be the ultimate carcinogen arising from vinyl chloride.

However, the fact that epichlorohydrin (6), which is used extensively as a solvent for paints and lacquers, is mutagenic when tested on human lymphocytes (Kucerova et al., 1976) lends some support to the epoxide theory, since oxiranes are themselves powerful alkylating agents, some of which can cause mutations and cancer.

$$\overset{\displaystyle O}{\overset{\diagup\,\diagdown}{CH_2-CH-CH_2Cl}} \qquad (6)$$

However, epichlorohydrin is not a mouse skin carcinogen, although it does induce a significant number of local malignant tumors by subcutaneous injection (Van Duuren et al., 1974). Inhalation studies should be made to determine whether this compound produces malignancies similar to those caused by vinyl chloride. It is also of interest that vinyl chloride induces recessive lethal mosaics in *D. melanogaster* (Magnusson and Ramel, 1976) and that waste products from plants manufacturing vinyl chloride (EDC-tar) were mutagenic in the *Salmonella* test system (Rannug and Ramel, 1976). When, however, a microsomal fraction from rat liver plus an NADPH-generating system was added, the EDC-tar exhibited a considerably stronger mutagenic effect. The results suggest that there are direct as well as indirect mutagens in the tar.

The *in vivo* formation of alkylating agents may not be the only reason for the carcinogenicity of vinyl chloride and related compounds. Its primary reaction in industrial use is free radical polymerization leading to the formation of PVC; this takes place by the following processes, where I· is a free radical initiator and T· is a chain terminator.

$$I\cdot \; + \; \cdot CH_2 - \overset{\displaystyle H}{\underset{\displaystyle Cl}{C}}\cdot \quad \longrightarrow \quad I - CH_2 - \overset{\displaystyle H}{\underset{\displaystyle Cl}{C}}\cdot \; + \; \left[\cdot CH_2 - \overset{\displaystyle H}{\underset{\displaystyle Cl}{C}}\cdot \right]_n$$

$$+ \; T\cdot \quad \longrightarrow \quad I - (CH_2 - CH - Cl)_{n+1} T$$

This hypothesis is given some support by the finding of Garro et al. (1976) that the mutagenic activity of vinyl chloride was stimulated by riboflavin in the presence of light, suggesting that free radicals may be involved. This effect was not observed if the riboflavin was shielded from the light.

Consequently, several mechanisms can be advanced to explain the carcinogenicity of vinly halides, none of which have been proved conclusively. However, there is little doubt that *in vivo* biological activation of the compound is probably required.

Trichloroethylene is also known to be carcinogenic (Anon., 1976c), but it was not mutagenic in tests conducted by Bartsch et al. (1976). However, it was slightly mutagenic when tested in a very sensitive test system with *E. coli* (Greim et al., 1975). This slight positive action was not anticipated since this compound is metabolized to chloral hydrate, trichloroethanol, and trichloro-acetic acid, which are not known to produce genetic effects. Thus there appears to be a borderline relation between the mutagenicity and carcino-genicity of this compound, which should be investigated further.

Chloroprene (7) is another vinyl halide that caused recent interest and some alarm.

$$CH_2 = \overset{\overset{\displaystyle Cl}{\displaystyle |}}{C}-CH = CH_2 \qquad (7)$$

It has been used by duPont for many years as a monomer for the production of neoprene, a synthetic rubber, and company records do not show any increase in the incidence of cancer in workers exposed to it. However, Khachatryan (1972a, 1972b) believed it to be carcinogenic based on an epidemiologic study made on factory workers in Russia. However, Lloyd (1976), after considering other contributory factors that were neglected in this study, is not fully convinced that Khachatryan's conclusion is correct.

Because of the suspicions aroused by these studies and the structural relationship of vinyl chloride to chloroprene, long-term animal studies have been initiated by the National Cancer Institute. It should be noted that chloroprene is mutagenic in the *Salmonella* microsome test (Bartsch et al., 1976; McCann and Ames, 1976). These preliminary results indicate that chloroprene is probably a far more powerful mutagen than carcinogen.

Two derivatives of haloethenes that definite can induce cellular transformations are diallate (8) and dichlorvos (9).

$$(CH_3)_2CH \diagdown \\ \qquad \qquad N-S-CH_2-CCl=CHCl \\ (CH_3)_2CH \diagup$$

$$\qquad (8)$$

$$CH_3O \diagdown \quad \overset{\displaystyle O}{\underset{\displaystyle \|}{}} \\ \qquad \quad P-O-CH=CCl_2 \\ CH_3O \diagup$$

$$\qquad (9)$$

Diallate, a herbicide, was shown to be carcinogenic to mice at a confidence level of $p < 0.01$ in studies conducted by Innis et al. (1969), while dichlorvos, an organophosphate insecticide, was shown to be mutagenic by several groups of workers (Wild, 1975; Shirasu et al., 1976) and is highly reactive with 4-(*p*-nitrobenzyl) pyridine, a reagent commonly used to measure alkylating power (Bedford and Robinson, 1972). Studies of the carcinogenesis of dichlorvos administered in rodent feed sponsored by the National Cancer Institute are underway, but test results are not yet available. However, an inhalation study conducted by Blair et al. (1976) in which Carsworth Farm Strain E rats were exposed to 0.05–5.0 mg/m^3 of compound for a period of 2 yr showed that no increase in dose-related tumor incidence was obtained on male or female rats.

While these two compounds contain groups other than vinylic halogens, it appears likely that the latter are probably responsible for the adverse effects produced in experimental test systems.

In relating chemical structure to carcinogenicity, it should not be assumed that all vinyl halides are unreactive because of the inertness of vinyl chloride in S_N1 and S_N2 reactions with nucleophilic substrates, since substitution with groups having a −M effect much larger than the +M effect on the halogen can lead to compounds whose reactivities are frequently higher than that of the saturated analog. Introduction of a nitrile group is such an example (Rappoport, 1969).

ACTIVE VINYLIC HALIDES

$$N{\equiv}C\text{-}CH{=}CH\text{-}\ddot{C}l \quad\longleftrightarrow\quad \bar{N}{=}C{=}CH\text{-}\overset{+}{C}H\text{-}Cl$$

$$(S_N1) \qquad\qquad (S_N2)$$

Vinylic compounds of this class are probably capable of reacting directly with metabolites in the absence of metabolic activation. Hence, vinyl halides could be carcinogenic by a number of mechanisms.

Oxygenated Haloalkanes

The introduction of an oxygen atom into an alkyl halide sometimes results in extreme activation of the halogen, depending on the position of substitution and whether an ether or carbonyl bond is formed (Table 6). Thus chloromethyl methyl ether (10) is 850 times more reactive with KI than 1-chloropropane because of the high electronegativity of oxygen and its attachment to the same carbon atom as the chlorine. It is probable that resonance forms involving carbonium or oxonium ions exist as follows:

$$\left[CH_3\text{-}O\text{-}\overset{+}{C}H_2 \right] Cl^- \quad\longleftrightarrow\quad \left[CH_3\text{-}\overset{+}{O}{=}CH_2 \right] Cl^- \qquad (10)$$

As a result, compounds of this class are capable of reacting spontaneously with nucleophilic substrates such as DNA without enzymatic mediation.

TABLE 6   Relative Reactivities of
Oxygenated Haloalkanes

Compound	Relative reactivity
$CH_3-CH_2-CH_2-Cl$	1
$CH_3-\overset{\overset{O}{\|}}{C}-O-CH_2-Cl$	250
CH_3-O-CH_2-Cl	850
$CH_3-\overset{\overset{O}{\|}}{C}-CH_2-Cl$	33,000
$CH_3-\overset{\overset{O}{\|}}{C}-Cl$	$\ll\infty$

Both **10** and the derivative in which both methyl groups are substituted with halogen atoms, bis(α-chloromethyl) ether (**11**) are highly toxic and mutagenic to *S. typhimurium* and *E. coli* (Mukai and Hawryluk, 1973). Compound **11** is a potent carcinogen, while **10** was not carcinogenic for mouse skin but showed pronounced initiating action in two-stage mouse skin carcinogenesis studies (Van Duuren et al., 1969).

$$Cl-CH_2-O-CH_2-Cl \qquad\qquad (11)$$

In other tests with **10** only one bronchogenic cancer and one esthesioneuroepithelioma were observed out of 74 animals (Laskin et al., 1975). It is tempting to ascribe the higher carcinogenicity of **11** to the fact that it is a bifunctional alkylating agent potentially capable of cross-linking DNA strands while **10** is monofunctional. However, Lawley and Brooks (1967) point out that in the Watson-Crick model for DNA the reactive groups of a bifunctional alkylating agent should be able to reach across a distance of approximately 8 Å. The relatively short distance between the reactive halogens of **11** renders cross-linking between the reactive sites of adjacent bases unlikely or impossible.

Compound **11** was first shown to be a potent carcinogenic alkylating agent when applied to mouse skin. Examining the effects of a single subcutaneous injection in newborn mice, Gargus et al. (1969) found a higher incidence of animals with pulmonary adenomas and more tumors per mouse in those receiving **11** than in those receiving **10** or in controls. In view of the fact that industrial exposure to these volatile compounds is more likely to be by inhalation than dermal contact, Laskin et al. (1971) exposed a group of 30 Sprague-Dawley rats to 0.1 ppm of **11** in air for 6 hr/day for a total of 101 exposures. Squamous cell carcinomas of the lung and esthesioneuro-epitheliomas (ENEs) of the olfactory epithelium were produced in high incidence in these animals. In a later study, Drew et al. (1975) exposed rats and hamsters to both **10** and **11** by inhalation. In these range-finding studies, the carcinogenicity of **11** was demonstrated by the induction of a skin cancer in a rat after three exposures, and a nasal tumor in a hamster after one exposure to 1 ppm of the compound in air.

These compounds are also carcinogenic to humans. Figueroa et al. (1973) found an eightfold increase in the incidence of lung cancer in workers exposed to **10** at a chemical manufacturing plant. Of 14 men in whom lung cancer developed, histologic confirmation was obtained in 13, and 12 had oat cell carcinomas. Three of the 14 men had never smoked. In a more recent study, Albert et al. (1975) compared 1,800 workers who had been exposed to **10** from 1948 to 1972 with 8,000 workers who had not been exposed. The age-adjusted death rate for respiratory cancer in the compound **10** group was 2.5 times that in the control group, whereas death rates due to other causes were comparable. There was also a gradation of lung cancer risk according to intensity and duration of exposure and the time elapsed since the onset of exposure. In a more limited study, Sakabe (1973) concluded that three factory workers died of lung cancer caused by exposure to **10**. Thus there is no doubt that **10** causes lung cancer in humans, the total number recorded being at least 47 (Nelson, 1976).

However, there are some ambiguities in the results. Although both compounds are toxic, **11** is by far the more potent carcinogen. Moreover, technical grade **10** contains as an impurity 2–8% of **11**, which could be the real culprit. Thus while the actual compound(s) that cause cancer are still unknown, for practical purposes **10** must be considered a carcinogen, although of a lower order of activity than **11**.

When the chlorine and oxygen atoms in chloroethers are separated by two or more carbon atoms, as in bis(β-chloroethyl) ether, alkylating power and carcinogenicity are greatly reduced. This compound had borderline activity in studies conducted by Van Duuren et al. (1972), but in lifetime feeding studies in mice it was found to be carcinogenic, the results being significant at the $p < 0.01$ level (Innis et al., 1969). The prinicpal concern here is that both bis(β-chloroethyl) ether and bis(β-isopropyl) ether have been found in waterways used as sources of drinking water and are present in the finished drinking water (Kleopper and Fairless, 1972).

Of six compounds related to **11** only two, bis(1-chloroethyl) ether and 2,3-dichlorotetrahydrofuran, initiated tumors by subcutaneous injections in mice (Van Duuren et al., 1972). Thus not all chloroethyl ethers cause cancer in mice in cutaneous tests.

Anticancer Drugs

Many drugs used in the treatment of cancer contain chlorine atoms or other reactive functional groups that can combine covalently with DNA or nucleoproteins. One special feature of these drugs is that they always contain two or more functional groups. This makes it possible for these compounds to cross-link DNA strands during mitosis and cause lethal mutations. They function as anticancer drugs because they are able to kill rapidly proliferating cancer cells by this process. However, they can also react with DNA in normal cells, causing mutations that can transform into cancer. This is because not all reactions with these compounds result in the formation of cross-links. One functional group could react with DNA, while the other could hydrolyze or otherwise combine with nongenetic material to cause a point mutation resulting in base pair substitution. If cross-linking occurred in all cases, these compounds would probably not be carcinogenic, since most of the mutants would be lethal. Even if cross-linking occurred in all cases, these drugs would still have toxic side effects through their ability to kill normal cells, although at much slower rates than rapidly proliferating cancer cells.

Anticancer drugs that can also induce cancer include dibromomannitol, dibromodulcitol, bis(2-chloroethyl) sulfide (mustard gas), uracil mustards, *N,N*-bis(2-chloroethyl)-2-naphthylamine, *N,N*-bis(2-chloroethyl)-4-aminophenyl acetic acid, *N,N*-bis(2-chloroethyl)-4-aminophenyl butyric acid (chlorambucil), DL-*N,N*-bis(2-chloroethyl)-*p*-aminophenylalanine, 2-chloroethyl methane sulfonate, and *N*-methyl-bis(2-chloroethyl) amine (nitrogen mustard) (Haddow, 1973; Harris, 1976). Neoplasias that can be induced by these agents include epitheliomas, leukemias, and mammary tumors in rats and mice.

Perhaps the best known and most widely studied of these compounds are the nitrogen mustards, which are reactive electrophilic compounds capable of alkylating a variety of substrates containing imino, amino, thiol, and hydroxyl groups. The nitrogen mustards (12), in neutral or alkaline solution, rapidly undergo intramolecular rearrangement to release chloride ion with the formation of a highly reactive quaternary immonium compound (Ross, 1962).

The immonium ion (13) will then react with an electron-rich site of a DNA base by a biomolecular reaction.

$$Cl-CH_2-CH_2-N(CH_3)-CH_2-CH_2-Cl \longrightarrow Cl-CH_2-CH_2-\overset{+}{N}(CH_3)\overset{CH_2}{\underset{CH_2}{\diagdown}}$$

(HN$_2$)

(12)   (13)

$$(DNA_1)-B \xrightarrow{} (DNA_1)-B-CH_2-CH_2-N(CH_3)-CH_2-CH_2-Cl \qquad (14)$$

The second functional group of the mustard can then cyclize and react with a base on another DNA strand, which would result in a lethal mutation. In the case of nitrogen mustard (12), the reaction product could be visualized as

$$\text{(DNA}_1)-B-CH_2-CH_2-N-CH_2-CH_2(DNA_2-B)$$

with CH_3 on the nitrogen.

(15)

The bases on the two strands may or may not be the same, but *in vivo* the favorite alkylation target is the 7-position of guanine.

However, if the second functional group merely reacts with water or a simple thiol, cross-linking would not occur, the effect might not be lethal, and a point mutation could take place that could subsequently lead to a cellular transformation resulting in malignancy in normal cells.

These are S_N1 reactions since the rate-controlling step is the unimolecular decomposition of the nitrogen mustard to form an immonium ion and chloride. This will take place at a constant rate regardless of the concentrations of reactive compounds in the immediate vicinity.

However, with other compounds reaction occurs through collision of a drug molecule with a metabolic substrate to form a transition state, which yields the product. Since two molecules are directly involved, the rate depends on the concentrations of both and the reaction is bimolecular (S_N2). It has been shown that some drugs closely related to nitrogen mustard react by the S_N2 mechanism.

The efficacy of these compounds as drugs and also as carcinogens is probably governed to some degree by the molecularity of the reaction. Chemicals reacting by an S_N1 mechanism will generate the toxic agent at a constant rate regardless of the concentrations and reactivities of nucleophiles in their immediate environment. Therefore, in theory at least, a compound reacting by an S_N1 mechanism should survive as long in blood as in pure water. On the other hand, a compound reacting by an S_N2 mechanism could be detoxified very rapidly by reactive compounds such as serum albumin before it reached a chromosomal target site. In a sense, compounds that react by the S_N1 mechanism are precarcinogens that do not require enzymatic mediation for activation.

These compounds are also mutagenic to a wide variety of organisms, including mice, *D. melanogaster, E. coli, Aspergillus* sp., maize, barley, and wheat (Fishbein et al., 1970).

The latency period of carcinomas caused by anticancer drugs could be

20-50 yr, which would still be within the life span of survivors of childhood cancer. However, the use of carcinogenic drugs for the treatment of cancer appears justified if other effective therapy is not available.

There is at least one important exception to this. Chlornaphazin is not only a powerful alkylating agent, but also a derivative of an aromatic amine that is on the OSHA list of the most dangerous carcinogens.

Hence, persons administered this drug would be potentially exposed to carcinogenic agents of two types. Three patients treated with the drug developed carcinomas of the urinary bladder 5, 6, and 10 yr following the intermittent administration of 70-100 g of compound (Shubik, 1972). With our increased knowledge of the relationship between chemical structure and carcinogenicity, it is unlikely that this kind of iatrogenic blunder will ever occur again in the future.

CHLORINATED HYDROCARBON INSECTICIDES

There is a satisfying if not complete correlation between alkylating power, carcinogenicity, and mutagenicity among haloalkanes, haloalkenes, and their oxygenated derivatives. Faith in this biologic trinity begins to waver when we consider geminally substituted polyhalides such as $CHCl_3$ and CCl_4: these are chemically unreactive, not mutagenic by presently known test procedures, but cause hepatocellular carcinomas and other tumors in mice.

This theoretical structure collapses completely, however, with the chlorinated hydrocarbon insecticides. These are specific neurotoxins that are not primarily biological alkylating agents, although some of them have this latent potential, or could be converted to electrophilic compounds by microsomal enzymes. As a group, they are sparingly volatile, lipid-soluble, and are stored in mammalian adipose and other tissues for long periods of time. In general, they are not mutagenic or only very weakly so. However, most of them cause tumors in mice during lifetime feeding studies, the most prevalent type being hepatocellular carcinomas.

Although these compounds have been mass-produced for the past 30-35 yr, there are no records of increased incidences of cancer among factory workers handling them, although safety precautions for the protection of personnel during the early days of their manufacture were very crude. In one factory operation, DDT was shoveled from a drying oven with a garden spade and ground by hand through ordinary window screen into 55-gallon drums. The only protection afforded the workers were canvas gloves and gauze face masks.

Cancer has been caused among workers engaged in the manufacture of vinyl chloride and chloromethyl methyl ether, although exposure was probably less because the volatility of these compounds and the irritant action of the ether required that they be handled in closed systems. Yet in its early days DDT was handled as casually as talcum powder.

TABLE 7 DDT and DDE Content (ppm) of Body Fat of
General Population in the United States[a]

Year	No. of samples	DDT	DDE	Total as DDT
1963	28	2.4	4.3	6.7
1964	282	2.9	8.2	11.1
1965	64	2.5	5.1	7.6
1965	25	2.3	8.0	10.3
1965	13	3.7	6.8	10.5

[a]Edmundson, 1972.

Because of its persistence in the environment and slow rate of metabolism, DDT has accumulated in the tissues of most of the world's population (Table 7). The amounts found in the tissues of people occupationally exposed to it are substantially higher (Table 8), but no differences in incidence of cancer between these groups have been reported. Unfortunately, because of the ubiquitous distribution of DDT, there is no large control group in the United States with zero DDT exposure and average exposure to other environmental chemicals. Thus there is no direct way to show that DDT and other chlorinated hydrocarbons cause cancer in humans. Yet the fact that these compounds cause tumors in mice must be given some weight. Even if they induce cancer in only 0.01% of the population during a 10 yr time span, this would result in 20,000 new cases per year in a population of 200 million, which would be unacceptable.

Thus the fate of DDT was sealed by its ubiquitous presence in human tissues and the fact that it causes tumors in mice. Yet not only is there no direct evidence that these compounds cause cancer in humans, the mechanisms by which they cause cancer in mice are completely unknown. The biological alkylating-mutagenesis hypothesis that in a general way accounts for the oncogenic properties of other groups of compounds seems to fail completely. However, this theory might be resurrected if it can be shown that compounds with long persistence and high cell permeation capacity coupled with weak

TABLE 8 DDT and DDE Content (ppm) in Body Fat of
Occupationally Exposed Persons[a]

Year measured	No. of persons	Occupation	DDT	DDE	Total as DDT
1965	30	Applicators	14.0	21.1	35.1
1965	14	Applicators	10.7	24.1	34.8
1953	1	Formulator	122.0	141.0	263.0
1956	1	Formulator	648.0	434.0	1,131.0
1956	6	Volunteers (35 mg/day)	234.0	24.0	258.0

[a]Edmundson, 1972.

alkylating power do, in the long run, produce the same cellular transformations as short-lived compounds that are powerful alkylating agents.

One thing seems certain: the mechanisms by which chlorinated hydrocarbons kill insects and are neurotoxic to mammals are probably in no way related to the processes by which they cause tumors in mice. In fact, in some cases the presence of chlorine in these compounds is only incidental to their activities as nerve poisons. Therefore several hypotheses concerning their modes of action as neurotoxins will be discussed.

Mechanisms of Insecticidal Action

It is easy to describe the overt physiologic effects that chlorinated hydrocarbons have on animals, but the mechanisms involved are more elusive. Many biochemical changes have been observed as the result of insecticide poisoning of arthropods and mammals, but it is difficult to determine whether these are the causes or results of death.

Although all of these compounds are nerve poisons, they interact with insects in subtly diverse ways. Evidence has accumulated over the past years that DDT acts on the peripheral nerves rather than the central nerves of insects. Lindane is a more rapid poison than DDT, and it appears to act primarily on the central nervous system, although opinions regarding peripheral involvement differ. Symptoms produced by cyclopentadiene insecticides are more similar to those of lindane than of DDT, although they develop more slowly. The effects of toxaphene appear to be on the central nervous system and are generally similar to those produced by the cyclopentadienes.

DDT and related compounds inhibit various enzymes involved in oxidative metabolism, but some nontoxic analogs (for example DDE) produce similar effects. Much work has been done on the Na^+-, K^+-, Mg^{2+}-, and Ca^{2+}-dependent adenosine triphosphatases (ATPases) of the nervous system, which may be involved in the regulation of ion transport through axon membranes, but it is by no means certain whether these enzymes are major targets for DDT and related insecticides. Although there have been many investigations on the effects of chlorinated hydrocarbon insecticides at the biochemical level in insects and mammals, the results cast little light on their modes of action, with one exception: most of these compounds appear to increase levels of acetylcholine in nerve tissues. This is the same basic mechanism by which organophosphate insecticides are known to act.

Acetylcholine is a chemical transmitter that is stored in vesicles at the ends of presynaptic nerve fibers. When a message carried by an electric impulse through an axon reaches the end of a nerve fiber, it triggers the release of acetylcholine, which diffuses across the synapsis and stimulates the neighboring cell to continue the message. The junction between excitable cells is commonly the site of an enzyme, acetylcholinesterase, that destroys the transmitter, ensuring that its action will be brief. If the enzyme is inhibited by an organophosphate, postsynaptic potentials are prolonged and enhanced, producing the neurotoxic effects typical of organophosphate poisoning.

Unlike organophosphates, DDT, lindane, and the cyclopentadienes do not inhibit acetylcholinesterase. However, it has been suggested that dieldrin causes excessive release of acetylcholine from its storage sites near the presynaptic membranes of cholinergic junctions (Shankland and Schroeder, 1973), and similar observations have been made for DDT (Metcalf, 1955; Richards and Cutcomp, 1945) and lindane (Sternberg and Hewitt, 1962), although the effects produced are not identical in all aspects. Nevertheless, the possibility exists that chlorinated hydrocarbons and organophosphates produce the same basic effect, namely an increase in acetylcholine concentrations at nerve synapses—the former by causing excessive secretion from bound reserves, and the latter by inhibiting the enzyme that normally destroys acetylcholine. In both cases, postsynaptic potentials would be prolonged and enhanced. A physiologic parallel is found in cats that have been poisoned by aldrin, which manifest peripheral parasympathetic disturbances, such as salivation and slowing of the heart, very much like those produced by organophosphate insecticides (O'Brien, 1967).

The existence of multiple sites of action and interactions between chlorinated hydrocarbon and organophosphate insecticides have been demonstrated directly by studies of inhibition of the photomigration of mosquito larvae by binary mixtures of insecticides (Storrs and Burchfield, 1954). When these materials are tested in mixtures, compounds that act jointly yield inhibition versus concentration curves that are concave; when they act independently the curves are convex (Fig. 1). The validity of this relationship has been demonstrated mathematically. Since the tests can be carried out in a short time, usually less than an hour, secondary interactions are minimized. Using this method, all mixtures of pairs of structurally analogous compounds— such as DDT-methoxychlor, chlordane-heptachlor, and malathion-parathion— were found to act jointly, as expected (Table 9). However, DDT was found to act independently of all other chlorinated hydrocarbons tested, which indicates different sites of primary activity. A key finding was that DDT acted jointly with parathion, indicating that both compounds probably increase levels of acetylcholine at the same synaptic junctions, although by different mechanisms. Thus binding by nerve tissues appears to be involved in the action of the major synthetic organic insecticides.

Two mechanisms have been suggested for the binding of organohalogen compounds to nerve tissues, based on molecular structure and dimensions. Mullins (1956) has calculated that lindane would fit into the pores of an axonic membrane consisting of cylindrical lipoprotein molecules 40 Å in diameter packed together in a hexagonal array so that they are 2 Å apart. An interesting extension of this concept is that the same interspaces could accommodate DDT. Holan (1969), after studying the toxicities of a number of DDT derivatives to houseflies, proposed that these compounds are bound at

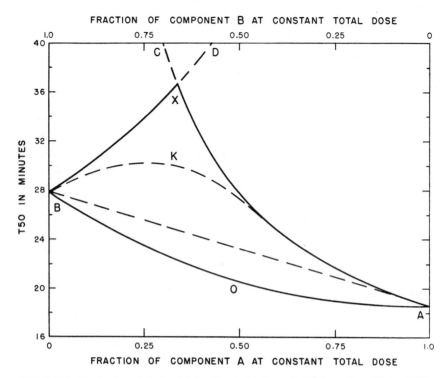

FIGURE 1 Illustration of similar joint action and independent joint action of insecticides.

bimolecular leaflets consisting of a protein layer and a lipid layer. The layers are spaced so that the aromatic rings of DDT form a complex with the protein layer, while the aliphatic portions of the molecule fit into recesses in the lipid layer, having the dimensions of a hydrated sodium ion. (This particular model is based on the assumption that DDT is toxic because it increases the permeability of axon membranes to Na$^+$.) Although these models are geometrically feasible, their equivalents have not been demonstrated to exist in nerve axons.

The nature of the chemical bonds that bind organochlorine compounds to nerves has been much discussed. O'Brien and Matsamura (1964) speculated that charge transfer complexes between DDT and components of nerve axons could be formed which would result in destabilization of the axons. However, this concept was later brought into doubt by the observation that similar interactions take place with nontoxic DDT analogs. Moreover, the concept would have limited applicability, since of the important chlorinated hydrocarbon insecticides, only members of the DDT group possess armoatic rings containing the π electrons necessary for the formation of charge transfer complexes. A more plausible explanation was suggested by Fahmy et al. (1973), who proposed that DDT and its analogs are bound to receptor sites

TABLE 9 Joint Action of Binary Mixtures of Structurally
Related and Unrelated Insecticides in Photomigration Tests

Group	Compounds	Reaction[a]	
		Expected	Obtained
1 + 1	DDT-methoxychlor	+	+
2 + 2	Heptachlor-chlordane	+	+
3 + 3	Dieldrin-aldrin	+	+
1 + 2	DDT-heptachlor	−	−
1 + 2	DDT-chlordane	−	−
1 + 3	DDT-aldrin	−	−
1 + X	DDT-parathion	−	+

[a]Plus = similar joint action; minus = independent joint action.

by van der Waals bonds, and that maximum insecticidal activity is obtained when these forces are optimal.

Formation of covalent bonds between organohalogen insecticides and metabolic substrates has never been proposed seriously as the basis for their primary biological activity. It has usually been assumed that low-energy bonds that dissociate readily are responsible for their bioactivities. This fits in well with the fact that the toxicity of DDT decreases with increasing temperature, which would not be expected except in the case of a loosely bound, thermally unstable complex (Hoffman and Lindquist, 1949; Guthrie, 1950). Lindane also has a negative temperature of toxicity (Guthrie, 1950), but its magnitude is much smaller than that observed with DDT.

The high stereospecificity required for insecticidal action also suggests that molecular configuration rather than chemical reactivity is primarily responsible for the insecticidal properties of these compounds: for example, DDT **(16)** is readily dehydrohalogenated to DDE **(17)** *in vitro* by alkalis and *in vivo* by enzymes. DDE is not insecticidal, and in fact this is a primary route for detoxication of DDT by resistant insects. By contrast, dianisylneopentane **(18)**, a structural analog of DDT that contains no chlorine, possesses high insect toxicity (Rogers et al., 1953).

DDT

active

(16)

DDE   inactive

(17)

Dianisyl-neopentane   active

(18)

It is obvious, then, that free rotation around a single carbon-to-carbon bond is more critical to the toxicity of DDT analogs than the presence of halogen atoms, which in fact do not appear to be required at all. While halogen substitution may greatly modify rates of cellular permeation, persistence in the environment, and biodegradability, it is apparently not basic to the intrinsic insect toxicity of the DDT group. On the other hand, the requirement for free rotation applies only to the DDT group. the cyclopentadienes are rigid molecules, and *cis-trans* isomerism is the key to the insecticidal activity of hexachlorocyclohexanes, the γ-isomer being the only member of the group having significant insecticidal activity.

Molecular Basis for Carcinogenicity

Cyclopentadienes. From the foregoing, it is evident that the chlorinated hydrocarbons are not insecticides because of their alkylating power. Nevertheless, some of these compounds and their proposed metabolites posses latent alkylating potential, which could result in mutagenesis or carcinogenesis because of their long residence times in mammalian tissues. For example, the chlorine attached to the 1-carbon of heptachlor (19) is allylic and is replaced by OH on heating with alkali. On biooxidation, heptachlor is converted to its expoxide (20). The epoxide groups of acyclic compounds are highly reactive, and compounds containing them are often both mutagenic and carcinogenic.

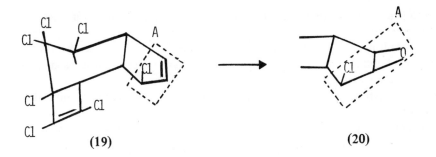

It is important to note, therefore, that a region (A) of the heptachlor molecule contains a group equivalent to a disubstituted derivative of allyl chloride, while in the epoxide the structure of this region is equivalent to that of epichlorohydrin. Both allyl chloride and epichlorohydrin are alkylating agents and the latter is a mutagen. However, when embedded in the cyclodiene framework they appear to become relatively inactive. This is probably caused in part by the greater size and complexity of the molecules.

The rate at which bimolecular reactions take place between two compounds is given in its simplest form by

$$k = PZe^{-E/RT} \tag{1}$$

where k equals the velocity coefficient, P is the probability factor, Z the collision factor, E the energy of activation, R the gas constant, and T the absolute temperature.

For descriptive purposes, Eq. 1 describes adequately why colliding molecules react at different rates. The factor Z is the frequency of collisions between reacting molecules, and can be calculated from elementary kinetic principles. However, not all high-energy collisions between molecules result in reactions. One factor that diminishes the frequency of successful collisions is the probability or P factor. Qualitatively, this factor is an expression of steric effects that tend to reduce reactivity between molecules. With small uncomplicated molecules, all collisions tend to occur in about the same way spatially so that P approaches unity. However, for large molecules some collisions with sufficient energies take place that do not lead to reactions. This is because the reactive centers may not approach one another closely enough on collision to permit the formation of a transition state. Groups that shield the reaction center from attacking molecules result in low probability factors. An illustration of this effect is that chlorocyclohexane is only about 1% as reactive as 1-chloropropane in reactions where chlorine is replaced by iodine. Other contributing factors may also exist. For example, chlorine substitution decreases water solubility while increasing lipid solubility. Hence these compounds are probably stored in fat globules, where they are isolated from hydrophilic reaction centers. Also, factors such as the ridigity of the cyclopentadiene structures in relation to bond angles and reaction rates need to be considered.

Aldrin is converted *in vivo* very rapidly to dieldrin, but the epoxide group of this compound is also unreactive, probably for the reasons given for heptachlor epoxide.

In effect, the cyclopentadienes possess latent alkylating groups whose activity is greatly diminished by steric and polar effects. Yet these compounds are not biologically inert, as shown by the fact that the allylic halogen of heptachlor can be replaced by a hydroxyl group, and dieldrin is converted to a *cis-trans* diol *in vivo* by an enzyme-mediated reaction. Therefore, it is possible that electrophilic intermediates with alkylating power could be formed during the extensive metabolic degradation of these compounds in the liver and other organs.

From the standpoint of relating chemical structure to chemical and biological activities, a study of heptachlor, epichlorohydrin, and chemicals intermediate in structure between them would be of great interest. Intermediate structures that should be evaluated include chlorocyclopentene, chlorocyclopentene epoxide, and other compounds containing methyl groups and chlorine atoms substituted in various positions on the rings. Information on *in vitro* chemical reactivities of these compounds with nucleic acids and proteins, partition, transport rates, covalent binding *in vivo* to metabolic substrates, mutagenicity, and carcinogenicity should shed light on the reasons why compounds of this class are carcinogenic to mice.

DDT. Although DDT has been studied more extensively than any other pesticide, additional information on this compound would be desirable in order to explain its observed carcinogenicity to rodents. The parent molecule does not contain aliphatic double bonds or active halogen. However, DDT **(21)** is readily dechlorinated enzymatically to yield DDD **(22)** or dehydrochlorinated to yield DDE **(23)**. Both of these compounds can be metabolized further to yield p,p'-DDMU **(24)**.

This compound has the potential of being epoxidized to yield **25**, which could be mutagenic or carcinogenic because of the alkylating power of the three-membered ring.

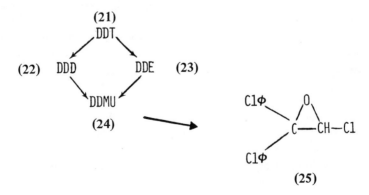

Compound **25** is, of course, immediately recognizable as a derivative of the unstable metabolic oxidation product of vinyl chloride, which probably accounts for its carcinogenicity. However, it is probable that **25** is more stable than the vinyl chloride intermediate because of steric and electronic effects. But first it must be determined whether the *p*-chlorophenyl groups interfere with or assist in epoxide formation.

Another possibility that exists that could account for the weak mutagenicity and carcinogenicity of many members of the DDT group of insecticides containing halogen atoms in the benzene rings. Bis(*p*-chlorophenyl)benzophenone **(26)** is a metabolite common to DDT, DDD, chlorobenzilate, and dicofol and is formed by the complete dechlorination and oxidation of the alkyl group. The primary valence bond structures of this compound can be written as **26A** and **26B**. Thus the resonance effect of the carbonyl group and the inductive effects of the chlorine atoms would result in formal positive charges at the *para* positions of the benzene rings. Therefore, **26** should be an active halogen compound capable of combining with nucleophilic substrates in S_N2 reactions with the elimination of chloride ion.

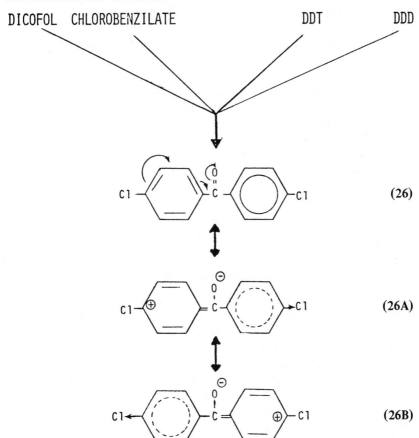

Thus it can be postulated that most, if not all, organohalogen insecticides can be transformed into potential alkylating agents by enzymatic dechlorination, dehydrochlorination, and epoxidation, or combinations of these reactions.

Steric and other effects. In discussing the insecticidal activities of organohalogens, primary attention was focused on molecular structure; in this section the emphasis has been on chemical reactivity, and it is probable that the mechanisms of action in the two cases are entirely different.

However, steric configuration cannot be dismissed altogether since acridine and phenanthridine dyes are mutagenic even though they are not alkylating agents. It is believed that these compounds are mutagenic because their dimensions are such that they easily become intercalated between base pairs in DNA molecules, and thus give rise to frame-shift mutations. Because the fused ring systems of these compounds are planar they can slide between adjacent base pairs of DNA, forcing them 6.8 Å apart, twice the normal 3.4 Å separation. Thus they become easily incorporated in genetic material without extensive distortion of the DNA double helices.

The organohalogen insecticides are not planar and have some highly specific requirements for insect toxicity, including free rotation in the case of DDT, specific *cis-trans* isomerism for lindane (the other *cis-trans* isomers of hexachlorcyclohexane are not insecticidal), and rigid three-dimensional frameworks for the cyclopentadienes. Relating these structural requirements to insect toxicity has defied the best efforts of pesticide chemists for the past 30 yr. Relating them to oncogenic activity may be even more difficult; therefore, it is expedient to initiate work on the complex problem of pesticide carcinogenicity with a study of metabolic activation to electrophiles, since these reactions have already been shown to be keys to the carcinogenicity of acyclic halogen compounds.

Of course these compounds could be tumorigenic to mice for reasons not yet explored. They are lipid-soluble, slow to metabolize, and persistent in tissues. It is conceivable that they could interact with cell membranes and other structures to cause the coalescence of adjacent cells to form multinucleate agglomerates. The possibility that this could occur and the oncogenic potential of multinucleate cells are, of course, unknown.

Carcinogenesis Bioassay Results

Organohalogen pesticides have been evaluated for carcinogenicity since the early 1950s. However, in many of these early tests the number of animals used was too small, the duration of the tests was too shcrt, routes of application were questionable, or the results were unacceptable for other reasons. In the mid-1960s, the National Cancer Institute initiated a comprehensive program to evaluate the tumorigenicity to mice of 120 selected pesticides and industrial compounds (Innis et al., 1969). The results of this study and all previous work done on the carcinogenicity of pesticides are summarized in a report made to the Secretary of Health, Education, and Welfare by a group of five expert Advisory Panels, one of which was concerned specifically with the carcinogenicity of pesticides (Mrak Report, 1969).

Since that time, the National Cancer Institute has instituted programs to test new compounds and retest others for which the previous results were questionable or the compounds were so important economically that confirmatory evidence was needed. In view of the superiority of these new data, the entire literature will not be reviewed. This summary will be based entirely on the publication by Innis et al. (1969), the Mrak report (1969), and technical reports issued by the National Cancer Institute on tests recently completed.

In the study by Innis et al. (1969), two hybrid strains of mice were used. At weaning, 18 mice of each sex from each strain were put on test. Thus, 72 animals were given each compound orally, with the exception of the positive control compound, ethyl carbamate.

The maximum tolerated dose (MTD) was used for each compound. This dose was given by stomach tube beginning when the mice were 7 days of age; after the mice were weaned at 4 wk of age the chemicals were mixed directly with the diet, which was provided *ad libitum*. The experimental design called for necropsy at 18 months of age. The logistics of performing necropsies in a study involving almost 20,000 animals were complex; therefore, the actual time of necropsy varied somewhat among the groups.

The postmortem procedure included an external examination and a thorough examination of thoracic and abdominal cavities, with histologic examination of major organs and of all grossly visible lesions. The cranium was not dissected. Thyroid glands were examined and sectioned in mice treated with amitrole and in one negative control group, but not in other groups. The entire carcass and all internal organs were fixed and saved. Blood smears were made on all mice before they were killed; they were examined only in cases showing splenomegaly or lymphadenopathy.

Statistical analysis showed that 11 of the 20 test compounds induced a significant elevated incidence of tumors, mostly hepatomas. This incidence was comparable to the mean tumor incidence of a group of control compounds known by previous work to be carcinogenic. The 11 positive compounds included five pesticides.

Therefore, additional work on pesticides was initiated by the National Cancer Institute under contract with several other organizations. The compounds assigned to Gulf South Research Institute included nine chlorinated hydrocarbon insecticides, seven organophosphate insecticides, four fungicides and herbicides, and three positive controls (amitrole, saffrole, and 2-AAF). The compounds were mixed with the feed.

For the long-term chronic studies, the MTD and half of the MTD were used as determined by a 6-wk preliminary study. B6C3F1 mice and Osborne-Mendel rats were used. In some investigations conducted at other laboratories, Sprague-Dawley rats were substituted. Fifty female and 50 male animals were used in each test group, so that each compound was tested on

400 rodents: 200 mice and 200 rats. Fifty control animals were used for each compound. The mice were scheduled for necropsy at 90 wk and the rats at 100 wk, but because of the logistic difficulties described by Innis et al. (1969), this schedule could not always be adhered to exactly.

At necropsy, the animals were examined for gross pathology, and macroscopic lesions, tissue masses suspected to be tumors, regional lymph nodes, and specimens from at least 41 different tissues and organs were preserved in formalin and subsequently examined histopathologically.

Although not all of the test results have been analyzed statistically yet, the number of chlorinated hydrocarbons that were found to be tumorigenic is formidable. There seems no doubt that unless tumors in mice cannot be correlated with cancer in humans (which at this time is very unlikely), chlorinated hydrocarbons as a class will be banned for use except in cases where human exposure is not involved, acceptable alternatives cannot be found, or the risk of death from infectious diseases carried by insects far exceeds the risk of increased incidence of cancer.

Several problems were encountered during these tests which will be corrected in future programs. Most important, the MTD as determined by a 6-wk preliminary study was in most cases too high. Pesticides are designed as economic poisons, and while they are usually species-specific, this specificity is not absolute. Consequently, some animals died of acute poisoning during the test, and dose levels had to be changed 175 times through the program to ensure survival of the remaining animals until the scheduled necropsy dates (Burchfield et al., 1975). Therefore, doses were calculated as time-weighted averages from the equation

$$D_t = \frac{C_1 D_1 + C_2 D_2 + \cdots + C_n D_n}{D_1 + D_2 + \cdots + D_n} \tag{2}$$

where D_t is the time-weighted dose, C is the concentration of compound in feed (ppm), and D is the number of days at that concentration level.

A more satisfactory procedure for the 2 yr studies would have been to use a fraction of the MTD found in preliminary studies, as proposed by Weil et al. (1969). Currently, 90 day preliminary studies are being used and the MTDs for 2 yr studies extrapolated from these.

Furthermore, metabolism studies made prior to the chronic tests at the

TABLE 10   Metabolism of Aldrin to Dieldrin
by Female Mice Fed 4 ppm of Aldrin
in Diet for 6 Wk

Tissue	Aldrin (ppm)	Dieldrin (ppm)
Adipose	0	7.8
Liver	0	2.9
Other viscera	0	1.1

TABLE 11   Metabolism of Heptachlor to Heptachlor Epoxide by
Rats Fed 20 ppm of Heptachlor in Diet for 4 Wk

Tissue	Heptachlor (ppm)	Heptachlor epoxide (ppm)
Adipose	0	15
Liver	0	2.6
Other viscera	0.003	2.9

proposed dose levels could have saved some duplication of effort. It has long been known that aldrin is biologically epoxidized to dieldrin, but the extent to which this would occur with the animal species and dose levels used was not known. Consequently, both aldrin and dieldrin were evaluated. In retrospective studies, it was found that practically all of the aldrin was converted to dieldrin by the test animals (Table 10). Hence, aldrin could have been eliminated from the study without loss of any significant information. Of lesser importance, heptachlor is oxidized to heptachlor epoxide. Heptachlor was evaluated, but its epoxide was not. Retrospective analytical studies showed that the heptachlor administered was converted almost entirely to the epoxide (Table 11). Therefore, the test results reported are representative of heptachlor epoxide, not the parent compound.

With some compounds administered at high dose levels, a mixture of metabolites might be formed, and the composition of this mixture could change with dose by overwhelming the capacities of metabolizing enzymes. The results of such a study would be very difficult to interpret in terms of which compound(s) in the mixture were the carcinogens, and whether they would occur at dangerous levels during ordinary human occupational or environmental exposure.

Finally, it is concluded that an insufficient number of control animals was used with each chemical group. In current practice, 600 animals are used for each test chemical, including 200 controls.

Mutagenicity

The correlation between the carcinogenicity of pesticides to rodents and their mutagenicity by a variety of tests is very poor. In bacterial and fungal tests with various strains of *S. typhymurium, E. coli, Serratia marcescens,* and *Saccharomysis cerevisiae,* DDT and its metabolites DDE, DDD, and DDA gave negative results (Fahrig, 1974). McCann and Ames (1976) reported that DDE was negative in their *Salmonella*/microsome test system. Other chlorinated hydrocarbons on which negative results have been obtained using microbial systems include chlorobenzylate, aldrin, dieldrin, endosulfan, and lindane. Shirasu et al. (1976) reported negative results on aldrin, BHC, DDT, dieldrin, and heptachlor using two strains of *B. subtilis,* two strains of *E. coli,* and four strains of *S. typhimurium.* Clearly, the chlorinated hydrocarbon insecticides as a class are not direct mutagens, and they are not easily metabolized to active compounds.

DDT, however, shows weak mutagenic activity in the X-linked recessive lethal test with *Drosophila*, induces chromosome aberrations in human lymphocytes, but gives ambiguous results in the dominant lethal test with mice (Fahrig, 1974). Metabolites of DDT also show weak mutagenic activity in one or the other of these test systems. Thus DDT appears at most to be a weak mutagen, and the results clearly show that negative results in *in vitro* systems can in no circumstances be regarded as evidence of nonmutagenicity in *in vivo* systems for this class of compound.

Almost all available tests indicate that dieldrin, and therefore its metabolic precursor aldrin, are not mutagenic (Bidwell et al., 1975). These include direct bacterial tests with and without microsomal activation, host-mediated assay, blood and urine analysis for active metabolites, micro-nucleus tests, metaphase analysis, dominant lethal tests, and heritable translocation tests.

The *Salmonella* tester strains used in all bacterial tests included excision repair-deficient mutants, partial and total lipopolysaccharide-deficient mutants, and both frame-shift and base analog mutation strains. No increase in the number of mutants was found in any of the five bacterial tests.

In most animal tests, dieldrin was administered at concentrations of 0.09, 0.8, and 8 mg/kg by gavage once per day for 5 days before mating for the dominant lethal and heritable translocation tests. Evaluation of the data obtained on mice showed that dieldrin was negative in all four animal tests.

Lindane has been tested *in vivo* in mice by Bauer and Frohberg (1972) by the dominent lethal test, and the results obtained were negative. Chlordane and heptachlor do not produce dominant lethal mutations in mice, according to unpublished work conducted at a commercial laboratory (Anon., 1976a). On the basis of this evidence, the manufacturer of these compounds believes it unlikely that they cause cancer, since most known carcinogens are also mutagens.

The limited evidence available thus far suggests that many chlorinated hydrocarbons may not be mutagenic *in vitro* or *in vivo*, with the possible exception of DDT, which has borderline activity *in vivo*. This finding raises two important questions: (1) Can mutagenicity be used as an indicator of carcinogenicity for *all* classes of compounds, although good correlations exist within others? (2) Are the hepatocellular carcinomas and other tumors produced in hybrid rodents during lifetime feeding studies an indication that these compounds will cause cancer in humans? These questions must be answered in order that regulatory agencies can make decisions on a sound scientific basis.

HALOGENATED ORGANOPHOSPHATE INSECTICIDES

Although this review is concerned primarily with organohalogen compounds, it must be taken into consideration that many organophosphates and carbamates also contain halogen atoms, among them being dichlorvos, trichlorfon, bromophos, chlorothion, and others. Of these, dichlorvos (27) has been worked on most extensively because of its intriguing structure, its use as a space fumigant, and the fact that it has been shown to alkylate DNA (Löfroth, 1970; Lawley et al., 1974). Moreover, the mutagenicity of this compound has been studied in numerous test systems, and a 2 yr study of its carcinogenicity to rodents is near completion. The structure of dichlorvos suggests that it can function as a phosphorylating or a methylating agent, or participate in reactions involving the dichloroethylene group. Undoubtedly, the insecticidal power of this compound is dependent on its ability to phosphorylate cholinesterases, the polar dichlorovinyl moiety (29) being the leaving group.

$$CH_3O \diagdown \underset{\overset{\|}{O}}{P} - OCH = CCl_2 \ + \ E \ \longrightarrow$$
$$CH_3O \diagup$$

(27)

$$CH_3O \diagdown \underset{\overset{\|}{O}}{P} - E \ + \ \underset{Cl \diagup}{\overset{Cl \diagdown}{C}} = CHOH \ \rightleftharpoons \ \underset{Cl \diagup}{\overset{Cl \diagdown}{C}} CH-CHO$$
$$CH_3O \diagup$$

(28)   **(29)**   **(30)**

The primary reaction product, other than the phosphorylated enzyme, would be 1,1-dichloro-2-hydroxyethene (29), which is tautomeric with dichloroacetaldehyde (30). The latter compound is an alkylating agent, and therefore could be a potential mutagen and/or carcinogen.

However, dichlorvos and other organophosphates, with or without halogen atoms, pose a secondary threat to the integrity of the genetic code. This concern arose in 1970 (Epstein, et al.), when it was found that the simple compound trimethyl phosphate is mutagenic in mice. This finding stimulated much work on the alkylation of DNA by dichlorvos both *in vitro* and in intact cells of *E. coli* (Lawley et al., 1974). Nucleic acid bases were methylated in both cases. In the *in vitro* experiments, between 63 and 85% of the total DNA methylation products was 7-methylguanine, with smaller amounts of other methylated bases, and in intact cells the primary reaction product was 7-methylguanine. This, at first thought, would appear to spell the doom of most organophosphates, since it is believed by many that alkylation of DNA bases results in point mutations, which some workers believe eventually lead to cancer. This concern has been alleviated to some extent by the finding that RNA or DNA isolated from heart, lung, liver, kidney, and other tissues of rats that were exposed to ^{14}C-labeled dichlorvos did not contain labeled 7-methylguanine (Shell Development Company Report to

EPA). Also, little or no 7-methylguanine was found in the rat urine. However, Wennerberg and Löfroth (1974) earlier reported that mice had received ^{14}C-labeled dichlorvos by ip injection or inhalation excreted 7-methylguanine in the urine. It is not clear whether methylation took place with guanine bound in nucleic acids, or by reaction with the free base. Until this point is clarified, it cannot be stated with certainty that organophosphates are not mutagens and potential carcinogens. An alleviating factor that is repeatedly stressed in this article is that dichlorvos reacts with proteins about 20–30 times more rapidly than with nucleic acids (Lawley et al., 1974; Wennenberg and Löfroth, 1974). In a recent study by Blair et al. (1975), the half-life of dichlorvos in male rat kidneys was found to be only 13.5 min. Thus rapid detoxication may often block the action of potential mutagens and carcinogens.

There is no doubt, however, that dichlorvos and other organophosphates are bacterial mutagens. Tester strains used included the streptomycin-dependent Sd-4 strain of *E. coli* (Löfroth et al., 1969), the tryptophan-requring WP2 strain of *E. coli* (Ashwood-Smith et al., 1972), *S. typhimurium* (Dyer and Hanna, 1973), *Klebsiella pneumoniae* (Voogd et al., 1972), and *Saccaharomyces cerevisiae* (Dean et al., 1972; Fahrig, 1973).

Dean et al. (1972) reported host-mediated assay studies with dichlorovos using the D4 strain of *S. cerevisiae*. Mice were administered the compound orally at doses as high as 100 mg/kg. The highest dose did not induce mitotic conversion in yeast cells kept for 5 hr in the treated animals. However, the dose was only 1/40 as great as the lowest dose producing mutations in the *in vitro* tests.

Negative results were obtained in tests with related compounds in *Drosophila* (Benes and Sram, 1969), mammalian cells in culture (Dean, 1972), or mammalian cells *in vivo* (Epstein et al., 1972). It is argued that these negative results may have resulted from the fact that dichlorvos is too toxic to exceed the concentrations employed in the bacterial assays for mutagenesis (Wild, 1975).

It is notable that dichlorvos was the most powerful mutagen in a group of 12 organophosphates tested (Wild, 1975). However, Bidrin, dimethoate, and oxydemeton methyl were almost as effective, and these compounds do not contain halogen atoms. Therefore, it is apparent that triesters of phosphoric acid are basically alkylating agents and potential mutagens, and that these functions will vary with details in structural and electronic configurations.

Another organophosphate that contains potentially reactive halogen is rebon (31). This compound could be hydrolyzed readily in the liver and other organs to yield dimethyl phosphate (32) and tetrachloroacetophenone (34).

The structure of this compound should incite suspicion because of the vinyl halide grouping and the well-known propensity of this moiety to epoxidize to yield an alkylating agent, which is presumed to be the mechanism by which vinyl chloride itself is converted *in vivo* to a carcinogen.

Certainly this possibility should be studied by using microsomal enzymes in combination with a trapping agent such as *p*-nitrothiophenol.

However, an alternative mechanism for carcinogenesis is also built into this molecule. The leaving group on enzymatic phosphorylation or hydrolysis is a derivative of ω-chloroacetophenone with three chlorine atoms substituted in the benzene ring. The parent compound is a powerful lachrymatory agent, war gas, and an ingredient of the crowd control agent MACE. The high chemical reactivity of the ω-chlorine atom is caused by its proximity to the electron-rich carbonyl group, which in turn is in resonance with the π electrons of the benzene ring. The three chlorine atoms substituted in the benzene ring are relatively unreactive. However, they could enhance the carcinogenicity of this compound by reducing volatility and increasing lipid solubility, thus increasing the residence time of the compound in vital tissues.

This is a striking example of potential biological activation. The vinyl halogen or rebon itself is quite unreactive, and the parent compound can probably be carried in the bloodstream to vital organs with a minimum of detoxication other than reacting with serum esterases. However, once it reaches a site of high enzyme activity, the liver for example, it could hydrolyze to yield a vinyl alcohol (33). This, of course, would immediately tautomerize to yield the highly reactive chloroketone (34). Thus four steps may be involved: (1) transport of a relatively unreactive compound to a vital target site, (2) hydrolysis to a vinyl alcohol, (3) isomerization to an active halogen compound, and (4) reaction of the latter with a nucleophilic substrate. Other insecticides with similar vinylic structures should also be capable of undergoing the same reactions.

In this section only two halophosphates have been discussed—dichlorvos and rebon. Many others are in use. However, these examples show that halogen atoms can play important roles in the mutagenesis and potential carcinogenesis of compounds that are ordinarily classified as phosphates. It would be unwise to make the generalization that most chlorinated hydrocarbons are carcinogenic and therefore should be banned, while all organophosphates are safe, except for a few unfortunate deaths caused by acute accidental poisoning.

FUNGICIDES CONTAINING ACTIVE
HALOGEN ATOMS

If the poor correlation between alkylating power, carcinogenicity, and mutagenicity among chlorinated hydrocarbon insecticides is often puzzling, the *apparent* weakness of such a correlation among fungicides containing active halogen compounds is little short of amazing. Perhaps the results of work now in progress and of future research will help to clarify many of these anomolies.

These compounds were, by change or by design, engineered to react with enzymes, cofactors, and nucleic acids containing ionized thiol, imino, and amino groups to remove them from the metabolic pools of fungus spores. The spores are then presumably killed by multiple inactivation of numerous metabolic pathways needed to sustain life processes.

The premise that these compounds are general protoplasmic poisons is supported by two well-documented observations. First, the amount of compound that must be taken up by spores in order to inhibit germination is of the order of 1,000–2,000 μg per gram of spores compared to a few micrograms per gram for most other biocides. Consequently, these compounds cannot be highly specific with respect to target sites. Second, attempts to produce strains of fungi that are highly resistant to these compounds by adaptation to increasing dose levels have failed, and strains of fungi resistant to the compounds have not developed in nature. This implies that a very large number of fungal mutations would have to take place to confer resistance to organohalogen fungicides, compared to the small number of mutations required to produce strains of insects resistant to chlorinated hydrocarbon insecticides. These facts suggest that active halogen fungicides dissipate themselves by forming covalent bonds with many metabolic substrates rather than attacking a small number of specific sites, which appears to be the case in the action of antibiotics and insecticides.

Structurally, these compounds can be aromatic, heterocyclic, alicyclic, or acyclic. However, they all possess one feature in common: they undergo nucleophilic substitution reactions with metabolic substrates to yield covalently bonded derivatives that are usually stable, in reactions of the general type:

$$FX + MZH \longrightarrow MZF + X^- + H^+$$

where FX is an active halogen fungicide and MZH a metabolite containing an electron-rich center. With the compounds studied thus far, the reactions have all been of the $S_N 2$ type, although there could be exceptions.

Therefore, even though most of these compounds contain ring systems of various types, it is convenient to classify them as biological alkylating agents, even though most of them do not contain alkyl groups. Moreover, many of them are bifunctional, and thus are potentially capable of cross-linking DNA. Some of the most widely known compounds of this class that have been studied include chloranil **(35)**, dichlone **(36)**, dyrene **(37)**, chlorothalonil **(38)**, captan **(39)**, folpet **(40)**, and captafol **(41)**. Although not used as a commercial fungicide, 2,4-dinitrofluorobenzene (FDNB) **(42)** is also included because it has fungicidal properties and has been used in many investigations of the mechanism of action of fungicides (Burchfield and Storrs, 1957, 1958), and because many laboratory workers have been exposed to it through its widespread use as a reagent for sequencing amino acids in proteins.

(35)   (36)   (37)

(38)   (39)   (40)

(41)   (42)

All of these compounds (FDNB excluded) are protectant fungicides. That is, they cover the surfaces of fruit and foliage, and kill invading spores by direct contact before they can germinate and send their mycelia into the plant tissues. Once disease has become established, it cannot be eradicated by use of these compounds.

These are direct alkylating agents, which presumably cannot be translocated. However, chloroneb (43) is a systemic fungicide which, when applied to plant seedling leaflets, moves acropetally in the treated leaflet, and can be detected in stem tissues above the treated leaf (Kirkpatrick et al., 1976). The structure of chloroneb suggests that it is not a direct alkylating agent. However, it has been shown that it can be converted to 44, 45, and 46 in vivo by demethylation followed by oxidation (Rhodes et al., 1971; Rhodes and Pease, 1971).

$$(43) \longrightarrow (44) \longrightarrow \text{conjugates}$$

(43): 1,4-dimethoxy-2,5-dichlorobenzene (OCH_3, Cl, Cl, OCH_3)

(44): (OH, Cl, Cl, OCH_3)

(45): (OH, Cl, Cl, OH)

(46): chloroquinone (O, Cl, Cl, O)

It will be noted that 46 is a chloroquinone, which probably reacts similarly to the direct alkylating fungicides chloranil (35) and dichlone (36) with metabolic substrates. However, its precursor, chloroneb (43), is an unreactive compound, which is probably why it can be transported through the vascular systems of plants, where it ultimately becomes metabolically activated to an alkylating agent. Compounds 35, 36, and 46 would probably be detoxified by spontaneous reactions with metabolites such as glutathione before they could diffuse to sites where they could react with nucleic acids. Thus prefungicides as well as precarcinogens may be more effective systemically than direct alklyating agents since they are not detoxified before they reach vital sites at which metabolic activation by microsomal enzymes can take place.

Active halogen fungicides react primarily with metabolic substrates that contain ionized thiol, amino, imino, and in some cases hydroxyl groups (Burchfield and Storrs, 1956). The rates at which these reactions take place are highly dependent on pH for groups that have pK_a values higher than the pH of the microenvironment in which the reactions take place. They vary in specificity for the groups with which they react. Thus dyrene reacts about 100 times more rapidly with thiols than with primary amines, FDNB and 1,000 times more rapidly with thiols than with primary amines (Table 12), while captan is almost completely specific for thiols. Dyrene is less substrate-specific than most other compounds of this class, but it can react with both RNA and DNA *in vitro*, although at lower rates than with other macromolecules (Table 13).

Hence, all active halogen fungicides are powerful biological alkylating agents, which is the main reason for their existence. Otherwise, they would not kill fungus spores. However, industrial and agricultural workers have been exposed to them for many years with no reported increases in incidence of cancer. Certain of these compounds, dichlone for example, can cause skin irritation, and some people become allergic to it, but there are no indications that it causes cancer in humans. Swine were fed chloranil for prolonged periods of time, and at the end of the experiment the pork was given to the laboratory employees for their personal use. No toxic effects were observed in either experimental group.

These casual observations do not constitute proof or disproof of the carcinogenicity of these compounds. They merely show that the most powerful group of alkylating agents to which factory and agricultural workers are regularly exposed are not highly visible carcinogens.

Unfortunately, scientific and public attention has not been focused on these compounds, so very little information is available on their carcinogenicities or mutagenicities in laboratory experiments. Also, the small amount of information available on them is conflicting. Certainly, all of these compounds would be expected to be mutagenic in simple bacterial tests, since they need not be activated enzymatically, and opportunities for detoxication should be minimal.

In tests employing the rec-assay procedure, a sensitive test utilizing H17 Rec^+ and M45 Rec^- strains of *Bacillus subtilis*, 23 pesticies out of a group of

TABLE 12 Comparison of the Rate Constants for the
Reaction of s-Triazine and FDNB with Compounds
Containing Various Functional Groups

Compound	pK'	Apparent rate $\times 10^3$ at pH 7.0 (mol liter^{-1} sec^{-1})	
		s-Triazine	FDNB
Glutathione	9.12	1,100	970
Proline	10.6	87	3.6
p-Hydroxybenzoic acid	9.40	28	1.3
R—NH$_2$ (average)	–	6.3	0.6
p-Aminobenzoic acid	4.92	320	6.7
Nicotinic acid	4.87	99	3.3

TABLE 13   Reactivity of 2,4-Dichloro-6-(o0chloroanilino)-s-triazine
with Macromolecules

Material	Concentration (mg/ml)	Half-time (min)	Relative reactivity (egg albumin = 1)
Edestin	5	$>10^3$	~0
RNA	10	~360	0.4
DNA	10	130	1
Egg albumin	10	130	1
Intestinal phosphatase	10	70	2
Pepsin	10	50	3
Lysozyme	10	50	3
Malt diastase	10	45	3
Pancreatic amylopsin	10	40	3
Trypsinogen	2.4	100	5
Urease	10	20	7

166 were shown to be positive (Shirasu et al., 1976). When these compounds were tested for reversion using *E. coli* and *S. typhimurium*, nine were found to be mutagenic. Microsomal activation was not used in these experiments, but this is not important since all of the compounds of interest in this group are known to be direct alkylating agents. Compounds of this class that were found to be mutagenic include captan, folpet, and captafol. These all belong to the chlorothiophthalimide group of fungicides. However, of great interest is the fact that both dyrene (37) and dichlone (36) were inactive. Perhaps this was caused by the fact that the liquid media used for the culture of all bacterial strains contained 10 g of meat extract and 10 g of polypeptone per 1,000 ml of water, and this same medium was solidified with 1.5% Difco agar for use in the rec-assay on plates. We have found that about one-half of the dyrene mixed with rodent chow at a level of 1,000 ppm disappears overnight, probably through reactions with feed components containing nucleophilic groups. Therefore, it is possible that the dyrene used in the mutagenesis experiment was detoxified by the meat extract and polypeptone before it could react at genetic loci.

Carcinogenesis bioassays with rodents are also inconclusive (Innis et al., 1969). Chloranil was found to yield an increased tumor incidence significant at the 0.01 level, but was deemed to be less of a hazard than DDT and other chlorinated hydrocarbon insecticides that are not alkylating agents. However, its close structural relative, dichlone, was found to be negative, which is entirely inconsistent with what is known about the chemical properties of these two compounds. This has no practical relevance since these two compounds are obsolete for use as fungicides in the United States. However, the disparity of the results makes one question the validity of the test procedure.

Captan yielded an increased tumor incidence significant at the 0.02

level, and was thus considered to be less dangerous than most of the chlorinated hydrocarbons. Carcinogenicity tests are now under way on dyrene (37), chlorothalonil (38), and captan (39). Some test results have not been analyzed and others are incomplete, so no specific comments can be made. However, in general it can be stated that active halogen fungicides are probably not highly potent carcinogens, although in carefully controlled laboratory experiments they should be mutagenic to most microorganisms.

This apparent discrepancy may arise from the fact that these compounds are not volatile and are sparingly soluble in water. When they slowly dissolve and permeate cells, they are probably detoxified by electron-rich molecules such as glutathione before they can cause serious genetic damage. Some of these compounds react at enormous rates with serum albumin, which may be the principal mechanism for their detoxication in mammals (Storrs, 1958).

One exception must be made to the above remarks. Quintozene (47) was found to be carcinogenic to mice at the $p < 0.01$ confidence level (Innis et al., 1969). It was not mutagenic to bacteria in the absence of microsomal activation (Shirasu et al., 1976). However, it differs from most polychlorinated fungicides in chemical reactivity. In the majority of these compounds, nitro, cyano, and other groups activate a halogen atom and cause it to be the leaving group in nucleophilic substitution reactions. However, with PCNB the chlorine atoms are the activating entities and the nitro group is the leaving group, as indicated by the fact that one of the principal metabolites of PCNB when it is fed to rabbits is a pentachlorophenol derivative of acetylcysteine (48).

(47) (48)

Hence, this compound may be the exception to the rule that polychlorinated fungicides are not highly carcinogenic, although they are alkylating agents that have a high mutagenic potential.

CONCLUSIONS

General conclusions on the carcinogenicity of organohalogen compounds cannot be made on the basis of present knowledge, and in fact probably could not be made if all basic facts regarding them were known, since their modes of action may be as diverse as the many manifestations of the disease itself. Alkyl halides are certainly alkylating agents, and by combining covalently with DNA cause mutations which, by mechanisms not yet clearly understood, induce cancer. Oxygenated alkyl halides, depending on the position of substitution, are generally more powerful alkylating agents and mutagens than the unsubstituted compounds. Bifunctional alkylating agents—bis(α-chloromethyl) ether, for example—are often more active than monofunctional agents, but paradoxically the former are among the most effective cancer chemotherapeutics.

The reasons for the carcinogenicity of chlorinated hydrocarbon insecticides to rodents are completely obscure. These compounds are not strong alkylating agents, and comparisons of the influence of chemical structure on insecticidal activity indicate that molecular configuration is probably far more important than chemical reactivity, as witnessed by the fact that only the γ isomer of the six isomers of hexachlorocyclohexane possesses significant insecticidal activity. With some of these compounds halogen might not be required at all, as shown by the significant insecticidal activity of bis(4-methoxyphenyl)-1,1,1-trimethylethane, a structural analog of DDT that does not contain chlorine. Conceivably, some of these compounds could be converted to alkylating agents by enzymatic dehydrochlorination, dechlorination, epoxidation, or a combination of these reactions. However, this has not yet been demonstrated experimentally.

Fungicides that contain halogen atoms activated by adjacent quinone, nitrile, nitro, and heterocyclic groups are powerful alkylating agents, and if tested under ideal conditions all of them probably would be mutagenic. The fact that some are not points to defects in the test systems. Some of these compounds may be detoxified rather than activated before they reach genetically vulnerable sites. Evidence on the carcinogenicity of these compounds to rodents is not complete. However, in general they appear to possess a relatively low order of carcinogenicity, possibly because they are detoxified before they can react with vulnerable target sites.

Aside from the basic chemical differences between these groups of compounds, some anomalies arise from the limitations of the test systems. For example bis(β-chloroethyl) ether had only borderline activity in cutaneous tests on mice, while it was carcinogenic at the $p < 0.01$ level in lifetime feeding studies.

Mutagenicity correlates well with carcinogenicity for many groups of compounds, but in the case of the organohalogen compounds this relationship breaks down badly. $CHCl_3$, CCl_4, dieldrin, and other chlorinated hydrocarbon insecticides are carcinogenic to mice but are not mutagenic when tested by any of the methods currently available. Perhaps in the future better techniques will be evolved for metabolic conversion of these compounds to ultimate electrophiles. However, it is equally possible that they are carcinogenic to rodents by entirely different mechanisms.

The validity of extrapolating results of tests made on rodents with high doses of chemicals to the environmental and workplace exposure levels of humans is still being hotly disputed, and the question may never be resolved. The most compelling evidence for accepting this relationship is the fact that all chemicals that are known human carcinogens cause cancer in experimental animals. However, the reverse side of this principle, that all chemicals that cause cancer in mice may have the potential of causing cancer in humans has not, and may never be, demonstrated.

REFERENCES

Abrahamson, E. and Lewis, E. B. 1971. The detection of mutations in *Drosophila melanagaster*. In *Chemical mutagens: Principles and methods for their detection*, ed. A. Hollander. New York: Plenum.

Albert, R. E., Pasternack, B. S., Shore, R. E., Lippman, M., Nelson, N. and Ferris, B. 1975. *Environ. Health Perspect.* 11:209.

Allen, J. W. and Latt, S. A. 1976. *Nature (Lond.)* 260:449.

Altanerova, V. 1975. *Neoplasma* 22:599.

Ames, B. N. 1971. The detection of chemical mutagens with enteric bacteria. In *Chemical mutagens: Principles and methods for their detection*, ed. E. A. Hollander, vol. 1, pp. 267–282. New York: Plenum.

Ames, B. N. 1972. A bacterial system for detecting mutagens and carcinogens. In *Effects of environmental chemicals*, eds. E. Sutton and M. Harms. New York: Academic Press.

Ames, B. N., McCann, J. and Yamasaki, E. 1975. *Mutat. Res.* 31:348.

Anon. 1976a. *Chem. Eng. News*, March 29:17.

Anon. 1976b. *Report on carcinogenesis bioassay of chloroform*. March 1. Carcinogenesis Program, Division of Cancer Cause and Prevention, National Cancer Institute.

Anon. 1976c. *Carcinogenesis bioassay of trichloroethylene*. Tech. Rep. No. 2, DHEW Publ. No. (NIH) 76-802.

Ashwood-Smith, M. J., Trevino, J. and Ring, J. R. 1972. *Nature (Lond.)* 240:418.

Bartsch, H. and Montesano, R. 1975. *Mutat. Res.* 32:93.

Bartsch, H., Malaveille, C., Barbin, A., Planche, G. and Montesano, R. 1976. *AACR Abstr. No.* 67:17.

Bateman, A. J. and Epstein, S. S. 1971. Dominant lethal mutations in mammals. In *Chemical mutagens: Principles and methods for their detection*, ed. E. A. Hollander, vol. 2. New York: Plenum.

Bedford, C. T. and Robinson, J. 1972. *Xenobiotica* 2:307.

Benes, V. and Sram, R. 1969. *Ind. Med.* 38:50.

Bidwell, K., Weber, E., Nienhold, I., Connor, T. and Legator, M. S. 1975. Comprehensive evaluation of mutagenic activity of dieldrin. In *Abstract of the 6th Annual Meeting of the American Environmental Mutagen Society, Miami Beach, Florida,* p. 314.

Blair, D., Hoadley, E. C. and Hutson, D. H. 1975. *Toxicol. Appl. Pharmacol.* 31:243.

Blair, D., Dix, K. M., Hunt, P. F., Thorpe, E., Stevenson, D. E. and Walker, A. I. T. 1976. *Arch. Toxicol.* 35:281.

Bridges, B. A. 1972. *Lab. Pract.* 21:413.

Bridges, B. A. 1974. *Mutat. Res.* 26:335.

Burchfield, H. P. 1958. *Nature (Lond.)* 181:49.

Burchfield, H. P. and Storrs, E. E. 1956. *Contrib. Boyce Thompson Inst.* 19:169.

Burchfield, H. P. and Storrs, E. E. 1957. *Contrib. Boyce Thompson Inst.* 18:395.

Burchfield, H. P. and Storrs, E. E. 1958. *Contrib. Boyce Thompson Inst.* 19:417.

Burchfield, H. P. and Storrs, E. E. 1976. Fungicide Toxicity and Metabolism Symposium. In *Proceedings of the Third International Biodegradation Symposium,* eds. J. M. Sharpley and A. M. Kaplan, pp. 1043–1055. London: Applied Science.

Burchfield, H. P. Storrs, E. E. and Kraybill, H. F. 1975. The maximum tolerated dose in pesticide carcinogenicity studies. *Environ. Qual. Saf.* 3:599.

Burreson, J., Moore, F. E. and Roller, P. P. 1976. *J. Agric. Food Chem.* 24:856.

Costa, A., Weber, G. and St. Omer, F. B. 1963. *Arch. De Vecchi Anat. Pathol.* 39:357.

Dean, B. J. 1972. *Arch. Toxikol.* 30:75.

Dean, B. J., Doak, S. M. A. and Funnell, J. 1972. *Arch. Toxikol.* 30:61.

Drew, R. T., Laskin, S., Kushner, M. and Nelson, N. 1975. *Arch. Environ. Health* 30:61.

Druckrey, H., Kruse, H., Preussman, R., Ivankovic, S. and Landschutz, C. 1970. *Z. Krebsforsch.* 74:241.

Dyer, K. F. and Hanna, P. J. 1973. *Mutat. Res.* 21:175.

Edmundson, W. F. 1972. Pharmacology of DDT–The background. In *Epidemiology of DDT,* eds. J. E. Davies and W. F. Edmundson, chap. 2. Mount Kisco, N.Y.: Futura.

Ehrenberg, L. 1971. Higher plants. In *Chemical mutagens: Principles and methods for their detection,* ed. A. Hollander, vol. 2. New York: Plenum.

Epstein, S. S., Bass, W., Arnold, E. and Bishop, Y. 1970. *Science* 168:584.

Epstein, S. S., Arnold, E., Andrea, J., Bass, W. and Bishop, Y. 1972. *Toxicol. Appl. Pharmacol.* 23:288.

Fahmy, M. A. H., Fukota, T. R., Metcalf, R. L. and Holmstead, R. L. 1973. *J. Agric. Food Chem.* 21:595.

Fahrig, R. 1973. *Naturwissenschaften* 60:50.

Fahrig, R. 1974. Comparative mutagenicity studies with pesticides. In *Chemical carcinogenesis assay,* IARC Sci. Publ. No. 10.

Fahrig, R. 1976. *Umschau* 76:224.

Figueroa, W. G., Raszkowski, R. and Weiss, W. 1973. *N. Engl. J. Med.* 288:1096.

Fishbein, L., Flamm, W. G. and Falk, H. L. 1970. Chemical mutagens. In *Environmental effects of biological systems,* p. 154. New York: Academic Press.

Franz, N. and Malling, H. V. 1975. *Mutat. Res.* 31:365.
Gargus, J. L., Reese, W. H., Jr. and Rutter, H. A. 1969. *Toxicol. Appl. Pharmacol.* 15:92.
Garro, A. J., Guttenplan, J. B. and Milvyn, P. 1976. *Mutat. Res.* 38:81.
Goethe, R., Calleman, C. J., Ehrenberg, L. and Wachmeister, C. A. 1974. *Ambio* 3:234.
Green, M. H. L. and Muriel, W. J. 1976. *Mutat. Res.* 38:3.
Greim, H., Bonse, G., Radwan, Z., Reichert, D. and Henschler, D. 1975. *Biochem. Pharmacol.* 24:2013.
Guthrie, F. E. 1950. *J. Econ. Entomol.* 43:559.
Haddow, A. 1973. *Perspect. Biol. Med.* Summer:503.
Harris, C. C. 1976. *Cancer, February Suppl.* 37:1014.
Heidelberger, C. 1973. *Cancer Res.* 18:317.
Hoffman, R. A. and Lindquist, A. W. 1949. *J. Econ. Entomol.* 42:891.
Holan, G. 1969. *Nature (Lond.)* 221:1025.
Innis, J. R. M., Ulland, B. M., Valerio, M. G., Petrucelli, L., Fishbein, L., Hart, E., Pallotta, A. J., Bates, R. R., Falk, H. L., Gart, J. R., Klein, M., Mitchell, I. and Peters, J. 1969. *J. Nat. Cancer Inst.* 42:1101.
Keplinger, K., Goode, J. W., Gordon, D. E. and Calandra, J. C. 1975. *Ann. N.Y. Acad. Sci.* 246:219.
Kirkpatrick, B. L., Kharbanda, P. D. and Sinclair, J. B. 1976. *Plant Dis. Rep.* 60:68.
Khachatryan, E. A. 1972a. *Gig. Tr. Prof. Zabol.* 18:54.
Khachatryan, E. A. 1972b. *Probl. Oncol.* 18:85.
Kleopper, R. D. and Fairless, B. J. 1972. *Environ. Sci. Technol.* 6:1062.
Kondo, S. 1973. *Genetics* 73:109.
Kucerova, M., Polivkova, Z., Sram, R. and Matousek, V. 1976. *Mutat. Res.* 34:271.
Laskin, S., Kuschner, M., Drew, R. T., Cappiello, V. P. and Nelson, N. 1971. *Arch. Environ. Health* 23:135.
Laskin, S. R., Drew, T., Cappiello, V., Kuschner, M. and Nelson, N. 1975. *Arch. Environ. Health* 30:70.
Lawley, P. D. 1974. *Mutat. Res.* 23:283.
Lawley, P. D. and Brooks, P. 1967. *J. Mol. Biol.* 25:143.
Lawley, P. D., Shah, S. A. and Orr, D. J. 1974. *Chem. Biol. Interact.* 8:171.
Lloyd, J. W. 1976. *Ann. N.Y. Acad. Sci.* 271:91.
Löfroth, G. 1970. *Naturwissenschaften* 57:393.
Löfroth, G., Kim, C. and Hussain, S. 1969. *EMS Newslett.* 2:21.
Magnusson, J. and Ramel, C. 1976. *Mutat. Res.* 38:115.
Maltoni, C. and Lefemine, G. 1975. *Ann. N.Y. Acad. Sci.* 246:195.
McCann, J. and Ames, B. N. 1976. *Proc. Natl. Acad. Sci. U.S.A.* 73:950.
McCann, J., Choi, E., Yamasaki, E. and Ames, B. N. 1975. *Proc. Natl. Acad. Sci. U.S.A.* 72:5135.
Metcalf, R. L. 1955. *Organic insecticides.* New York: Wiley, Interscience.
Mohn, G., Ellenberger, J. and McGregor, D. 1974. *Mutat. Res.* 25:187.
Mrak report. 1969. In *Report of the Secretary's Commission on Pesticides and Their Relationship to Environmental Health, Part I and II.* Washington, D.C.: Government Printing Office.
Mukai, F. H. and Hawryluk, I. 1973. *First International Conference ASILOMAR, No. 33,* p. 228.
Mullins, L. J. 1956. Publ. No. 1, American Institute of Biological Sciences, Washington, D.C.
Nelson, N. 1976. *Ann. N.Y. Acad. Sci.* 271:81.

O'Brien, R. D. 1967. *Insecticides, action and metabolism*, p. 165. New York: Academic Press.
O'Brien, R. D. and Matsamura, F. 1964. *Science* 146:657.
Olson, W. A., Habermann, R. T., Weisburger, E. K., Ward, J. M. and Weisburger, J. M. 1973. *J. Nat. Cancer Inst.* 51:1993.
Poirier, L. A., Stoner, G. D. and Shimkin, M. B. 1975. *Cancer Res.* 35:1411.
Powers, M. B., Voelker, R. W., Page, N. P., Weisburger, E. K. and Kraybill, H. F. 1975. *Abstract of the 14th Annual Meeting of the Society of Toxicology, Paper No. 123*, p. 99.
Rannug, U. and Ramel, C. 1976. *Mutat. Res.* 38:113.
Rannug, U., Gothe, R. and Wachtmeister, C. A. 1976. *Chem. Biol. Interact.* 12:251.
Rappoport, Z. 1969. Nucleophilic vinyl substitution. In *Advances in physical organic chemistry*, ed. V. Gold. New York: Academic Press.
Reuber, M. D. and Glover, E. L. 1967a. *Arch. Pathol.* 83:267.
Reuber, M. D. and Glover, E. L. 1967b. *J. Natl. Cancer Inst.* 38:891.
Reuber, M. D. and Glover, E. L. 1968. *Arch. Pathol.* 85:275.
Reuber, M. D. and Glover, E. L. 1970. *J. Natl. Cancer Inst.* 44:419.
Rhodes, R. C. and Pease, H. L. 1971. *J. Agric. Food Chem.* 19:750.
Rhodes, R. C., Pease, H. L. and Brantley, R. K. 1971. *J. Agric. Food Chem.* 19:745.
Richards, A. G. and Cutcomp, L. K. 1945. *J. Cell. Comp. Physiol.* 26:57.
Rogers, E. F., Brown, H. D., Rasmussen, I. M. and Heal, R. E. 1953. *J. Am. Chem. Soc.* 75:2991.
Ross, W. C. J. 1962. *Biological alkylating agents*, p. 11. London: Butterworth.
Rubin, H. 1976. *Science* 191:241.
Sakabe, H. 1973. *Ind. Health* 11:145.
Selikoff, I. J. and Hammond, E. C., eds. 1972. *Ann. N.Y. Acad. Sci.* 246:1.
Shankland, D. C. and Schroeder, M. E. 1973. *Pestic. Biochem. Physiol.* 3:77.
Shirasu, Y., Moriya, M., Kato, K., Furuhashi, A. and Kada, T. 1976. *Mutat. Res.* 40:19-30.
Shubik, P. 1972. Iatrogenic cancer. In *Environment and cancer*, pp. 142-156.
Simmon, V. F. and Poirier, L. A. 1976. *Cancer res.* 35:1411.
Slor, H. 1973. *Mutat. Res.* 19:231.
Smith, R. H. and Von Borstel, R. C. 1971. Inducing mutations with chemicals in Habrobracon. In *Chemical mutagens: Principles and methods for their detection*, ed. A. Hollander, vol. 2. New York: Plenum.
Sternberg, J. G. and Hewett, P. 1962. *J. Insect. Physiol.* 8:643.
Storrs, E. E. 1958. The interactions of the mercaptalbumin fraction of bovine serum albumin with 2,4-dichloro-6-anilino-*s*-triazine derivatives. M.S. thesis, New York University.
Storrs, E. E. and Burchfield, H. P. 1954. *Contrib. Boyce Thompson Inst.* 18:69.
Uehleke, H., Greim, H., Kramer, M. and Werner, T. 1976. *Mutat. Res.* 38:113.
Van Duuren, B. L. 1969. *Ann. N.Y. Acad. Sci.* 163:633.
Van Duuren, B. L., Goldschmidt, B. M., Katz, C., Langseth, L., Mercado, G. and Sivak, A. 1968. *Arch. Environ. Health* 16:472.
Van Duuren, B. L., Sivak, A., Goldschmidt, B. M., Katz, C. and Melchionne, S. 1969. *J. Nat. Cancer Inst.* 43:481.
Van Duuren, B. L., Katz, C., Goldschmidt, B. M., Frenkel, A. and Silva, A. 1972. *J. Nat. Cancer Inst.* 48:1431.

Van Duuren, B. L., Goldschmidt, B. M., Katz, C., Seidman, I. and Paul, J. S. 1974. *J. Nat. Cancer Inst.* 53:695–700.

Viola, P. L., Biogotti, L. A. and Caputo, A. 1971. *Cancer Res.* 31:516.

Voogd, C. E., Jacobs, A. A. and Van der Stel, J. J. 1972. *Mutat. Res.* 16:413.

Waxweiler, R. J., Stringer, W., Wagoner, J. K. and Jones, J. 1976. *Ann. N.Y. Acad. Sci.* 271:40.

Weil, C. S., Woodside, M. C., Bernard, J. R. and Carpenter, C. P. 1969. *Toxicol. Appl. Pharmacol.* 14:426.

Wennerberg, R. and Löfroth, G. 1974. *Chem. Biol. Interact.* 8:339.

Wild, D. 1975. *Mutat. Res.* 32:133.

Williams, G. M. 1976. *Cancer Lett.* 1:231.

Chapter 11

REFLECTIONS ON THE ART OF BIOASSAY FOR CARCINOGENESIS

Michael B. Shimkin

Department of Community Medicine
University of California at San Diego
La Jolla, California

The year 1938 was a very good one for me. I got married, received a research fellowship, and acquired an abiding interest in cancer.

The year 1938 was also good for cancer research. The National Cancer Institute was established, and the solution of the cancer problem loomed just behind a corner. Kennaway and his London group had isolated the carcinogenic polycyclic hydrocarbons (Shimkin and Triolo, 1969). A. Butenandt and E. A. Doisy had defined the chemical structure of estrogens. Both groups of compounds looked as if they were related to cholesterol. Then methylcholanthrene was synthesized from bile acids. Cancer could now be conceived as an inborn error of metabolism, in which cholesterol became converted to carcinogens. Relating chemical structure to carcinogenic activity was an important approach to this hypothesis, especially in those preisotope, prechromatography days. The centers for research on polycyclic hydrocarbons were in London, where J. W. Cook synthesized analogues, and at Harvard, where L. F. Fieser was the prime organic chemist. In London the chemicals were tested for carcinogenic activity by painting random-bred mice with benzene solutions, with cutaneous carcinomas as the end point. At Harvard a collaborative arrangement with the Office of Cancer Investigations was made for biologic testing. M. J. Shear implanted 5-10 mg of the crystals, moistened with glycerol, subcutaneously in mice and watched for the appearance of sarcomas at the site of injection.

Then, as now on rereading the summary papers (Cook and Kennaway, 1940; Fieser, 1938), I was struck by the sophisticated chemistry and the crude biology of the investigations. To a pharmacologist, the absence of quantitative design was particularly apparent. The bioassay contributions of J. H. Gaddum and of C. I. Bliss were already in the literature, and their methods were obviously applicable to studies in carcinogenesis. W. R. Bryan and I went to work and performed a model analysis of three active hydrocarbons. Our papers (Bryan and Shimkin, 1941, 1943) are still referred to honorably. To be brutally frank, however, they did not elucidate any key questions of carcinogenesis. More bioassays over a wide range of compounds could well have been informative. But by then research attention had turned in other directions.

One newer area was azo dye carcinogenesis introduced by T. Yoshida and other Japanese workers. Its relation to dietary factors and metabolic conversions offered attractive research possibilities. Biochemists embraced the easily accessible liver as the material for their studies, comparing adult, fetal, and regenerating livers with livers at various stages after exposure of rats to hepatocarcinogens and with hepatomas. This work was done without much reference to formal quantitative bioassay procedures. Large doses of carcinogen were usually given in order to accelerate the effects, and cirrhosis preceded carcinogenesis. These two reactions were dissociated by a neat quantitative study of Eschenbrenner and Miller (1945–1946), who used carbon tetrachloride in mice for their investigation.

Quantitative bioassay was developed primarily as a technique for estimating by means of animal responses the content of an active ingredient in different samples of crude material, such as digitalis in leaf decoctions. Bioassay procedures became unnecessary when pure alkaloids replaced crude preparations, and dosages could be based on weight alone.

Comparison of crude mixtures for carcinogenic activity, chemical or viral, remains a prime area of application for quantitative bioassay. During the 1930s, it was noted that lung cancer rates were increasing, especially in larger cities. Carcinogens in atmospheric contaminants were suspected as a causative factor. Air samples were gathered from several sources, extracted, and injected into mice. Sarcomas were elicited in 18 of 291 mice during 12 months of observation (Leiter et al., 1943).

Circumstances did not permit extension of the investigations to quantitative comparisons between samples from different localities. Such comparisons became important in evaluating samples of another crude environmental carcinogen, tobacco smoke condensate, especially when it was decided to invest in the development of less hazardous cigarettes. Bioassay procedures will continue in this role until the chemical carcinogen in tobacco smoke is definitely identified. Then, as with digitalis, direct chemical determinations will replace bioassay estimates for the carcinogenic chemical.

Compounds of the polycyclic hydrocarbon type are deemed to be "direct-acting" carcinogens and are assayed by their response at contact with skin or subcutaneous tissues. The amino azo and aminofluorene compounds require metabolic conversion; their response is most evident in the liver. Urethane, encountered as a carcinogen in 1943, exerts its most striking neoplastic effect on the lung of mice. This major-response concept, however, was obliterated by the discovery of the carcinogenic nitroso compounds in

1954. The work of Magee and Barnes (1967) seems to negate any single neoplastic response as a basis for a single satisfactory or even internally consistent bioassay procedure.

Then, with the world's attention aroused by the thalidomide tragedy, the Food and Drug Administration had added the Delaney clause to their regulations; this amendment prohibits the inclusion of any amount of any carcinogenic material in food. The industrial technology of our civilization invents new chemicals at a rate that exceeds even the breeding capacity of rodents and certainly the facilities they would require. And no one is satisfied in using only one species, or extrapolating data obtained on mice to humans.

What are our options? Among the unacceptable ones are to throw up our hands and ignore the problem or to prohibit any more chemicals to be made until we catch up with the backlog. Among the acceptable ones are to invest in research that might lead to simpler, faster, and more informative indices of dangers that we wish to define and to eliminate.

In regard to simpler methodology, a major research investment is being made on *in vitro* tests. It is intriguing to imagine that someday, instead of roomfuls of smelly animals, all one would need would be cell cultures in neat retorts in shiny incubators. Much has been learned and much more will be learned from *in vitro* investigations. There are already interesting permutations. One is the *in vivo*-mediated *in vitro* test, in which pregnant animals are injected with test substances and the embryo-derived cells observed for transformations (DiPaolo et al., 1973). Another is the priming of cells with a virus before exposing the cells to the chemical to be tested (Freeman et al., 1970).

These investigations are important. But it will be a long time before *in vitro* methods are acceptable and accepted. Problems of stability, reproducibility, and interpretation of changes in cell populations deprived of the homeostatic mechanisms of the host appear to be more formidable with cell populations than with populations of animals.

There are' many suggestions of the use of nonneoplastic determinations for carcinogenic activity. The hair-follicle atrophy reaction to polycyclic hydrocarbons and to ionizing radiation is an old example and is still useful within its limitations. More recently, the appearance of fetoproteins and of antigens associated with the activation of latent viruses has gained attention. Tests for the inhibition of immune mechanisms also should be mentioned. All are interesting and worth further investigations. The very nature of these approaches, which measure the host mechanisms rather than the stimuli, suggests that they will lack specificity.

Despite the numerous permutations and varieties of the impudent overgrowths of tissues that we call cancers, there must be a common thread that unifies them as neoplasia. At the present state of our knowledge, it can be proposed with some confidence that carcinogenesis involves an alteration in DNA. The alteration must be small enough to retain cellular viability and must be stable and permanent so that it can be transmitted in subsequent genetic copies. The carcinogen must get into the cell, and must interact with and cause damage to DNA, and there must be repair of the DNA. Such a conceptual sequence is independent of whether a latent virus or a protovirus is contained in the DNA. The eventual alteration in DNA may not be of only one type but must be specific rather than random.

This concept brings together the reactions of carcinogenesis and of mutagenesis. Demerec in 1948 showed a close relationship between mutagenicity and carcinogenicity in tests on *Drosophila*. More recently, Ames et al. (1973) extended the use of bacterial indicators of mutation by combining liver homogenates to induce metabolic conversion of chemicals.

The study of DNA damage and repair in cells exposed to carcinogens seems a fruitful approach. Not only mammalian cells, but also other bacterial and viral models need to be explored. Even with these *in vitro* systems, however, the tests would represent bioassay procedures. The eventual goal would be to use DNA as a chemical and to identify the interaction between the DNA molecule and carcinogens. Such chemical tests would obviate the use of biological systems for primary screening of chemicals and other potential environmental hazards for carcinogenic activity.

The elucidation of the DNA molecule and the changes in the molecule produced by carcinogens is worthy of support and encouragement. A major research investment in this area is valid regardless of outcome.

The precision of chemical tests for carcinogenesis is a mere theoretical possibility for the future. Today we must contend with the realities of animal systems for bioassay of chemicals suspected of having carcinogenic activity.

There is no royal road to such tests. There is no single test that will answer all problems, there are no shortcuts that are safely taken, and interpretations of all but the most obvious positive effects will include humanly fallible judgments. The tests, no matter how carefully conceived and monitored, will reflect the state of the art at the time and must be continually improved by new information. There is definite danger in standards and procedures that become prematurely frozen. This freezing process is hard to avoid if certain methodologies become accepted as standards by regulatory agencies.

Thoughtful reviews and reports on testing for carcinogenic activity are available in the literature. Two papers by the Weisburgers (1967, 1973) are particularly commendable. The proceedings of a conference on carcinogenesis testing of chemicals held in 1973 form a useful document (Golberg, 1974). The deliberations of an international committee on the subject, edited by Berenblum (1969), deserve reading to emphasize the difficulties in reaching agreements even on points that seem almost obvious. An informative paper by Bliss (1957) should be required reading for anyone who undertakes bioassay.

All bioassays involve the *material* to be tested and the *biological system* on which the test is to be performed. Both should be as stable as possible and be kept under as definably stable environmental conditions as possible. The end point of the test should be quantitatively defined.

Carcinogenesis is but one of many chronic toxic reactions of a host to a noxious stimulus. The end point is the appearance or acceleration of one or more neoplasms in animals with a known neoplastic background. Other physiologic and pathologic effects should not be ignored; gross abnormalities of tissues, as an example, of course should be investigated by microscopy. It is easy, however, to overload pathology resources by sectioning "all" tissues and so dilute the main objective. By the same token, tests for teratogenic effects are best carried out separately from tests for carcinogenesis. They have their own considerations, procedures, and difficulties.

Reasons for testing for carcinogenic activity are many and will influence the choice of the bioassay procedure. At one end are studies aimed at correlating chemical structure to carcinogenesis and on the other, determinations of environmental exposures for carcinogenic hazards. The first is usually carried out on defined, chemically pure materials. The second may require testing of crude mixtures of unknown constitution. In both, the collaboration of organic chemists is essential. For the pure chemicals, relation of structure to known carcinogens, data on stability, solubility, and other physical factors are useful. Possible dangers to the investigator working with the material must be defined. For the crude mixtures, chemical determinations for suspected carcinogens are in order, as well as references such as nitrogen content by which the sample can be compared with other samples.

Environmental exposures are usually to many substances at low levels, whereas most bioassay testing is done at high doses of single compounds. There is no way to predict whether combinations in complex mixtures will have additive, synergistic, or antagonistic effects. And limitation of tests to highest tolerated levels of single compounds encounters the possibilities of such effects as metabolic overloading (Kraybill, 1974) and immunologic depression. It would be nice to have data on multiple chemical exposures, but the design of such experiments leads to frightening numbers of animals, and it is not clear what such data really would contribute. This is one of those experiments one suggests be done by someone else, somewhere else than in one's own facilities. An instructive example, published by Gardner et al. (1970), shows that nonneoplastic events may obscure the issue despite prodigious work.

If there are any solutions to this species of problem, they include the suggestions that to study an environment, study it as it is as well as in some laboratory copy, and with any chemical, a wide dose range should be explored. Pharmacology or bioassay devoid of dose-response design is neither.

As to the animals to be used for carcinogenesis bioassays, arguments will cease about the choice when bioassays are replaced by chemical techniques.

Of course more than one species is desirable. Of course *Mus musculus* is not *Homo sapiens*. Of course lifetime observations are needed for chronic effects. Of course controls are irreplaceable. There must be parallel controls as well as historical ones and vehicle-injected as well as untreated groups. "Positive controls," to assure the reactivity of the animals, are also desirable.

Having said all that, the choice of the animal depends upon the purpose of the experiment and is determined by available information and available stocks. For most purposes in carcinogenesis there is no known substitute for that convenient little beast, the mouse, with its many "strains" of defined genetic background, of defined microbial flora, and of defined neoplastic responses. This information has been accumulated for over half a century, and no other species has as rich a base for our manipulations.

There still appears to be the need, nevertheless, to speak for the use of genetically defined animals. Investigators who agree that the food, water, environmental conditions, and care of the animals need to be uniform and defined, sometimes still press for noninbred stocks. The point is not the inbreeding but the defined genetic constitution that yields reduced variability and closer definition of the biological "background noise." For practical purposes of animal procurement, pen-bred inbred mice may serve the purpose of the experiment. However, to contend that non-genetically defined animals are to be preferred over genetically defined animals is as illogical as to neglect dietary and other environmental conditions.

As to route of administration, schedule of administrations, and similar important matters, these must be individualized to the requirements of the investigations. Simplicity and economy should be favored. If the design of the experiment does not necessitate intravenous injection, the intraperitoneal route is much simpler and surer. If the design of the experiment indicates that groups of 20 animals at three dose levels will answer the question, the allocation of 50 per group is a waste. The oral route for materials that are usually ingested seems reasonable but should relate to the aims of the specific experiment. Most hepatotoxins probably are best given to rats by being mixed with food, but this does not preclude other approaches or the need for dose-response design.

The end point of carcinogenesis testing on animals is the appearance of malignant neoplasms, preferably in the absence of such neoplasms among the untreated controls. Induction, therefore, is inferred, although experience shows that induced tumors usually represent the earlier appearance of tumors encountered "spontaneously" at later times and in smaller numbers among the untreated population.

A significant acceleration and increase of neoplasms that occur spontaneously seem to be only quantitatively different from the presumed induction end point. A neoplastic reaction of this type that has served well in quantitative bioassay procedures for carcinogenesis is the adenomatous primary pulmonary tumor of susceptible mouse strains, especially strain A. The type 2 cell of the alveolus of mice is sensitive to neoplastic transformation by a wide variety of carcinogens. The response is rapid as *in vivo* tests for carcinogenesis go; 4 months is adequate for stronger carcinogens and most tests can be completed by 6 months. The number of tumors per lung provides a particularly quantitative measure of response. An intriguing and useful feature of the response is that the slopes of dose to number of tumors are parallel over a wide range of dissimilar chemical compounds, allowing direct comparisons of relative activity (Shimkin et al., 1966; Shimkin and Stoner, 1975).

Biometric design of bioassay experiments should be taken for granted these days, and certainly this includes analysis and presentation of the results. Collaboration with statisticians should be developed and is often instructive, if they stick to biology at least as closely as to mathematics and computers.

In the end, however, except for the most obvious results, some interpretation will be necessary and some disagreement among those who pose as experts is unavoidable.

Chemicals tested for carcinogenic activity are usefully classifiable by more characteristics than only as positive or negative. One subclassification might be by the predominant tissue in which the carcinogenic response is elicited. Polycyclic hydrocarbons, with cancers induced at point of contact of cutaneous and subcutaneous tissues, are of a different class of carcinogens than those primarily evoking cancers of the liver.

The dose and time required to elicit a neoplastic response should array compounds from rapidly acting ones to weak ones. Here the slopes of the dose-response curves are informative. Chemicals that elicit cancers rapidly and with but fractions of a milligram deserve scientific and practical considerations that differ from chemicals that after prolonged administration of larger doses finally produce a few tumors.

A third consideration is whether the carcinogenic response is elicited in many species and tissues or is restricted to specialized conditions. Aflatoxin, for example, is a potent carcinogen by all definitions. It should be categorized differently from, say, griseofulvin, which increases the frequency of hepatomas in newborn male mice.

We come back to our societal and political attitudes, the arena in which all temporarily final decisions are reached. In carcinogenesis, the Delaney amendment is our present guide, and it seeks absolute prohibition of carcinogens in foods. Absolutes are permissible philosophical abstractions but are not to be found in the real world we inhabit. The Delaney amendment should stand, as a goal, so that all kinds of peculiar exceptions and relaxations do not creep in under the guise of economic and other needs (Epstein, 1974). But the determination of what is and what is not carcinogenic, especially when extrapolated from animals to humans, must be a judgmental matter. Such judgments are based on group considerations, with spokesmen for divergent viewpoints.

Spokesmen are people, and people have motivations; it is useful to attempt to identify both. In our mercantile culture, we do our utmost to avoid the important question of who owns, distributes, and profits from commodities that are simultaneously our pride of progress and the cause of our concerns. Spokesmen for industry, with vested economic stakes, should be in the role of witnesses rather than of jurors (Shimkin, 1969). Environmentalists and ecologists, however, also have motivations that lead to challengeable conclusions. It again comes down to the Socratic question of who selects the judges. In a democracy, we are back to the leaky raft that does not sink, to the worst form of government except for every other form, and to the endless tedium of public persuasion.

We must do the best we can with our limited information and our even more limited wisdom. Part of that wisdom is to continue to expand our knowledge and not to seek absolute solutions. This fable is applicable to carcinogenesis bioassays:

> In olden days, a Prince of Araby returned from an unsuccessful lion hunt in the desert and summoned his Seer. "Wise man," said the Prince, "devise for me an infallible method of catching a lion in the desert." The Seer thought and finally spoke, "My Prince, get a net of steel, 20 feet across and 20 feet deep, with meshes of six inches. Now sift all the sands of the desert through the net, and infallibly you will catch a lion."

REFERENCES

Ames, B. N., Durston, W. E., Yamasaki, E. and Lee, F. D. 1973. Carcinogens are mutagens: A simple test system combining liver homogenates for activation and bacteria for detection. *Proc. Natl. Acad. Sci. U.S.A.* 70:2281–2285.

Berenblum, I., ed. 1969. *Carcinogenicity testing*, UICC Technical Reports Series, vol 2. Geneva: International Union Against Cancer.

Bliss, C. I. 1957. Some principles of bioassay. *Amer. Scientist* 45:449–466.

Bryan, W. R. and Shimkin, M. B. 1941. Quantitative analysis of dose-response data obtained with carcinogenic hydrocarbons. *J. Natl. Cancer Inst.* 1:807–833.

Bryan, W. R. and Shimkin, M. B. 1943. Quantitative analysis of dose-response data obtained with three carcinogenic hydrocarbons in strain C_3H mice. *J. Natl. Cancer Inst.* 3:503–531.

Cook, J. W. and Kennaway, E. L. 1940. Chemical compounds as carcinogenic agents. *Amer. J. Cancer* 39:381–428, 521–582.

Demerec, M. 1948. Genetic potencies of carcinogens. *Acta Unio Intern. Contra Cancrum* 6:247–251.

DiPaolo, J. A., Nelson, R. L., Donovan, P. J. and Evans, C. H. 1973. Host-mediated *in vivo–in vitro* assay for chemical carcinogenesis, *Arch. Path.* 95:380–385.

Epstein, S. S. 1974. Environmental determinants of human cancer. *Cancer Res.* 34:2425–2435.

Eschenbrenner, A. B. and Miller, E. 1945–1946. Liver necrosis and the induction of carbon tetrachloride hepatomas in strain A mice. *J. Natl. Cancer Inst.* 6:325–341.

Fieser, L. F. 1938. Carcinogenic activity, structure and chemical reactivity of polynuclear aromatic hydrocarbons. *Amer. J. Cancer* 34:37–124.

Freeman, A. E., Price, P. J., Eigel, H. J., Young, J. C., Maryak, J. M. and Heubner, R. J. 1970. Morphological transformation of rat embryo cells induced by diethylnitrosamine and murine leukemia virus. *J. Natl. Cancer Inst.* 44:65–78.

Gardner, M. B., Loosli, G. G., Hanes, B., Blackmore, W. and Teebken, D. 1970. Pulmonary changes in 7,000 mice following prolonged exposure to ambient and filtered Los Angeles air. *Arch. Environ. Health* 20:310–317.

Golberg, L., ed. 1974. *Carcinogenesis testing of chemicals.* Cleveland, Ohio: CRC Press.

Kraybill, H. F. 1974. Unintentional additives in food. In *Environmental quality and food supply,* ed. P. L. White and D. Robbins, pp. 173–184. New York: Futura.

Leiter, J., Shimkin, M. B. and Shear, M. J. 1943. Production of subcutaneous sarcomas in mice with tars extracted from atmospheric dusts. *J. Natl. Cancer Inst.* 3:155–165.

Magee, P. N. and Barnes, J. M. 1967. Carcinogenic nitroso compounds. *Adv. Cancer Res.* 10:163–246.

Shimkin, M. B. 1969. Summary of the conference on biological effects of pesticides on mammalian systems. *Ann. N. Y. Acad. Sci.* 160:418–422.

Shimkin, M. B. and Stoner, G. D. 1975. Lung tumors in mice: Application to carcinogenesis bioassay. *Adv. Cancer Res.* 21:1–58.

Shimkin, M. B. and Triolo, V. A. 1969. History of chemical carcinogenesis: Some prospective remarks. *Progr. Exp. Tumor Res.* 11:1–20.

Shimkin, M. B., Weisburger, J. H., Weisburger, E. K., Gubareff, N. and Suntzeff, V. 1966. Bioassay of 29 alkylating chemicals by the pulmonary-tumor response in strain A mice. *J. Natl. Cancer Inst.* 36:915–935.

Weisburger, J. H. 1973. Chemical carcinogenesis. In *Cancer medicine,* ed. J. F. Holland and E. Frei, pp. 45–90. Philadelphia: Lea & Febiger.

Weisburger, J. H. and Weisburger, E. K. 1967. Tests for chemical carcinogens. In *Methods in cancer research,* ed. H. Busch, vol. 1, pp. 307–398. New York: Academic Press.

INDEX

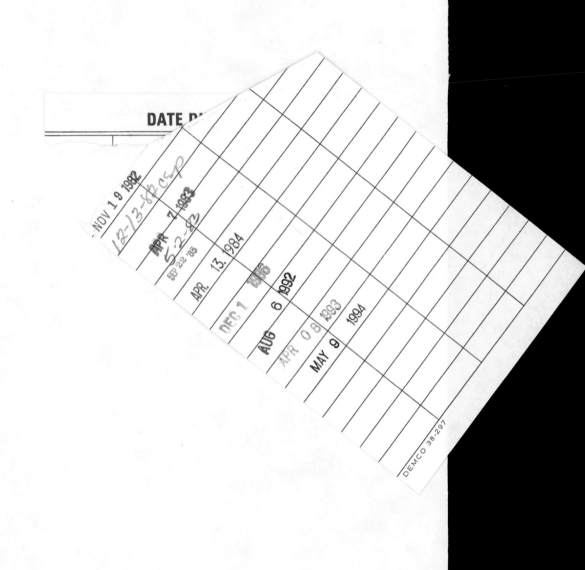